HIP SURGERY
An Odyssey

HIP SURGERY
An Odyssey

Augusto Sarmiento MD

Former Professor and Chairman
Department of Orthopedics
Universities of Miami and Southern California, USA
Past President of American Academy of Orthopedic Surgeons

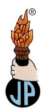

JAYPEE BROTHERS MEDICAL PUBLISHERS (P) LTD

New Delhi • Panama City • London

Jaypee Brothers Medical Publishers (P) Ltd

Headquarter
Jaypee Brothers Medical Publishers (P) Ltd
4838/24, Ansari Road, Daryaganj
New Delhi 110 002, India
Phone: +91-11-43574357
Fax: +91-11-43574314
Email: jaypee@jaypeebrothers.com

Overseas Offices

JP Medical Ltd
83 Victoria Street London
SW1H 0HW (UK)
Phone: +44-2031708910
Fax: +02-03-0086180
Email: info@jpmedpub.com

Jaypee-Highlights Medical Publishers Inc.
City of Knowledge, Bld. 237, Clayton
Panama City, Panama
Phone: 507-317-0160
Fax: +50-73-010499
Email: cservice@jphmedical.com

Website: www.jaypeebrothers.com
Website: www.jaypeedigital.com

© 2012, Jaypee Brothers Medical Publishers

Inquiries for bulk sales may be solicited at: jaypee@jaypeebrothers.com

This book has been published in good faith that the contents provided by the author contained herein are original, and is intended for educational purposes only. While every effort is made to ensure a accuracy of information, the publisher and the author specifically disclaim any damage, liability, or loss incurred, directly or indirectly, from the use or application of any of the contents of this work. If not specifically stated, all figures and tables are courtesy of the author. Where appropriate, the readers should consult with a specialist or contact the manufacturer of the drug or device.

Publisher: Jitendar P Vij
Publishing Director: Tarun Duneja
Editor: Richa Saxena
Cover Design: Seema Dogra, Sumit Kumar

Hip Surgery: An Odyssey

First Edition: 2012

ISBN 978-93-5025-360-1

Printed at Replika Press Pvt. Ltd.

Dedication

I dedicate this book to the many people who throughout my professional career provided me with a desire to improve my understanding of conditions affecting the hip joint. Amongst them are the hundreds of residents I had the privilege to assist in their education. However, I owe the deepest gratitude to Austin T Moore, under whom I had two-thirds of my orthopedic residency, and who for the rest of his life treated me with special affection. In addition to Dr Moore, I extend my gratitude to Sir John Charnley, for his frequent personal advice and for his commitment to excellence; to Frank Stinchfield for his insistency on focusing on the "big picture", and his personal encouragement to sustain academic pursuits; to Mark Coventry for his views on sharing knowledge; and to Maurice Muller for his organizational skills.

My family deserves special recognition, for without their tolerance, patience and love it would have been impossible for me to dedicate so much time to my work while depriving them of closer attention.

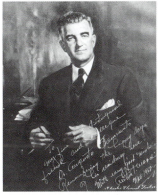

Austin T Moore

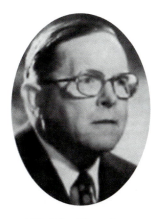
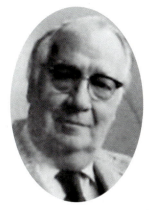
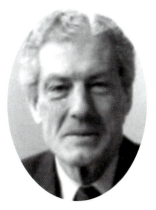
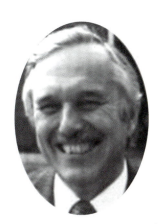

Sir John Charnley   **Frank Stinchfield**   **Mark Coventry**   **Maurice Muller**

Preface

This text is not intended to be a history of hip surgery. It is simply a recollection of my personal experiences with hip surgery over nearly half a century. The narrative dwells, in various degrees, with ideas and procedures that have, thus far, either survived the test of time or have vanished from the scene. Experiencing successful as well as the unsuccessful events has allowed me to better appreciate the evolution of the discipline and the manner in which old ideas spawned new ones.

Without any doubt, total hip arthroplasty represents one of the most important and impressive technological developments in the history of orthopedics and one that still attracts the attention of the orthopedist. Orthopedists had tried for hundreds of years to surgically relieve the pain and disability that accompany the arthritic hip joint with nothing more than occasional clinical successes. With the advent of anesthesia and later more sophisticated metallurgical advances, major progress began to take place.

Having witnessed the birth of a number of innovations which were initially heralded as the final solution to the replacement of the arthritic hip, but soon to be found wanting and then replaced by either improved or new techniques or implants, were lessons of great importance. To ignore the continuous evolution of hip surgery and to assume that we have finally found a permanent solution is not only wrong but rather naïve. It will be a long time before perfection is attained. This is why, I have structured this book in a manner that identifies the likely reasons for the failures of so many different approaches to the "hip problem" hoping that our enthusiasm with "new" techniques will be tempered by the lessons of history.

The encouraging results obtained with the use of a Vitallium cup, designed by Smith-Petersen from Boston, the acrylic cement prosthesis of Judet from Paris, and similar ventures into the field early in the twentieth century gave impetus to further experimentation. These two implants gained great popularity, but within less than a couple of decades their usage was discontinued—the Smith-Petersen because of failure to provide long-lasting relief of pain and loss of motion; and the Judet implant because of mechanical failure of the material and boring of the head into the acetabulum.

Austin Moore and Fred Thompson's endoprostheses developed in the 1940s suggested that effective replacement of the hip joint had become a realty. Their implants, however, failed to provide consistent good results since complete and permanent relief of pain became elusive. Over time, the prosthetic heads often bored into the acetabulum producing pain and disability. Their use in the care of femoral neck fractures found wider applications.

It was not until the late 1950s and early 1960s that it became evident that more successful replacement of the arthritic hip was within sight. The pioneer work of McKee and Farrar from England, was a major breakthrough. They used opposing metallic surfaces to replace the arthritic cartilage of the acetabulum and femoral head. Peter Ring, from England, several years later, attempted to improve the McKee-Farrar concept by developing an implant that replaced the acetabulum with a screw-in cup, and the femoral component with an Austin Moore endoprosthesis. Neither the McKee-Farrar nor the Ring implants survived, since either loosening of the components or wear of the articulating metallic surfaces became frequent complications.

Charnley, in the 1960s, used Teflon, a plastic material, to replace the socket and a metal ball made of stainless steel to replace the femoral head. Although surgeons, like Habush from New York and Leon Wiltsi, from California, had done some work with acrylic cement, it was John Charnley from England, the first one to successfully use it to stabilize the parts. Charnley's initial spectacular success with Teflon was short lived. The massive bone lysis around the prosthetic components that developed in virtually all of his patients necessitated removal of the prostheses, leaving the patients with flail, disabling joints. The Teflon material, under *in vivo* weight-bearing conditions, underwent significant wear. The particles of debris traveled into the medullary canal and all areas around the femur and acetabulum created havoc.

Charnley readily recognized that Teflon, though heralded as the ideal material to tolerate weight-bearing stresses, did not do well in the human body. Undeterred by the major tragedy and professional failure, he proceeded to search for a better material. He found it: high-density polyethylene; a material that 50 years later is still felt by many to be the preferred material to oppose the metallic head. Recent work with improved cross-linked polyethylene, metallic designs and ceramics has raised questions regarding the permanent acceptance of the traditional polyethylene as the preferred bearing surface. Within the next few years, we may have an answer to this.

As soon as the word spread out that Charnley's results with the new material were very good, the world's orthopedic community embraced the concept. People from all over the world traveled to England to learn about the new procedure. I personally made my pilgrimage to John Charnley's Mecca and spent three months observing his operation and learning about his overall philosophy of hip disease.

Some orthopedists, desirous to make additional contributions to the field, or blinded by the sight of possible overnight fame, modified the design of Charnley's implant even before they had an opportunity to learn and appreciate Charnley's teachings. One of them, after spending a few days at Charnley's Hip Center, designed upon his return to the United States, his own prosthesis, made minor modifications to the original design and attached his name to the new implant. He, however, chose the wrong material and his implant was promptly discredited.

Industry saw enormous market opportunities and began, with the aid of physicians, to further modify the Charnley's prosthesis since his design was protected with a patent. By the mid-seventies, there were dozens of different total hip prostheses available in the market. They differed in length, width, shape, texture and every conceivable geometric variety. Some had grooves, others notches; some were longer, others shorter. Larger and smaller collars were designed and some prostheses not even had a mark where the old collars once existed. Some advocated matted surfaces while others claimed that polished surfaces were better. Some implants had larger heads in millimeters increments. The sockets were also modified. Some were reinforced with metal-backed shells or had projections to better make the column of cement equal in thickness. Modularity was introduced in order to best accomplish gains during leg length equalization. In some instances, these modifications resulted in improvements, but in other instances, retarded progress. The excessive commercialization of orthopedics has done harm to the profession and patients as well.

A variety of innovations were made in the technique of cement injection: plugging, water picking, rasping and pressurizing. These variations became known as the second generation of cementing techniques. The cement itself was then offered with different speeds of polymerization. Some were more viscous than others.

The osteotomy of the trochanter, essential component of Charnley's original operation, began to loose popularity and, within a few years, virtually disappeared from the scene. I, for one, referred to it as an unnecessary "masochistic ritual".

New materials were introduced and efforts were made to discredit stainless steel after occasional stem fractures were reported. Cobalt-Chrome alloys replaced stainless steel implants. I personally became involved in the frenzy of improvement and thought that a material with a lower modulus of elasticity would eliminate the stress shielding of the proximal femur that the stiffer stainless steel and Cobalt-Chrome alloys seemed to have created. I designed the first Titanium prosthesis used in the United States, anticipating improvement in the radiological and clinical results. My expectation was not fulfilled in spite of initial encouraging results.

In the early 1980s, after thousands of orthopedic surgeons throughout the world had performed millions of hip arthroplasties, reports of complications with the operation began to flood the medical journals. Loosening of the components was the main problem. Acrylic cement was blamed for those complications and "cement disease" became a familiar term among orthopedic surgeons.

Efforts made to eliminate the "evil cement" from the surgical procedure, gave birth to the noncemented prosthesis. To the best of my knowledge, the first such implant was conceptualized by Emmet Lunceford from Columbia, South Carolina. He had been a fellow-resident of mine and later an associate of Austin Moore. He named the experimental implant as AML (Austin Moore-Lunceford). Lunceford died tragically a few years later and never had the opportunity to observe the clinical results with his prosthesis. With alacrity and without waiting for good documentation of the superior qualities of the noncemented implant, the use of the new technique became an epidemic. It was heralded as the answer to all the problems created by the cement. The noncemented prostheses had porous surfaces into which the bone would grow.

It did not take very long, however, for the orthopedic community to find itself disappointed by the lack of consistent good results. Thigh pain appeared to be a very frequent sequella that either did not be spontaneously disappear or persisted for a long period of time. Furthermore, and more disturbing, was the appearance of lysis, both in the pelvis as well as in the femur.

Postmortem examinations demonstrated that bone ingrowth did not occur in all instances or throughout the entire porous surface. Even in patients who had remained asymptomatic during their lives, only small areas of bone ingrowth were found. Femoral osteopenia around the implant, sometimes of worrisome degrees, was encountered in some instances.

Hoping to eliminate complications, the extent of porosity on the surface of the metallic components was modified. Arguments were advanced in favor and against the degree to which the stem should be covered with porous material, and soon we witnessed the manufacturing of prostheses with porous surfaces throughout their entire length; others only to mid-level or proximal third, and even just over a small area below the collar of the femoral implant.

Surgeons found themselves having serious difficulties removing porous implants, which though well-fixed in the medullary canal or acetabulum needed to be revised for a variety of reasons such as recurrent dislocation, disabling pain, infection, and fractures of the components of the femur. Bone had grown into the pores making their removal difficult if not impossible.

Wear of the polyethylene socket continued to be a concern with both cemented and noncemented arthroplasties. Wear was originally found to be higher with the noncemented ones for reasons, which are not yet clear. It is believed that one reason for the higher wear observed with uncemented implants was the increased number of foreign body elements arising either from motion between the stem and the surrounding bone, from the outer surface of the acetabular cup, the plastic-metal articulation, the Morse taper head fixation, or from other modular components. These phenomena occurred more frequently with titanium alloy implants because the material is softer and, therefore, has a propensity to scratching.

The initial dissatisfaction with the cementless implants prompted a solution: the use of a noncemented acetabulum and a cemented femoral component. This modification was allegedly inspired by the finding that cementless acetabula had experienced a very low failure rate, while the femur had not performed as well. Although this "hybrid" model is still popular at this point, I have doubts about its future. I have personally documented a higher incidence of radiological complications in patients who had "hybrid" titanium prostheses than comparable cohorts of totally cemented titanium arthroplasties.

Experiences with implants with ceramic heads and acetabulum, rather than metal on polyethylene appear at this time, are encouraging. The success is explained by the reduced wear of the material as documented in laboratory conditions and in mid-term clinical series. However, ceramics are brittle and fractures of the implants have been reported. It is too early to categorically state that ceramics will replace metal on polyethylene. More recent reports have indicated that wear debris from these implants may initiate osteoclastic activity leading to loosening.

Similar concerns can be extended to metal-on-metal articulations. Metal-on-metal prostheses are beginning to show metallosis increasingly in large numbers. This development should be a source of concern in light of the finding of chromosomal abnormalities found in tissues at the site of metallosis, as reported by Professor Patrick Case from Bristol. Others, in the United States and in other countries, have expressed concerns about metal debris in the body, such as Jonathan Black from Philadelphia, and Joshua Jacobs from Chicago.

While the new approaches to weight-bearing surfaces are being evaluated, significant improvements are being made on the wear performance of new cross-linked polyethylenes. It will be a while before the true superiority of the cross-linked polyethylene is definitively proven.

The use of hydroxyapatite as a coating of the prosthetic implants, designed to further ensure bone ingrowth, has been reported to render better results. This perception is not universally shared at this time. When first recommended, a high failure rate was encountered, apparently due to the grains of the material being either too large or too small.

Recently, a great deal of enthusiasm has been generated with the concept of "minimally invasive" surgical approaches to total hip replacement. It is claimed to be a recent innovation, however, it was first introduced in Buenos Aires over 40 years ago by Dr Fermin Garcia. I visited him forty years ago and had the opportunity to observe the performance of the arthroplasty through a small incision. I returned home and tried the procedure. It was successful. However, I detected from the outset possible limitations of the system and the possibility of unexpected complications. The procedure is more difficult to perform and intraoperative complications more likely to occur.

At the time of this writing, acetabular osteotomies are being re-introduced into the armamentarium of the orthopedic surgeon, as well as concepts regarding the etiology of some types of osteoarthritis, such as the "lump" that grows on some femoral heads creating the now called "impingement syndrome". These ideas and procedures are being marketed with a great deal of enthusiasm, but it is much too premature to declare them effective. The same applies to the use of "navigation" to facilitate the most appropriate position of the various prosthetic components. This very appealing concept is already being discredited in some quarters because of a higher incidence of complications. I suspect that within the next few years, the system may become a part of history.

Despite the progress made in hip replacement, I feel it has not been proportional to the efforts made in this regard. I suspect the slow progress we have made is due to the fact that the orthopedic community relinquished many of its responsibilities to industry. Its control is so great that I have been able to state on numerous occasions that "the education of the orthopedist is structured primarily to satisfy the marketing needs of industry". The same can be said about research.

Two different episodes summarize eloquently the reasons for my deeply rooted concern over the extreme role the industry plays in the life of the orthopedist and the control of his education. The president of a major implant manufacturing company, whom I had known for quite some time, invited me a number of years ago to visit his factory to discuss my ideas regarding the future of total hip replacement. During the course of the visit, he said, "By the time we release a new prosthesis, we are already working on a new implant, in order to meet the competition given by their new implants." A few years later, the vice president of another company said to me, "The philosophy behind implant development is not the making of a better one, but a different one. The orthopedists seem to believe that a different implant is always better than the one it replaced." If these two experiences are not good eye-openers, I do not know what will it take to remove the blinders we have found so comfortable. These two episodes explain why is it that today we have on the market several hundred different total hip prostheses.

Had we retained control of our destiny, and maintained a balanced working relationship with industry, rather than accepting a subservient position, it is possible that we would have been in a better position to identify important issues and set aside ones which have only marketing value. The more recent trend of direct-to-patient marketing is making matters worse. At this moment, one can see elaborate ads on television advertising total joint prostheses using an athlete kicking a soccer ball and doing rock climbing after having his hip or knee surgically replaced. Such a marketing technique is misleading, dishonest and totally unprofessional. It should be forcefully opposed by our representative organizations. However, until now they have remained silent, much to the detriment of patients and the profession as a whole.

John Charnley warned us that wear was the biggest problem looming on the horizon and suggested that a concerted effort should be made in that direction. We ignored his words and today we find ourselves confronting problems that should have been solved long ago.

After limiting my surgical practice entirely to total hip replacement for 35 years, I stopped doing surgery and went back to teaching in outpatient clinics devoted to the indigent, where enormous deficiencies exist. Contrary to expectations, I did not find it difficult at all to stop doing hip surgery. Five years have gone by and have not once regretted my decision. I do, however, miss seeing patients and observing the unfolding of clinical events. This lack of enthusiasm for surgery was precipitated by the gradual realization that the operation was no longer challenging. It had become a routine where the appropriate use of techniques was the "name of the game". I compared this reaction with the continued challenges that traumatic conditions of the skeleton still make the subject so fascinating.

The progress that has taken place in the management of the fractured hip during the last few decades has been, in my opinion, limited. Fractures of the femoral neck, which have been known for a very long time to be associated with a high frequency of nonunion and avascular necrosis continue to occur despite the development of a multitude of differently fixation devices. The same can be said about the management of idiopathic avascular necrosis, which despite better diagnostic tools and techniques, remains an unsolved problem. Efforts to revascularize the necrotic head through a variety of techniques, such as core decompression, vascularized bone grafts and osteotomies, have rendered disproportionably unsatisfactory results. Prosthetic replacement of the necrotic head is being performed with greater and greater frequency in preference to osteotomies, grafting and other techniques. Prosthetic replacement has virtually become the only reasonable approach to the condition. This trend can be justified, not only in light of the frequency of bad result from reconstructive procedures but also because the good results from primary total hip replacement arthroplasty are being obtained.

The intertrochanteric and subtrochanteric fractures have fared better. The introduction of the closed intramedullary interlocking nail has revolutionized the care of these fractures. There is still much to be learned about the place and role of this technique. Suffices to say, however, that early results are encouraging to the point that its use has become the most popular and effective method of fixation of many, if not all, intertrochanteric and subtrochanteric fractures of the femur.

My interest in hip disease began very early in my career. My first experience took place during my internship. It happened in the Radiology Department at the Colombian Military Hospital in Bogota, where an elderly woman was lying on the table. She had sustained a fracture of the femoral neck the night before. The treating surgeon injected Novocain into the joint as well as over the subtrochanteric region. Once the anesthetizing was completed, he manipulated the extremity, following which an X-ray was obtained. Apparently happy with what he had seen, he picked up an instrument that held at its end what I was then told was a Smith-Petersen nail. With a single blow of a hammer, he drove the nail into the neck and head of the femur. An X-ray showed him that the placement of the nail was correct. The procedure had taken just a few minutes.

A couple of weeks later, I assisted Dr Guillermo Vargas in the reduction and nailing of a femoral neck fracture that a young soldier had suffered during a long march, shortly after his entry into the military. The experience this time was quite different. The reduction was impossible to obtain through manipulation, so an open reduction became necessary. Even though the femoral head and neck were being held reduced by the assistant surgeon, the driving of the nail into the head proved to be a major undertaking. The hard femoral head separated from the neck with every blow of the hammer. The bone seemed to be as hard as marble. I do not know what happened to the young man. I suspect, however, that his femoral head experienced avascular necrosis. These experiences prompted my desire to become an orthopedist.

Fate took me shortly afterwards to Columbia, South Carolina, where Austin T Moore, an already recognized giant in the field of hip surgery, had his practice. I became his resident and obtained from him, for a three years period, enormous love for hip surgery. His overall philosophy about patient care, his innovating ideas, and his restless and passionate commitment to the subject, did nothing but to reinforce my desire to become an active participant in the further development of the subspecialty.

Upon leaving South Carolina, I spent an additional year of residency in Orlando, Florida. The third program where I took my extended residency was at Jackson Memorial Hospital, the main teaching hospital for the University of Miami. From many of the attending surgeons, I also learned a great deal. However, Miami in the late 1950s did not have any one surgeon who could be considered a hip expert. Despite that absence, or perhaps because of the absence of such a person, I found myself deeply involved in efforts to raise the standards of care of the hip and to conduct investigative studies.

With élan and enthusiasm, and what appeared to be boundless energy, I delved into the subject of hip fractures. I performed the first Moore endoprosthetic replacement in the city. My interest in the intertrochanteric fracture led me to conduct studies in postmortem specimens and to gain insight into this very interesting fracture. I managed to arrange being notified every time a patient who had a hip fracture expired in the hospital or a nursing home in the community. I removed their hip joints and subjected them to crude testing. Eventually I published my findings and described an I-Bream nail for the treatment of those fractures. The new device, however, was promptly eclipsed by the sliding nail that had been developed by Kay Clawson, then Chief of Orthopedics in Seattle.

Suddenly, John Charnley came into my life. In the late 1960s, in the United States, very few people knew much about him. Some had read his masterful small book on fractures and had heard of his method of fusing hip joints. With skepticism, we learned of his experiences with hip arthroplasty and of his efforts to develop an implant, which contrary to the endoprosthetic replacement of Moore, would replace both sides of the joint. Our reluctance to embrace his new idea was further aggravated when it was learned that many of his patients had experienced catastrophic complications. Teflon, the plastic material that Charnley had used to replace the acetabulum, had poor wear properties. Bone lysis readily took place and massive damage to the surrounding tissues required removal of the implants.

Undeterred by the horrifying experience, Charnley continued his work. He had realized that he had made the mistake of choosing the wrong plastic, and began a desperate search for a better one. In polyethylene he found the right one. To this day, 60 years later, though not perfect, polyethylene remains the gold standard.

Upon learning of Charnley's success with the new plastic material, I issued him an invitation, on behalf of the American Academy of Orthopedic Surgeons, to attend a postgraduate course in Miami, which I, as chairman of the course, was organizing. I had asked him to participate by discussing his operation, and the results he was obtaining. His response was a dry and pithy one. "Total hip replacement should not be taught in an auditorium," he said. Then, he added, "Only those surgeons who have been trained under me for a period of one year and commit themselves to the frequent performance of the procedure, should do this type of surgery."

Somewhat offended by his remarks "since by that time I considered myself a fledgling hip surgeon". I asked him if he would accept me in his hospital for a period of three months, which was the longest time I could be away from my work at the University of Miami. His response was a positive one.

The next two and one-half months proved to have been one of the most exciting periods in my entire academic life. I was absolutely overwhelmed by Charnley's personality and his knowledge of the hip joint. Upon my return to the United States, I committed myself entirely to total hip replacement. It was the only surgical procedure I was to perform during the next 35 years.

Forever, fixed in my memory was the brief conversation I had with him the day I went to his office to say good-bye and to thank him for the opportunity he had granted me. I asked him, what was the next frontier in hip replacement. Without hesitation, he responded, "This is it. The only obstacle yet to be overcome is improving the articulating surfaces to prevent the production of debris and the resulting lysis."

I do not wish to describe his remark as hubris. However, his belief that his operation was the final word (though it could have been the case) left me a bit uncomfortable. Despite his greatness, he was human after all.

My interest and involvement in traumatic and degenerative conditions of the hip caught the attention of Dr Frank Stinchfield, the Professor of Orthopedics at Columbia University in the 1960s and 70s, who invited me to be among other 19 orthopedists to be a founding member of the Hip Society in 1968. In 1976, the International Hip Society was also founded by Dr Stinchfield, to which he invited me to be a founding member. I served as President of the Hip Society in 1976-1978 and have remained active in the functions of both societies. For eight years, I was the historian of the Hip Society.

Throughout the text, I based my comments primarily on my own personal experiences and conclusion, though vicariously learned in many instances. I am keenly aware many of my expressed views have been or will be proven to have been erroneous. That should not matter to the reader. No human being has had or will ever have the monopoly of knowledge. As far as I am concerned, what is important is the effort involved in seeking the truth. Not reaching that goal is not a crime; quite the contrary, the best part of the quest. It was Socrates, the immortal Athenian Philosopher who said, "An unexamined life is not worth living."

There will be some amongst the readers of the book who will readily argue the book dwells too heavily on subjects that have only historical interest, which are not worth knowing about; and that new ideas and techniques have permanently replaced the old ones. To some extent, they are correct; however, they ignore the fact that this is not the only time the orthopedic community has welcomed new ideas and expected them to become infallible, eventually realizing that those new ideas were soon replaced with "newer and better" ones. To question and investigate the reasons for their failure should help us in the charting of future ideas and the developing of newer techniques. It was Winston Churchill who said, "The longer you look back, the more you can see further."

I question the wisdom of those who dismiss history, and pay attention only to contemporary attitudes and trends. They are the ones who argue that it is irrelevant for the young to learn the role the ancient Indians, Chinese, Egyptians, Mesopotamians, Greeks and Romans played in the foundation of our civilization. To them, it is a waste of time to read the classics, and argue that modern ideas and literature is all that is needed to reach success in our materialistic society. Those people have been extremely successful in removing the reading of Shakespeare, Dante and Cervantes from the curriculum of so many of our colleges and universities, and have equally declared that the music of Back, Mozart or Beethoven should be replaced with the incoherent noise that currently pollutes the air.

At the risk of being criticized for listing a references composed exclusively of articles, commentaries, books and lectures I have published and/or delivered, I have choosen this route upon realizing that I have neither the talent nor the patience to quote the thousands of publications dealing with the subjects at hand. This book, therefore, is neither a scholarly written document nor a *manifesto* proposing a definitive plan of action. It simply is a personal attempt to bringforth personal experiences and vicarious experiences accumulated over a long professional career devoted to the study of hip diseases and traumatic conditions.

Augusto Sarmiento

Contents

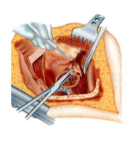

SECTION 1: RECONSTRUCTIVE SURGERY

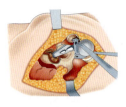

SECTION 2: SPECIFIC PATHOLOGICAL CONDITIONS

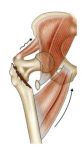

SECTION 3: THE FRACTURED HIP

SECTION 4: ANNEXURES

Section 1

Reconstructive Surgery

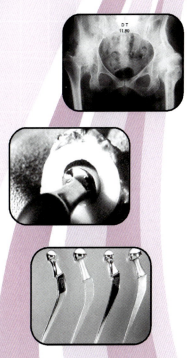

1

Thromboembolic Disease

Infection used to be the complication surgeons who performed total hip arthroplasty feared the most. More effective prophylactic antibiotics have made the procedure much safer. Thromboembolic disease following hip surgery has been identified as today's number one problem; so much so that it is virtually impossible to find a surgeon who does not use some type of chemical prophylactic whenever he or she performs any major surgery around the hip joint.

Is the danger of thromboembolic disease as great as we have been led to believe? Is chemical prophylaxis the most effective way to prevent it? I doubt both premises. No one denies the fact that pulmonary emboli and/or thrombophlebitis can complicate major hip surgery but, in my opinion, their incidence has been greatly exaggerated. Interested pharmaceutical companies (the Pharmaceutical lobby) have unduly, and sometimes irresponsibly, promoted chemical prophylaxis as an indispensable adjuvant under all circumstances. In order to frighten the lay and medical community, data from experiences that took place four of five decades ago are presented. This is misleading, since in the early days of total hip replacements patients were kept in bed for several weeks following the surgical procedures. Today, they are mobilized either the first or second postoperative day, with obvious beneficial results. This factor has made a major difference.

I doubt the current popularity of prophylactic anticoagulants has had a positive influence in the incidence of thromboembolic disease. As far as I am concerned we have "made a mountain out of a mole" and have allowed industry to skillfully manipulate the issue.

Can I support my views on the issue? I think so. Doctor Lorraine Day, during her tenure as chief of orthopedics at the San Francisco General Hospital in the 1980's, allegedly reported on 1000 patients who underwent nailing of intertrochanteric fractures, and who did not receive chemical prophylactic of any kind. The incidence of thromboembolic disease she found was virtually nonexistent.

I was very intrigued by her report when I first heard it. It prompted me to look more carefully into the issue. Today, based on careful analysis of my own data and the review of the world literature, I am convinced that the problem, though a potential one, is being approached by most people without solid scientific support.

In the case of total hip arthroplasty, it is very likely that vascular damage, caused at the time of surgery, might eventually lead to the formation of clots and their possible dislodgment into the systemic circulation. This observation was first made by surgeons in New Zealand, whose names unfortunately I do not recall. Others in this country have repeated the New Zealanders' studies and some of them have claimed originality. The initial studies were performed using venography during surgery. *It indicated that the femoral vessels experience severe kinking during extreme degrees of flexion and rotation of the hip.* This kinking may be significant enough to injure the vessels. *They also demonstrated that the degree of kinking was greater when the surgical procedure was performed through an anterior approach that calls for flexion and external rotation of the hip. The kinking was less when the posterior approach was used, which requires flexion and internal rotation.* Our clinical experiences have supported this view, since the incidence of thromboembolic complications was higher when the anterior approach was used.

Since, I have virtually performed all of my total hip replacements through a posterior approach with the exception of the first one thousands, for which I used the anterior approach—I have adhered to an intraoperative protocol consisting of avoidance of extreme rotation and flexion of the hip and knee, and the *frequent passive mobilization of the hip, knee and ankle during the surgical procedure*. Since, it is necessary during surgery to hold the hip joint in flexion and internal rotation during the preparation of the femoral side, when the posterior approach is used, the length of time for such a position should be shortened as much as possible. There is no need to hold the knee in full flexion and internal rotation of the hip for more than the few minutes necessary to obtain the proper orientation.

I am also convinced that physical exercise is a most effective means of prophylaxis; better than any chemical or physical method. In my practice, I insist that patients begin active isometric and isotonic exercises of their gluteus maximus, the quadriceps and ankle and toes muscles as soon as possible. I also recommend deep breathing and trunk and abdominal exercises.

When I first visited Sir John Charnley's Hip Center in England in 1970, I heard him discuss the problem of thromboembolic disease in total hip surgery. *At that time he kept his patients in bed for a very long time following surgery.* He had tried various methods of prophylaxis with ambivalent results. At that particular time he was experimenting with ReoMacrodex. When I returned to the United States I used it in a large number of patients. I was disappointed by the high incidence of extensive swelling of the extremity that accompanied its use. I then proceeded to use aspirin as prophylaxis. For the last thirty-five years it has been my preferred chemical agent. The results have been satisfactory; however *I suspect that it is not the aspirin that led to those results but the program of intraoperative and postoperative exercises.*

Doctor AK Goswami, a former Fellow in our department in Los Angeles and now a surgeon in the United Kingdom, reviewed all my total hip arthroplasties and made some very interesting observations. For example, the incidence of fatal pulmonary embolism in nearly 1800 patients was 0.1%. *There was no difference in results in relation to gender or age of the patients; the same was true for the type of stockings used, compressive elastic or intermittent compression devices. There was also no difference in the rate of complications between those patients who had the surgery performed on the East and West coasts of the United States. Epidural anesthesia, however, was associated with a lower incidence of complications as well as the posterior approach when compared with the lateral, transtrochanteric one.*

The American literature is virtually empty of reports where no chemical prophylaxis was used. The British literature has seriously addressed the issue and some have claimed that prophylaxis is not needed. Some investigators have demonstrated, using controlled populations, that the incidence of thromboembolic disease was the same in patients receiving placebos and those receiving chemical prophylaxis. It is not likely that similar reports will be forthcoming from surgeons in the United States. The fear of litigation in the event of a fatality scares all of us. The power of the pharmaceutical industry is awesome. One method the pharmaceutical industry uses to enhance its power is the use of orthopedists to serve as peddlers of its products, who travel from city to city singing the praises of the respective medications. These peddler, needles to say, are in the direct or indirect payroll of the sponsoring firms. Their testimony against anyone who fails to administer the product they market is likely to bring about the guilty verdict of malpractice.

A pharmaceutical firm has offered between $800 and $1000 per patient to orthopedic surgeons willing to use low-molecular heparin and complete forms indicating demographic information and short post-surgical data. Recently, an internist in our hospital received $50,000 for the inclusion of 15 patients into the "study" being conducted by the industrial concern.

Paying kickbacks to orthopedic surgeons for the use of marketing of surgical implants by industrial concerns has reached the degree that called for the Justice Department to officially investigate egregious abuses. The Justice Department refers the issue as being full of "serious transgressions and corruption."

Obviously, aspirin in combination with exercise is not the only effective protocol against thromboembolic disease. Good results have been reported using other methods such as Coumadin. However, this method is complicated. The incidence of associated bleeding is relatively high and its use requires daily laboratory tests, which increase the cost of care. However, the cost is not nearly as high as it is with the use of low-molecular heparin (Lovenox). The hospital charge for the daily injections in the Miami area is over $100. The need to continue the daily injections (as recommended by the makers of the product) for either twenty or thirty days further raises the ultimate cost. Low-molecular heparin precludes the use of spinal and epidural anesthesia because of the reported danger of intraspinal bleeding. Instances of paraplegia secondary to the administration of heparin have appeared in the literature.

We have recently published our results in 1835 hip arthroplasties performed in 1585 patients where the prophylactic protocol consisted of intra and postoperative exercises followed by the rectal administration of 10 grains of aspirin immediately after surgery and 325 mg of the medication orally twice a day for the length hospitalization.

The surgical approach to the hip was a posterior one, and was carried out under general anesthesia in 459 instances, and regional anesthesia in 1376 instances. Graduated elastic stockings were used in 1117 instances and intermittent compression stockings in 718 instances. Passive exercises to the major joints of the operated extremity were carried out intra-operatively, and active exercises postoperatively. *Fatal pulmonary embolism developed following 2 (0.10%) surgical procedures. Nonfatal pulmonary embolisms were diagnosed in 17 (0.9%) instances, and deep venous thrombosis in 18 (0.9%) instances.*

These well-documented experiences strongly indicate that the simple and inexpensive method of prophylaxis is superior to more expensive methods that have associated complications, some of which serious.

A recent publication by Forward et al, conducted in Baltimore MD but published in the British edition of the Journal of Bone and Joint Surgeons, documented that aspirin and exercise render results superior to those with low-molecular heparin. This publication vindicates our work and that conducted by many others.

References*

15, 80, 82, 92, 96, 98, 99, 102, 103, 106, 109, 110, 116, 120

---

* References provided at the end of the book after annexures.

2

Fat Embolism

We dread the situation when a patient suffering from some type of musculoskeletal condition develops signs of fat embolism, since we know the condition may be fatal. A number of measures to treat the syndrome have been advocated over the years. I am not qualified to comments on the merits of the various approaches. All I know is that the management of this complication is more successful today that it was a few decades ago.

The syndrome is extremely rare following elective hip surgery, so much that we seem to take for granted it does not occur. We rarely mention it to our patients as a possible complication.

It is believed the pathophysiology of fat embolism is that of a sudden introduction of fat into the systemic circulation reaching the lungs and other organs. That is how we explain it when it follows a fracture of the femur. The rich marrow of the bone releases the fat when the fracture occurs. Why is it that the syndrome does not develop more often after hip replacement, when theoretically, it should be a common occurrence?

My interest in the subject began in the early seventies while working with Doctor Tomas Kallos, an anesthesiologist at the University of Miami. He closely monitored patients on whom I was performing total hip surgery. Prior to beginning the surgical intervention he had placed catheters into the major vessels leading to the heart. He was not the first one to notice that at the time of insertion of the cement and prosthesis into the medullary canal there was an audible "gurgle" coming from the vicinity of the heart. The sound was easily detected through the stethoscope. He identified a large amount of bone marrow fat flowing into the systemic circulation at the time of injection of the cement and prosthesis in the medullary canal. In spite of that, patients did not develop symptoms or signs of fat embolism. Intrigued, he took the project to the animal laboratory, where he carried out a procedure similar to the cemented prosthetic replacement. His findings reproduced the ones observed in the human situation: the experimental animals did not show any of the clinical symptoms or findings of fat embolism.

He was able to create the syndrome by making the animals hypovolemic prior to the injection of the cement. When the animals were subsequently sacrificed and studied, there was evidence of massive amounts of fat in organs throughout the body. If the animals were maintained normovolemic no complications occurred.

From his experiences we learned that appropriate oxygenation and maintenance of blood volume are essential for the prevention of the intraoperative fat embolism that leads to the clinical syndrome.

I have extrapolated from the total hip replacement observations to trauma. It has been said that early intramedullary stabilization of fractures of long bones reduces the incidence of fat embolism. *The proponents of this approach argue that the early fixation with intramedullary nails stops the leakage of medullary fat into the systemic circulation.*

I find the argument, in my opinion, runs contrary to common sense. The nailing of a femur brings a massive shower of fat into the systemic circulation, even greater that the one experienced immediately following the original insult. Theoretically, the nailing should make matters worse. *However, patients do better. I submit, not because the amount of released fat has been reduced but because the patient, prior to and throughout the surgical procedure, is maintained normovolemic and properly oxygenated by the anesthesiologist. The* anesthesiologist wants to be certain that the patient's oxygenation and hemoglobin levels are appropriately maintained by transfusing blood and administrating oxygen.

The patient with a femoral fracture who is kept in traction is likely to lose blood and fat into the tissues around the fracture bone and continues to do so for a period of time until tamponade occurs or spontaneous hemostasis takes place. It is during this relatively early period of time of progressive hypovolemia that the patient develops the symptoms and signs of fat embolism. The early nailing prevents the undesirable environment.

3

Acetabular and Femoral Osteotomies

Prior to the introduction of total hip replacement, osteotomies of the femur or acetabulum were, along with fusion, the most common procedures used in the treatment of disabling osteoarthritis of the hip. Muscle releases (the "hanging hip"), drilling of the femoral head and neurectomies were used with less frequency. Large numbers of different types of fusions were described in the literature, each one having its strong supporters. It was Freika, the Czechoslovakian surgeon who said, "For the care of the chronically painful hip any operation brings about relief".

Osteotomy of the acetabulum was quite popular, but the results obtained from it were not frequently long-lasting, and within a few years a recurrence of symptoms was usually observed. Most acetabular osteotomies consisted in procedures where grafts taken from the iliac bone were anchored to the lateral aspect of the acetabulum in an effort to enlarge the cavity and obtain greater contact between the femoral head and the bony socket. The Chiari acetabular osteotomy was different, and was for quite some time the most popular osteotomy, and in retrospect a physiological one. The procedure basically consisted of a pelvic osteotomy, followed by manual displacement of the distal component in a medial direction, resulting in coverage of the femoral head and a major change in the distribution of stresses in the hip joint. The operation is no longer performed in the adult, though the lessons learned from it are vital to the

understanding of more contemporary osteotomies, as well as that of replacement arthroplasty.

I personally performed a few Chiari osteotomies and had the opportunity to convert failed ones to total hip arthroplasty. I also had the opportunity to listen to Chiari report on his long-term experiences. In the mid-70s, at a meeting of the International Hip Society in Berne, Switzerland, I witnessed the memorable event I will cover in the chapter dealing with the International Hip Society. (See Addendum: *The International Hip Society*).

My personal experience with femoral osteotomies is also limited. The popular femoral osteotomies of a couple of decades ago, were aimed at realigning the femur in order to increase or decrease the varus, valgus or rotation of the proximal femur. They were performed primarily for the treatment of osteoarthritis following congenital hip dysplasia (Figs 3.1A and B). In other instances the operations were carried out in order create a better mechanical environment for nonunion of femoral neck fractures. The last of the popular femoral osteotomies was the varus one described by Renato Bombelli, form Italy. His enormous experience with congenital hip disease gave him the opportunity to study the subject in great depth. Ultimately, total hip arthroplasty (Fig. 3.2) appears to have relegated his procedure to the heap of history, as it was the case with the vast majority of other procedures performed about the hip. I suspect this

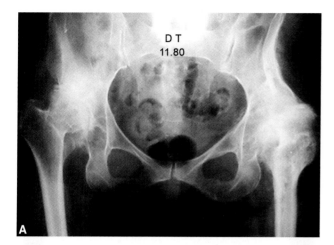

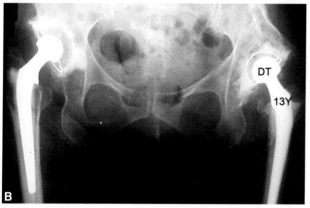

FIGS 3.1A AND B

(A) Bilateral congenital hip dysplasia treated by manipulation and casting. At a later date the left hip had an acetabular osteotomy. (B) Radiographs obtained 13 years after bilateral cemented titanium arthroplasties

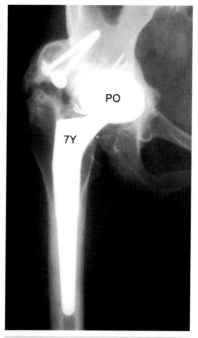

FIG. 3.2

Radiograph of a noncemented total hip arthroplasty showing a graft built laterally, allegedly in an attempt to provide good acetabular coverage. *One can see that the graft was not necessary since good coverage was accomplished simply by deepening the shallow acetabulum*

adverse reaction will prove to have been premature. *A careful review of the literature proves that femoral osteotomies have a very definite place in the care of the osteoarthritic hip in the younger age group.* Despite the great advances made in total hip surgery, there is no evidence as yet that the clinical results from the procedure will last the 60 or 70 years the "optimists" are predicting.

I suspect acetabular osteotomies will gain greater popularity as their value becomes better known within the orthopedic community, and the surgical technique is made easier. At this time it is said that the periacetabular osteotomy offers a good prognosis only if the radiological changes are minimal. There are some hip surgeons, however, who are attempting to enlarge the indications for the osteotomy, who are reporting increasingly gratifying results. I see no reason as to why the trend should soon die, since osteotomies, like the Chiari one, proved to be successful in many

patients, who at the time of surgery had advanced degenerative disease. If these surgeons find their results from osteotomies performed in moderately advanced osteoarthritis to be satisfactory, a major advancement in reconstructive hip surgery would have been accomplished.

I address at this time only my experiences with revision of failed osteotomies into total hips.

The little bit I know today about acetabular osteotomies is based on vicarious information, primarily from observing Joel Matta, from Los Angeles, perform the operation several times and following some of his patients for several years (Figs 3.3 and 3.4). *I noticed in a few patients that had periacetabular osteotomies ended up with final limitation of internal rotation. I was concerned that such an abrupt limitation of motion might lead to later osteoarthritic changes (Figs 3.5A and B).* Doctor Matta, however, has given me reassurance that such limitation of motion improves with time and that it can be prevented by proper adherence to technical details. I assisted Doctor Matta in surgery a few times hoping to be able to learn the technique. It did not take me very

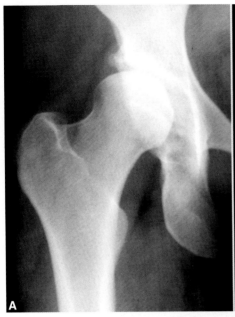
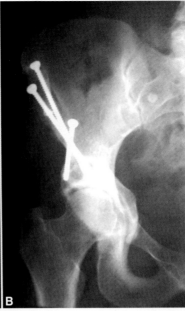

FIGS 3.3A AND B
(A) Radiograph of the left hip of a 35-year-old woman who suffered from bilateral congenital hip dysplasia. Radiologically, the osteoarthritic changes were minimal and clinically the symptoms and findings were mild. (B) Radiograph obtained 3 years after acetabular osteotomy. Notice the good coverage of the femoral head, and the absence of pathological findings. The range of motion of the hip was normal. (*Courtesy:* Joel W Matta, MD)

FIGS 3.4A AND B
(A) Preoperative radiograph of dysplastic hip. The clinical symptoms and radiological findings were minimal. (B) Radiograph of post-acetabular osteotomy obtained 8 years later. There was a long delay in obtaining union of the pubic osteotomy, however, it eventually took place. (*Courtesy:* Joel Matta, MD)

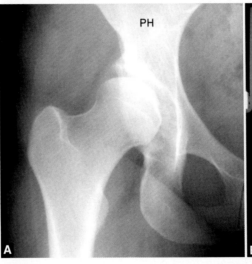
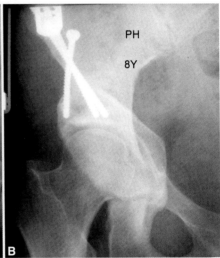

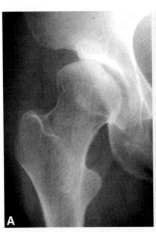
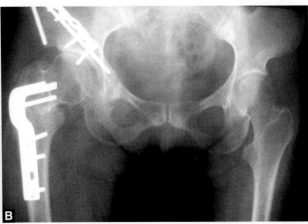

FIGS 3.5A AND B
(A) Radiograph of dysplastic painful hip showing moderate osteoarthritic changes. (B) Radiographs showing the final result from the osteotomy. The resulting severe varus shortened the extremity and altered the muscular balance necessary to walk without a limp

long to realize that I lacked the three-dimensional vision required for its performance.

Total hip arthroplasty for failed osteotomies may be difficult as a result of the distorted anatomy, the frequent presence of limitation of motion and the shorter limb. It is not uncommon to see patients, following the replacement arthroplasty, regain motion very slowly, and oftentimes end-up with permanent limitation of motion. That limitation of motion, I suspect, may be highly responsible for the loosening of some of these implants. *This is likely to be similar to the loosening of prostheses in other parts of the body where limitation of motion is present.* One can extrapolate that the abrupt blocking of motion of the joint transfers stresses to the artificial implants, which are not easily tolerated. Perhaps, an analogy can be established with the patient with a fused hip, who after receiving a total knee implant frequently develops early loosening of the knee implant.

4

Cement Pressurization

When the concept of pressurization of cement into the cancellous bone of the acetabulum was introduced, I felt uncomfortable, because of the possible damage that the deep penetration of cement into cancellous bone might do. *I speculated that though it is obvious that the deeper the penetration of the cement into the cancellous bone would provide better mechanical fixation, a greater amount of cancellous bone is immobilized by the stiffer cement. That degree of unphysiological immobilization could result in eventual atrophy of the now nonstressed cancellous bone.*

We took the idea to the laboratory where we injected cement deep into the greater trochanter and in the distal femoral condyles of rabbits. The animals were sacrificed at regular intervals and the injected areas were studied microscopically. We found that, at first, there was a burst of capillary reaction suggesting an inflammatory response. We also noticed that with the passage of time the capillary activity decreased, the walls of the cancellous bone got thinner and the viability of the remaining bone was significantly lost (Figs 4.1 to 4.5).

I see no need to describe in great detail the findings obtained form the study. Let it suffice to say that, as expected, when the higher pressures were used for the injection of the cement, its penetration into the cancellous bone was greater. We had chosen to apply the forces normally used in the human during routine performance of total hip arthroplasty.

When vascular studies were conducted, it was notices that one week after the injection of the cement a major capillary reaction took place.

As expected the thickness of the bony trabecular observed after the injection of the cement was that of a normal bone. However, when the animals were

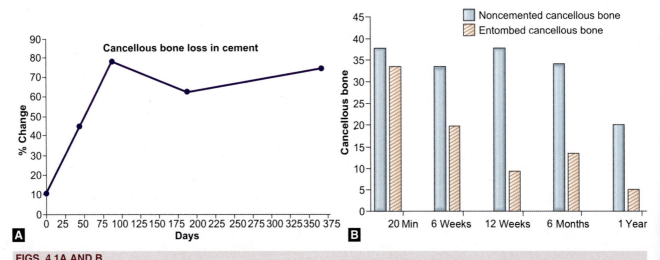

FIGS 4.1A AND B

Cement that penetrates deep into cancellous bone produces a larger area of bone death, probably due to the immobilization of bone created by the foreign material

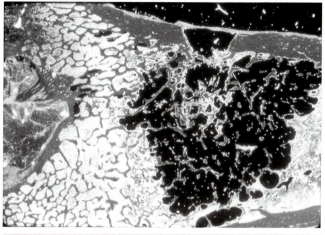

FIG. 4.2

Illustration of deep penetrating cement into the cancellous bone of the femoral condyle

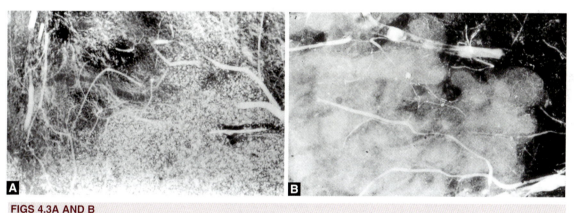

FIGS 4.3A AND B

Illustration of the vascular reaction that follows the injection of the cement into the cancellous bone

sacrificed at later dates it was observed that the trabecular thickness had gradually decreased (Figs 4.4A to E).

The length of the study was limited to one year. We have no idea what the biological changes in the area would have been if the animals had been followed for a longer period of time. *We concluded, however, that the deeper the penetration of cement into the bone, the greater the degree of bony atrophy and death of bone.* We speculated that the weak mechanical area present at the junction between normal could partially explain the late loosening of some cemented acetabular components.

I am not suggesting that this is the only mode of failure of cemented acetabular cups. To conclude this is the only cause of loosening would be foolish, since we know that other mechanical and biological phenomena may also play a role. Our findings however, should not be dismissed too quickly.

It is well-known that as we age, the medullary canal of our bones expands at the expense of the cortical bone. The inner diameter of the canal increases and the cortex gets thinner. This normal phenomenon suggests that over the years all cemented implants should get loose as the inner diameter of the cortex increases. However, this does not seem to be the case. It is possible that the reduced bending, tensile and compressive forces on the cortical bone are compensated by previously non-existing hoop stresses.

I had long been greatly interested in the subject of fracture healing and the role of motion and stresses at the fracture site, and had participated in numerous studies that strongly suggested that immobilization was detrimental to fracture healing. The changes that occur under a plate that rigidly immobilizes a fracture are highly undesirable. The thinning of the cortical bone and the overall demineralization of the bone under the plate were explained by its advocates as being the result of impaired local circulation. This explanation did not withstand the test of time or further scientific studies. It is now recognized that the

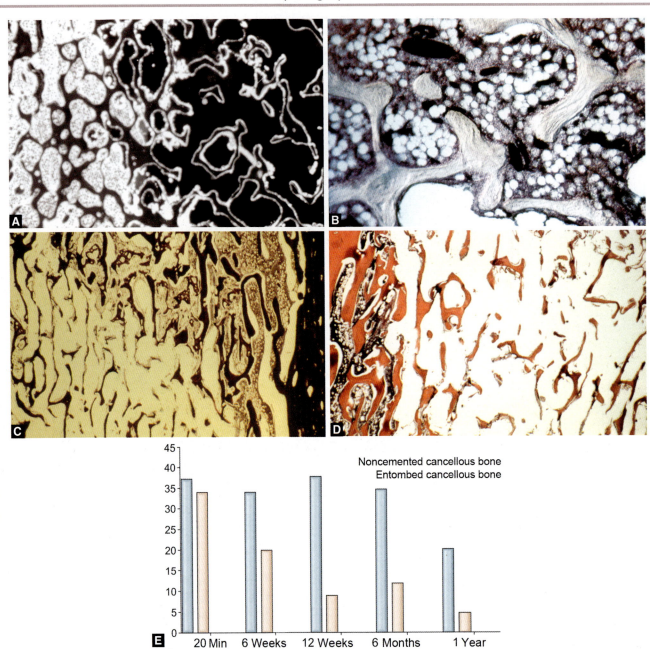

FIGS 4.4A TO E

(A and B) Microscopic pictures of the normal thickness of the trabecular bone seen shortly after the injection of acrylic cement. (C and D) With the passing of time, the bone trabecular becomes thinner. (E) Barograph demonstrating the progressive thinning of the trabecular bone as time passes. It compares the changes that occur in the low-pressure of the cement injection with the higher pressure. Notice that the atrophy of the trabecular occurs in both groups, the greater atrophy seen in the high-pressure group

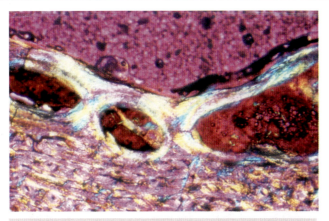

FIG. 4.5

An inflammatory reaction takes place at the bone-cement interface.
It gradually subsides

real reason for the adverse changes under the immobilizing plate is the lack of motion at the fracture site.

Efforts to explain the slow healing that takes place when diaphyseal fractures are treated with plates have included the thesis that damage to the periosteum is the main culprit. However, this myth that surrounds the power of the periosteum vanishes when one considers that plates inserted with meticulous avoidance of periosteal stripping do not show any evidence of periosteal callus. By the same token, the absence of periosteal callus in fractures managed with rigid external fixators, further undermines the long-held belief in the role of the periosteum in fracture healing. Shortly after a diaphyseal fracture occurs, a massive invasion of capillary is seen. The perithelial and endothelial cells of these capillaries have the ability to undergo osteoblastic metaplasia. Therefore, the greater the number of capillary the bigger and stronger the callus. If the fracture is rigidly immobilized the capillary invasion never takes place, and the repair of the fracture is provided by the endosteum through a so-called primacy healing; healing without external callus, which is weaker and develops slowly.

References*

47, 115, 121

* References provided at the end of the book after annexures.

5

Radiolucent and Sclerotic Lines

The presence of a fracture of the cement provokes a logical reaction of concern in the mind of the surgeon. Such a development is usually interpreted as a sign of early failure. The recognition of a fracture is not necessarily a reflection of impending failure and can very well be a normal phenomenon of an inconsequential nature. In our laboratories, several investigators conducted sophisticated studies on the subject and reached very interesting conclusions regarding the mechanism that accompanies the subsidence of cement into the medullary canal and the fact that some degree of debonding is not in itself an unhealthy development.

Some surgeons have categorically stated that a fracture of the cement below the tip end of a prosthesis is an ominous sign, since further pathological changes inevitably follow. Though it is true that the presence of a fracture of the cement can be an early sign of failure, *I have seen a number of radiographs demonstrating a distal cement fracture, without showing any further changes over a period of years (Figs 5.1A to C).*

I do not wish to belittle and underestimate the presence of cement fractures. I simply wish to share with the readers my personal observations regarding their appearance, suggesting that their appearance should not be taken necessarily as being ominous. However, they should be monitored on a regular basis, since often times their progression can lead to complete failure.

A debate raged in the orthopedic arena regarding the importance of the width of those lines (Figs 5.2A to E). Some felt that, for example, radiolucent lines between bone and cement were of no consequence if

they measured less than one millimeter. Having worked very closely with Thomas Gruen, he eventual guru of total hips reading, we began to realize that there was nothing scientific or logical to justify excluding thin lines from consideration. After all, they all represent a process that though it may be inconsequential sometimes, it might be an expression of impending future problems.

Our zealously, however, may have gone too far, and we may have failed to see the forest for the trees. Nothing suggests to me that the final word has been written. Much too often I have followed patients whose radiographs demonstrated the gradual onset of bone-cement or meta-cement radiolucent lines that reached a certain thickness never to progress any further. Other times, I have seen radiolucent lines that within a very short time progressed rapidly.

This variance might be due to the fact that the etiology of radiolucent lines does not always has the same etiology. Some may be the product of chemical changes brought about by chemical phenomena initiated from wear debris, cellular reaction for which we do not as yet have clear understanding, or simply mechanical alterations in the acrylic cement resulting from modified distribution of stresses.

Many have studied the content of newly created bone-cement interfaces and have been able to advance information suggesting chemical/cellular changes capable of explaining the etiology of those lytic lesions. I insist, however, that all increased bone-cement interfaces cannot be explained in a universal and

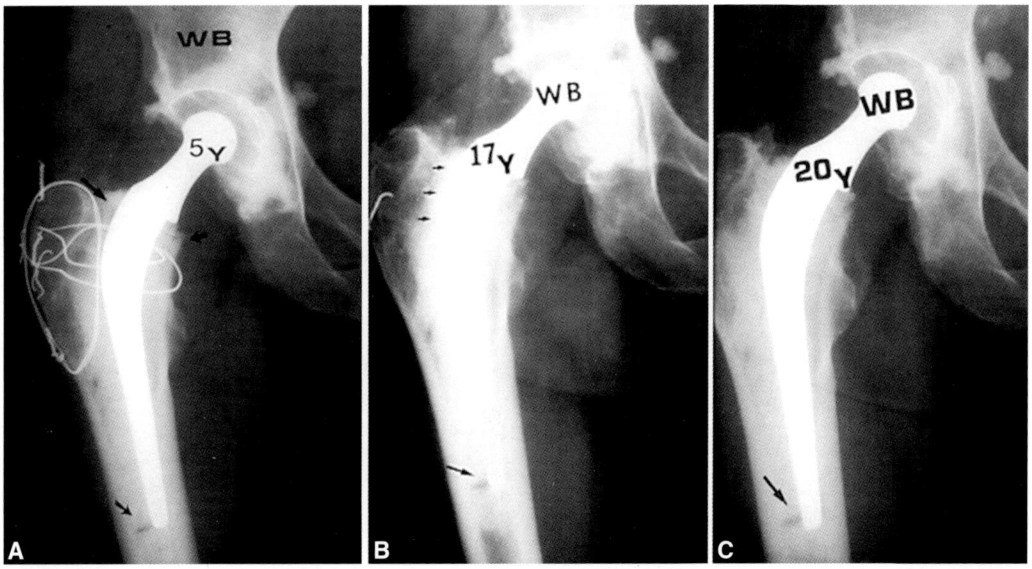

FIGS 5.1A TO C

(A) Radiograph showing a fracture of the cement distally 5 years after surgery. The patient was a very active, tall and heavy man. (B) Radiograph obtained 17 years after surgery. A cement/metal radiolucent line is seen in zone one. (C) Radiograph showing no evidence of progressive loosening 20 years postsurgery

simple manner. Putting it bluntly, our knowledge is still very limited in this area and it may be a long time before we can understand the issue and find solutions.

The presence of sclerotic lines, which are more likely to be seen in noncemented femoral implants have always been considered an expression of loosening of the metallic stem. This simple and often logical and valid explanation seemed to satisfy our limited curiosity and did not permit us to challenge the concept.

However, if one looks carefully at the development and behavior of some of the sclerotic and lytic lines present in noncemented implants, one must be puzzled by their geometry and distribution. Loosening cannot explain some of them. For example, many surgeons, including myself, have explored surgically non-cemented femoral components, having a proximal porous surface, which we had diagnosed as being loose, based on the presence of gradual increase in the with of the space between the end on the prosthesis and the medial wall of the femur. The gap had gotten larger, and the stem had migrated into the lateral femoral cortex, oftentimes bulging into it. Pain usually accomplished the drifting prosthesis.

At the time of surgery, however, it is discovered that the implant is rigidly fixed to the bone and the porous surface of the stems unequivocally shows bone ingrowth. Having made this mistake more than once, and having discussed the issue with surgeons who had

similar experiences, *I concluded that the radiological changes were on occasion, an expression of bending of the bone below the tip of the prosthesis rather than the anticipated move of the prosthesis toward the bone.* It does not take much thought to justify this explanation. The difference in the modulus of elasticity of the bone versus that of the implant is enormous, particularly in the osteoporotic individual. The bone normally bends when it is subjected to vertical loading in a degree that decreases as the bone ages. The child falls a hundred times a month and may never sustain a fracture. His/ her bones bend under the impact, something that cannot happen to the bones of older people, since they have become less flexible and more brittle.

Under the constant vertical forces to which the femur is subjected at every step the bone bends but the implant does not since it is too stiff. *The fulcrum for the bending is located at the end of the prosthesis. In some instances, for reasons not well-understood, the femur continues to bend, undergoing permanent deformation.* Through this mechanism one can explain, in those instances, the displacement of the distal stem toward the lateral cortex.

To reinforce the logic of the argument, one must also consider the fact that the separation between the stem and the cortex does not seem to occur throughout the entire length of the implant, only very distally. *If the space were to be explained as a windshield wiper motion of the stem, a gap between the bone and the implant would have to be*

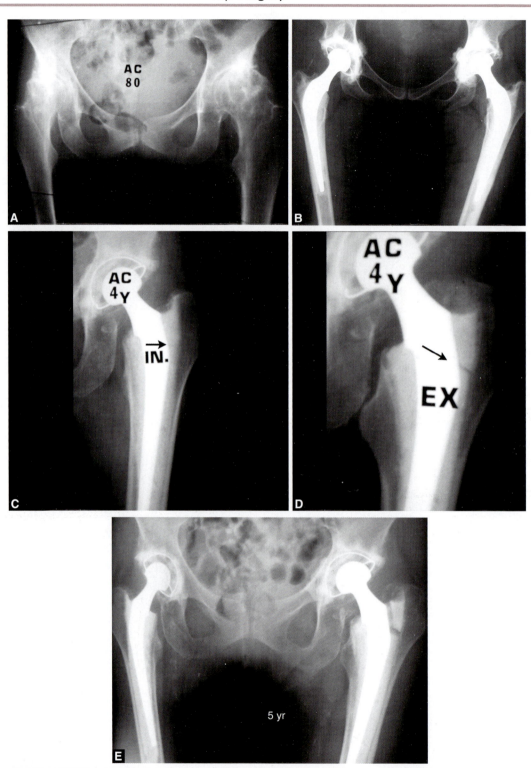

FIGS 5.2A TO E

(A) Bilateral osteoarthritis. (B) Bilateral cemented titanium alloy arthroplasties. (C and D) Radiograph taken with the leg in internal and external rotation. (E) Radiograph obtained five years after surgery. The patient was still asymptomatic and died a year later

necessarily present also around the proximal end of the implant. This does not happen, simply because proximally bone ingrowth has taken place, preventing any pendulum motion (See *Late Onset of High Pain*).

It is not uncommon to find loose endoprostheses that radiologically show the presence of an involucrum-like structure forming along the length of the stem. Upon removal of the implant the involucrum remains intact. As the canal is reamed for the insertion of a new stem,

and unless a deliberate effort is made to remove the involucrum, the newly injected cement remains inside the narrow tunnel, never becoming in contact with the true femoral cortex (See *Late Onset of Thigh Pain: Page 266*).

References

20, 43, 70, 72, 76, 104

Section 1

---
* References provided at the end of the book after annexures.

6

The Charnley Prosthesis

When it comes to discussing total hip replacement, the name of John Charley should appear first, for without his pioneering work the field would be today virtually empty. His work in the 1960s set the stage for the subsequent attempts made by many others to finally crystallize the long dream of successfully replacing the hip joint. He was indeed not the first one to try but, very definitely the first one to make the dream a reality.

It should remember that it took the genius of Charnley, his tenacity and integrity, to make replacement of the hip joint successfully. His first experience with the new procedure was a devastating catastrophe, since he wrongly chose Teflon as the material to the acetabulum. Under laboratory conditions Teflon had proven most suitable for implantation in the body, however, that was not the case. Within a very sort time he found out that Teflon underwent rapid wear that created harmful debris. This debris formed granuloma that produced severe lysis of the surrounding tissues (See *Wear*).

If I am not mistaken Charnley found it necessary to remove the implants in all of the several hundred patients on whom he had performed the procedure. I happened to be a few months at Charnley's Hip Center when the last of his patients was admitted to the hospital to have the implants removed. One could easily see the granuloma bulge under the skin of the thigh and the lower abdomen. The pelvis as well as the femur had undergone massive destruction.

A person of a lesser stature would have stopped any further attempts to solve the problem. John Charnley decided to turn the defeat into a challenge; and he confronted the new challenge it with the same passion and enthusiasm that had displayed with Teflon. He immediately realized that the acrylic cement that he had used to anchor the parts in place was not the culprit. He then began a furious search for a better material to replace the Teflon. He found in high density polyethylene that material he was looking for. The rest is history.

Charnley had undertaken his investigations in the most sophisticated manner possible in his days. Contrary to the intuitively more desirable large heads to replace the large human femoral heads, he concluded that a small prosthetic head made more sense. He recognized the fact that a small head (22,2 mm) would show a higher linear wear than a bigger head, but would produce more volumetric wear. He knew that polyethylene, though of much better wear properties than Teflon, would eventually wear, and in the process create lysis. He categorically stated that a total hip arthroplasty would not last 30 years in an active individual. He was wrong in this pronouncement, but served the orthopedic community in restraining from performing the procedure in very young people.

His cautious prognosis of failure, provides a stark contrast with pronouncements made by others, who today state that the new cross-linked polyethylenes will be successful in patients of any age and under all circumstances. Despite early good results with these polyethylenes, several reports have described complications, suggesting, among other things, problems with the loss of mechanical properties with the aging of the material.

Laboratory studies strongly supported his concept that small prosthetic heads reduce friction

or approaching the hip anteriorly but posteriorly, and using a Titanium alloy instead of stainless steel. He responded saying that he appreciated my sharing with him my changing surgical and philosophical approach to total hip replacement. However, he felt, " I had missed my call' by approaching the hip from behind

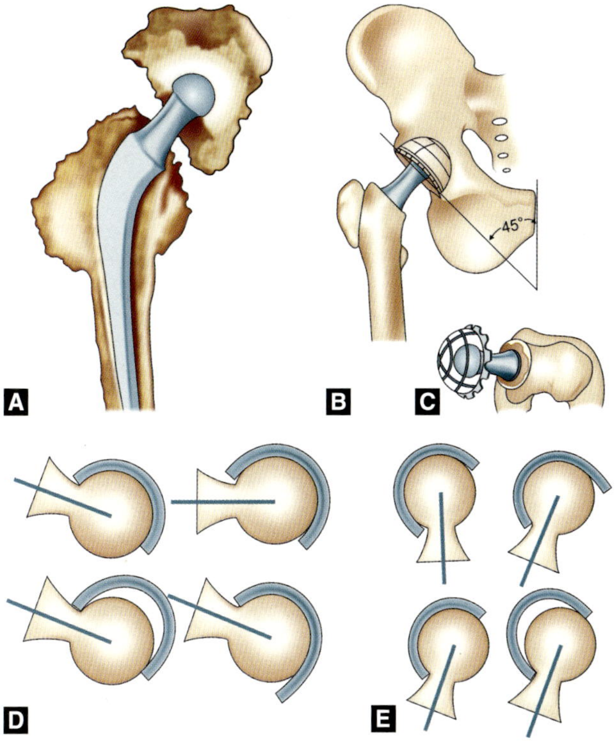

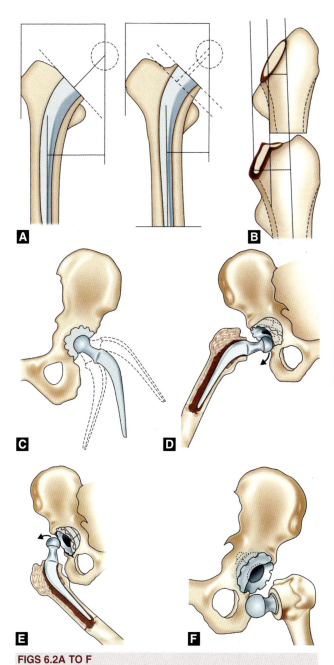

FIGS 6.1A TO E

(A) Photograph of one of Charnley's prosthesis recovered during autopsy. (B and C) Schematic drawing of the appropriate 45 degree angle of inclination of the acetabular component. (D and E) Schematic drawings demonstrating the stability of a small prosthetic head

(Figs 6.1A to E). He felt that the risk of dislocation was not increase with the smaller head and that the osteotomy and reattachment of the greater trochanter would provide a stable environment. The seminal issue in his studies was the prevention of wear and lysis. The importance of trochanteric osteotomy also occupied his fertile mind until the end of his days. Despite strong disagreement with the osteotomy, frequently associated with breaking down of the fixating wires, did not alter his belief in the value of this surgical step. I for one, abandoned the performance of the trochanteric osteotomy, and call the surgical exercise a "masochistic ritual".

Charnley, who was not the most elegant surgeon, did believe that the success of the procedure was predicated in adherence to technical details. He described methodically the many steps involved in the surgery. He advocated an anterior approach to the hip in preference to a posterior one, which had been the most popular in America for quite some time, particularly in the performance of hemiarthroplasty.

I still have the letter that Sir John sent to me in response to mine, in which I had informed him that I was no longer osteotomizing the greater trochanter,

FIGS 6.2A TO F

(A and B) Schematic drawing illustrating the appropriate level of osteotomy of the femoral head in order to obtained the desirable length of the extremity, according to the treated condition. (C, D, E and F) Drawings depicting the importance of alignment and orientation of the acetabular component, as well as the avoidance of impingement of the neck of the femur on the pelvic wall. Carefully adherence to these features reduces the incidence of dislocation

Section 1

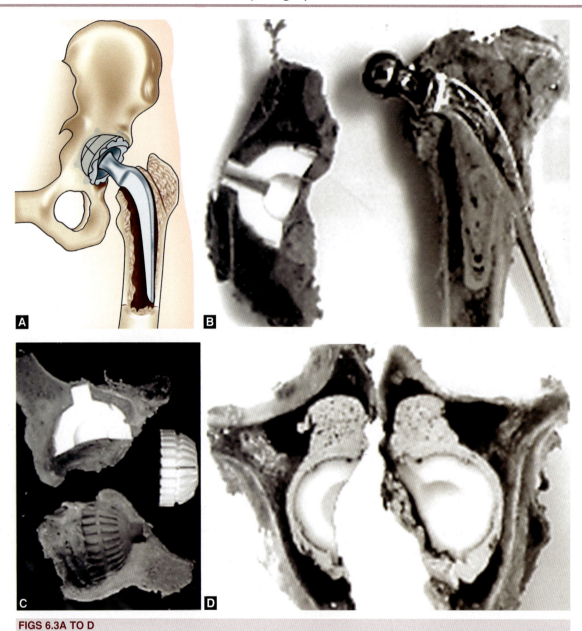

FIGS 6.3A TO D

(A) Drawing of a stem placed in varus; a position that increases the risk of failure. (B) Specimen of an early Charnley prosthesis. The stem was inadvertently left out of the femur. (C and D) Specimens of early Charnley arthroplasties illustrating the implants as well as their relationship with the cement and adjacent bone

rather than from the front. To him this meant that I did not have the mentality of an orthopedist but that of a "gynecologist". Eventually he forgave my trespasses and freely discussed our differences.

Charnley had felt that the transfer of the greater trochanter more distally and anteriorly favorably reduce the length of the medial lever arm of the hip, while increasing the length of the lateral one. We conducted studies in our laboratory and found out that his argument was correct, but I concluded that the minimal gain was not sufficient to offset the disadvantages (Figs 6.2 to 6.5).

We reviewed our experience with the Charnley prosthesis and drew some interesting conclusions, which I will describe in some detail. The Charnley arthroplasty was the only one I performed from 1970 through 1975. After that time, I began to use a Titanium alloy implant that we had developed, very similar in shape to the Stainless Steel Charnley implant. *It was the first time Titanium was used as a total hip implant in the United States, and was manufactured by Zimmer.* Recently it has been publicized that *Biomet*, another major manufacturing company, was the first company to introduce a Titanium alloy in total joint surgery. It

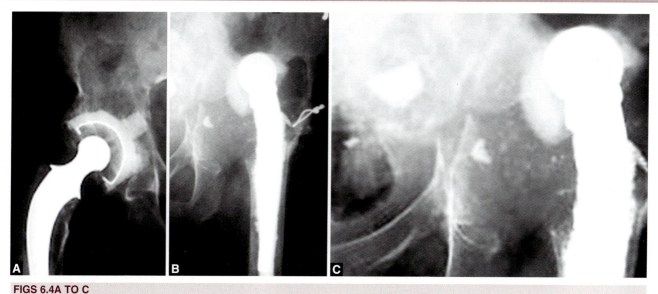

FIGS 6.4A TO C

(A) Radiograph of Charnley's Teflon acetabulum showing extensive lysis of the acetabulum. (B and C) Radiograph of Teflon acetabular component, illustrating the massive destruction of surrounding bone in the acetabulum and femur

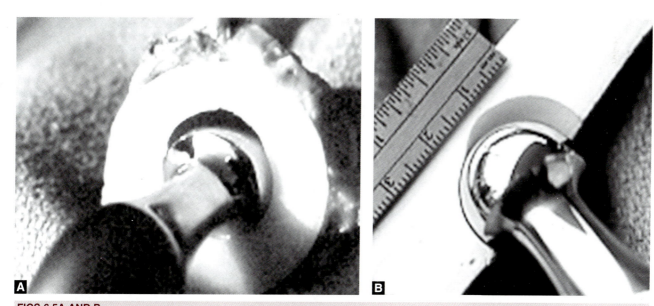

FIGS 6.5A AND B

Wooden replica of a worn acetabulum with a small 22 mm femoral head. Charnley described the phenomenon as "boring"

is true, however, that Dane Miller, founder and president of Biomet, did most of the original investigative work with Titanium, while working as an engineer with Zimmer.

Though, I anticipated clinical and radiological advantages with the titanium implant (STH), my expectations never crystallized. Implants with body and head made of Titanium alloy proved to be a bad idea. Titanium is too soft and therefore prone to be scratched, creating debris that once it reaches the metal head/polyethylene articulation produces damage to the plastic material and ultimately lysis if the surrounding tissues. What kept me from abandoning the Titanium implant sooner was the fact that many such implants functioned extremely well in the body, so much that at this time I have a number of active patients on whom I had performed the procedure 30 years earlier (See *Titanium Prostheses*).

References*

17, 19, 33, 40, 46, 51, 55, 58, 61, 70, 76, 77, 113

_____

* References provided at the end of the book after annexures.

Section 1

7

Long-term Follow-up of Charnley Arthroplasties

The following chapter is based on a document that we have published in a peer–review journal. It relates my experiences with the Charnley arthroplasties I performed from 1970 to 1975. The paper had been denied publication primarily on the basis that it was not a prospective study; and did not provide clear information on the number of patients lost to follow-up or those who had their hips revised. I will try to answer those questions, no matter how difficult they are. Having moved from Miami to California, where I performed all the Charnley arthroplasties, and then to Scotland, and once again to Miami, made it very difficult to obtain information in all patients. This, despite the fact that ever since I performed the first Charnley arthroplasty 37 years ago I have written to every patient a "boiler plate letter" accompanied with a personal note requesting follow-up information. Despite that effort, many did not respond either because they probably felt I was no longer in the same city or had found another orthopedist to follow them; or had moved into nursing homes and no longer had the intellectual capacities or the means to obtain new X-rays; had moved out of the area where they had lived, or had simply died. Making up false information in order to satisfy some journals was out of the question.

From a group of 383 patients who had 470 Charnley arthroplasties (87 bilateral), performed between July 1970 and July 1975, 39 (8.29%) joints were known to have been revised; their mean age was 62 ± 13 years and their mean weight 67 kg. The mean follow-up until revision was 122 ±months with a maximum of 270 months. 244 (63.7%) patients were lost to follow-up prior to their reaching 15 years after surgery. I assume that many of them had expired or that the loss to follow-up was due to other reasons, such as revision surgery performed elsewhere or simply patients' unwillingness or inability to respond to our requests. Four (1%) patients were alive but their X-rays could not be obtained. We conducted analysis of radiographs in the 135 hips of the 109 (28%) patients who were available for review between 15 and 35 years after surgery.

I had performed the Charnley total hip replacements through a lateral approach with trochanteric osteotomy. Nonpressurized finger packing of the cement was followed by insertion of the components. No medullary canal plugging was used in any instance. The original 50 mm acetabular cup was used in all patients. The femoral component consisted of the classical monoblock smooth, polished 22 mm Charnley implant made of stainless steel (Zimmer); 368 (78%) arthroplasties had curved stems; 36 (7.6%) had straight stems; and 66 (14%) had the Cobra style stems. The Cobra prostheses had matted surfaces.

From the total group of 383 patients, 287 (74%) had a primary diagnosis of osteoarthritis. In this subgroup, 299 (72.8%) patients had idiopathic osteoarthritis; 68 (23.6%) patients had osteoarthritis secondary to hip dysplasia, and 10 (3.4%) patients had osteoarthritis secondary to other conditions, i.e. Perthes disease, slipped capital femoral epiphysis; 53 (13.8%) patients had rheumatoid arthritis; 10 (2.6%) patients had a painful endoprosthesis; 21 (5.4%) patients had idiopathic avascular necrosis of the femoral head; 9 (2.5%) patients had post-traumatic avascular necrosis of the femoral head, 2 (0.5%) patients suffered from ankylosing spondylitis; and one (0.2%) patient had an spontaneously fused hip secondary to head injury.

Weight bearing began within a few days after surgery, but full, unprotected weight bearing was postponed for six weeks. All patients were contacted on a yearly bases at which time they were either seen personally or were asked to obtain radiographs of their operate hips and to complete a simple questionnaire concerning the presence or absence of pain and the need and type of assisted ambulation.

The 109 patients available for radiographic follow-up had 135 arthroplasties performed. Twenty-seven (24.7%) patients had bilateral replacements; 21 (77.7%) of these arthroplasties were performed at different times; and 6 (22.2%) arthroplasties were performed simultaneously. 115 (85%) stems were curved; 6 (4%) stems were straight; and 14 (10%) stems were of the cobra type. Forty-two (38.5%) patients were males and 67 (61.4%) patients were females. The mean weight of the patients who had curved stems was 67 kg; in the patients who had straight stems the mean weight was 65.5 kg; and in the patients who had cobra stems the mean weight was 68 kg. Among the patients who had unilateral replacement, 49 (44.9%) procedures were performed on the right hip, and 32 (29.3%) procedures were performed on the left hip.

The age of these 109 patients at the time of surgery ranged from 16 to 71 years. Three (2.7%) patients were between 16 and 20 years of age; two (1.8%) patients were between 21 and 30 years of age; 8 (7.3%) patients were between 31 and 40 years of age; 17 (15.5%) patients were between 41 and 50 years of age; 29 (26.6%) patients were between 51 and 60 years of age; 45 (41.2%) patients were between 61 and 70 years of age and 5 (4.5%) patients were 71 years of age (Table 7.1).

The immediate postoperative radiographs were studied concerning the coverage and inclination of the acetabular component, the attitude of the femoral stem in the medullary canal, the thickness of the cement at the level of the calcar, the distal extension of the cement in reference to the tip-end of the femoral stem, and the ratio between the diameter of the stem and the diameter of the medullary canal seven centimeters below the base of the neck of the prosthesis.

TABLE 7.1	Age range 16-71 years at the time of surgery		
Age (years)	Number of patients	Mean weight (kg)	Weight range (kg)
16-20	3 (2.7%)	56	52-57
21-30	2 (1.8%)	59	56-69
31-40	17 (15.5%)	63	61-78
41-50	45 (41%)	67	57-89
51-60	29 (26.6%)	61	54-76
61-70	8 (7.3%)	62	55-70
> 70	5 (4.5%)	60	55-68

This study does not include clinical data regarding pain or mode of ambulation of the studied patients. I concluded that the information available was incomplete and to a great extent unreliable, since there were no means to determine in many instances whether patients lost to follow-up had died, their hips had been revised elsewhere or simply were not interested or capable of responding to requests made to them for additional information. In some instances it was chosen to consider certain patients as having expired because of their very advanced age at the time of the last follow-up visit. In addition, the project was strictly a radiological evaluation of films taken of patients who had a minimum follow-up of 15 years.

From the final group of 109 patients with follow-up ranging between 15 and 33 years, who were available for radiological review 94 (86.2%) had the surgery performed for osteoarthritis; their mean age at the time of surgery was 64 years and their mean weight was 66 kg. From this subgroup, 75 (75.5%) patients had idiopathic osteoarthritis, 20 (21.1%) patients had osteoarthritis secondary to hip dysplasia, and three (3.1%) patients had osteoarthritis secondary to slipped capital epiphysis or Perthes disease. Four (3.6%) patients had rheumatoid arthritis; their mean age at the time of surgery was 35 years and their mean weight was 62 kg. Five (4.5%) patients had failed endoprostheses; their mean age at the time of surgery was 63 years, and their mean weight was 62 kg. Four (3.6%) patients had avascular necrosis of the femoral head. In this sub-group 2 (50%) had idiopathic avascular necrosis. Their ages were 27 and 38 years respectively; and their weight at the time of surgery was 63 and 69 kg respectively; two (50%) patients had post-traumatic avascular necrosis of the femoral head; their ages at the time of surgery were 29 and 38 respectively; and there weight was 62 and 70 kg. respectively. One (0.9%) patient had ankylosing spondylitis; her age at the time of surgery was 25 years and her weight 62 kg. One (0.9%) patient had a post-traumatic spontaneous fusion of the hip; her age at the time of surgery was 16 years and her weight was 52 kg (Table 7.2).

The mean weight of the 3 patients who were between 16 and 20 years of age at the time of surgery was 56 kg (Range 52-57 kg). In the 21-30 age group was 59 kg (Range 56-69 kg); in the 31-40 age group was 63 kg (Range 61-78 kg); in the 41-50 age group was 67 kg (Range 57-89 kg); in the 51-60 age group was 641 kg (Range 55-70); in the 61-70 age group was 62 (range 55-70 kg); an in the >70 age group was 60 kg (Range 55-68 kg).

Forty-three (32%) hips were followed between 16 and 20 years; 38 (28.3%) hips were followed between 21 and 25 years; 44 (32.8%) hips were followed between 25 and 29 years; and 10 (7.6%) hips were followed between 30 and 33 years after surgery (Table 7.3).

Review of the initial and latest radiographs indicated that one hundred and twenty six (93.4%) hips had one hundred percent coverage of the acetabular component, while 9 (6.6%) hips had between 80 and 90 percent coverage. The inclination of the acetabular component was between 40 and 50 degrees in 88 percent hips.

The orientation of the femoral component was neutral in 112 (82.9%) hips; in varus in 13 (9.6%) hips; and in valgus in 10 (7.4%) hips.

The percentage of medullary canal occupied by the femoral stem 7 centimeters below the collar of the prosthesis was more than 50 percent in 110 (81.4%) femurs; in 13 (9.6%) femurs the prosthesis filled less than 50 percent of the canal and in 12 (8.8%) femurs 50 percent of the canal was occupied by the femoral component.

The cement in the femoral canal did not reach the tip-end of the prosthesis in 12 (9%) radiographs; the cement came to the level of the tip-end of the prosthesis in 9 (7%) radiographs; and the cement extended distally to the tip-end of the prosthesis in 113 (84%) radiographs.

The thickness of the column of cement at the level of the transected femoral neck measured between 3 and 5 millimeters in 84 percent radiographs; between 0 and 3 millimeters in 11.8 percent radiographs; and more than 5 millimeters in 3.7 percent radiographs (Table 7.4).

Metal/cement radiolucent lines in the femur were seen in 3 (2.3%) radiographs; while no metal/cement lines were seen in 132 (97.7%) radiographs.

No migration of the acetabular component was seen in 130 (96.2%) radiographs; migration of less than

TABLE 7.2	Diagnoses		
Diagnoses	Number of patients	Percentage	Mean weight (kg)
Osteoarthritis	94	86.2%	66
Idiopathic	71	75.5%	
Dysplasia	20	21.1%	
Others	3	3.1%	
Rheumatoid arthritis	4	3.6%	62
Failed endoprostheses	5	4.5%	62
Ankylosing spondylitis	1	0.9%	60
Avascular necrosis	4	3.6%	63
Idiopathic	2	50%	
Trauma	2	50%	
Hip fusion	1	0.9%	52

TABLE 7.3	Follow-up range: 16-33 years	
Follow-up brackets	Number of patients	Percentage
16-20 yr	43	32.7%
21-24 yr	38	28.3%
25-29 yr	44	32.8%
>30 yr	10	7.6%

TABLE 7.4	Technical features	
Description of feature measured	Measure	%
Acetabular coverage	100%	93.5%
	80-90%	6.5%
Acetabular inclination	40°-50°	88%
Femoral component alignment	Neutral	82.9%
	Valgus	7.4%
	Varus	9.6%
Ratio of stem/medullary canal (At 7 cm)	> 50%	81%
	50%	8%
	< 50%	9.6%
Cement thickness	0-3 mm	3.7%
Proximal femur	3-5 mm	84.5%
	> 5 mm	11.8%
Cement extension	Above tip	9%
	Tip level	7%
	Below tip	84%

5 millimeters was measured in 4 (2.9%) radiographs; and in one (0.7%) radiograph migration of more than 5 millimeter was recorded.

A continuous bone/cement radiolucent line in the acetabulum was seen in 8 (5.9%) radiographs while no continuous lines were seen in 127 (94%) radiographs.

Bone/cement radiolucent lines in the femur, measuring more than 1 millimeter, were seen in 6 (4.4%) radiographs; while no bone/cement radiolucent lines were seen in 129 (95.5%) radiographs.

Fractures of the cement in the femoral side were seen in 5 (3.7%) radiographs; while no fractures were observed in 130 (96.2%) radiographs.

Acetabular lysis measuring as much as 5 millimeters was seen in 6 (4.4%) radiographs; 95.6 radiographs did not have acetabular lysis. Lysis (resorption) of the neck of the femur was seen in 6 (4.4%) radiographs, ranging from 3 to 6 mm. The two groups represented different patients.

Wear, measured according to Charnley's original technique, indicated that 30 (22.2%) polyethylene sockets had no evidence of wear; 89 (66%) sockets measured between 1 and 3 millimeters of wear; 13 (9.6%) sockets measured wear between 3 and 5 millimeters; and 3 (2.2%) sockets measured more than 5 millimeters (Table 7.5).

Despite the plethora of different total hip prostheses brought into the market during the past four decades, it is not possible at this time to state categorically that any one system or implant is significantly superior to all others. The noncemented system of hip arthroplasty came into being on the belief that acrylic cement was associated with complications such as loosening and lysis. However, for some time after the popularization of the original noncemented arthroplasty, it became evident that bone lysis was more likely to develop with these implants. Modifications in the geometry of the implants and the distributions of the porous area have significantly improved the results.

Reviews of clinical and radiological results with the Charnley implant have suggested that certain details influence the long-term outcome of the surgical replacement, for example, the degree of coverage and inclination of the acetabular component; the attitude of the stem in the medullary canal, i.e. varus, valgus, neutral; the thickness of the column of cement at the level of the proximal/medial femoral cortex; the ratio between the diameter of the femoral implant and that of the femoral component; the patients age at the time of surgery and the disease for which the surgery is performed.

TABLE 7.5	Abnormal changes	
Description of changes measured	Measure	% patients
Acetabular migration	None	96.2%
	<5 mm	2.9%
	> 5 mm	0.7%
Acetabular bone-cement radiolucent lines	None	94.1%
	>1 mm	5.9%
Femoral bone-cement radiolucent lines	None	95.5%
	>1 mm	4.4%
Femoral metal-cement radiolucent lines	None	97.7%
	Present	2.3%
Cement fracture	None	96.2%
	Present	3.7%
Polyethylene wear	None	30 (14.8%)
	1-3 mm	89 (66%)
	3-5 mm	13 (9.6%)
	>5 mm	3 (2.2%)
Broken wires	None	85.5%
	Broken	14.5%
Acetabular lysis	None	95.6%
	< 5 mm	4.4%
Femoral lysis (Neck resorption)	None	95.6%
	< 5 mm	4.4%

Based on the above information we elected to review our Charnley arthroplasties that had survived between fifteen and thirty-three years to determine if the radiological and clinical features that have been previously identified were present in the long-surviving hips.

This review indicated that the vast majority of patients had met the previously identified observations.

1. 93.3 percent hips had 100 percent coverage of the acetabular component.

2. 88 percent hips had the acetabular component inclined between 40 and 45 degrees and 8.8 percent hips between 45 and 50 degrees.

3. 82.9 percent hips had the femoral component in a neutral attitude and 9.6 percent in a valgus attitude, while only 7.5 percent had the implants in varus.

4. 84.4 percent hips had a column of cement at the level of the transected femoral neck a thickness between 3 and 5 millimeters.

5. 81.4 percent hips had femoral stems that occupied more than 50 percent of the diameter of the medullary canal.

6. 84 percent hips had a column of cement that extended below the tip of the prosthesis.

Section 1

Review of the radiographs of this group of patients with long-term follow-up demonstrated a low incidence of findings commonly known as being of an undesirable nature, some of which are generally considered to be signs of early failure.

1. Absence of measurable acetabular migration was documented in 96.2 percent hips.
2. 94.7 percent hips did not have continuous acetabular bone/cement radiolucent lines.
3. 95.5 percent hips did not show continuous cement/bone radiolucent lines.
4. 97.7 percent hips did not have femoral metal/cement radiolucent lines.
5. 96.2 percent hips did not have fractures of the femoral cement column.
6. Wear of the acetabular polyethylene component was found in most hips; only 14.8 percent hips did not have measurable wear.
7. Minimal femoral lysis was present in 4.4 percent radiographs; and acetabular lysis was documented in 2.5 percent patients. It is interesting to note that neither the age nor the weight of the patients at the time of surgery seem to correlate with acetabular wear, bone-cement or metal cement radiolucent lines. The small number of patients in the series and particularly in each category of "abnormal changes" precluded the statistical analysis that is possible with larger series.

The data we gathered suggest that the patient's weight may not be important in view of the fact since it was similar in analyzed parameters, such as disease categories, i.e. osteoarthritis, avascular necrosis, rheumatoid arthritis (Tables 7.1 and 7.2).

Clinical data was not reported in the current review despite the fact that attempts to gather pertinent information was made on a yearly basis. The patients' clinical performance was not discussed because we considered the information obtained from question-naires to be frequently unreliable. For example, the use of external support or ability to walk long distances. We had long-realized that elderly people, for reasons frequently unrelated to the operated hips, use a cane or walker, not because of pain in the hip, but because associated degenerative conditions require their use. Often, elderly patients afflicted with multiple physical or mental problems do not appropriately respond to questions asked in written questionnaires, and frequently report the presence of pain. Subsequent telephone conversation with them makes it obvious that quite often the alleged symptoms are due to spine and other joints' pathology rather than to hip disease.

It is likely that patients whose radiographs do not show certain abnormal changes are likely to have asymptomatic hip joints.

It is not uncommon to see patients whose radiographs show significant abnormal changes who, nonetheless have minimal discomfort or are totally asymptomatic. Therefore, one may conclude that revision surgery is not an accurate end-point criterion in determining success or failure of total hip arthroplasties. There are also times when painful arthroplasties are never revised for a variety of reasons, such as the presence of medical conditions that preclude surgery or patients' unwillingness of undergo additional surgery.

The data obtained from this study does not provide information regarding the impact that the described technical features may have had in the degree of wear of the polyethylene acetabular component.

This review does not intend to imply that long-term success of Charnley arthroplasties can be assured if the technical details identified in the text are carefully implemented. However, the information obtained strongly suggests that successful radiological long-term results from Charnley arthroplasty—and perhaps also from other types of cemented arthroplasties—may be significantly dependent on adherence to the details identified in this study.

The method of measuring the various parameters presented in the report has been widely reported in the literature. The following 2 illustrations (Figs 7.1A and B) depict the method use to evaluate the ratio between the diameters of the femur and femoral stem.

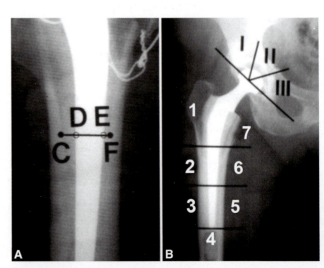

FIGS 7.1A AND B

Illustration of the method used to determine the ration between the diameters of the femoral canal 7 centimeters below the cut in the neck of the femur and the diameter of the femoral stem at that level

The following (Figs 7.2 to 7.20) are additional representative examples of Charnley arthroplasties performed for a variety of conditions. I admit form the outset that I have experienced every possible complication and had my share of bad results. I do not use the frequently heard excuse that the initial series of patients do not count because they represent the excusable learning curve. Though it is true that the first few arthroplasties were not performed with the ease that came with further experience, I do not know how to define the "learning curve". Should be the first 10, 20, 30 or 100 procedures be part of the nonreportable "learning curve"? Since I had the opportunity to learn the technique from John Charnley himself during the less than 3 months I spent in his hospital, where I saw him and his associates perform six arthroplasties every

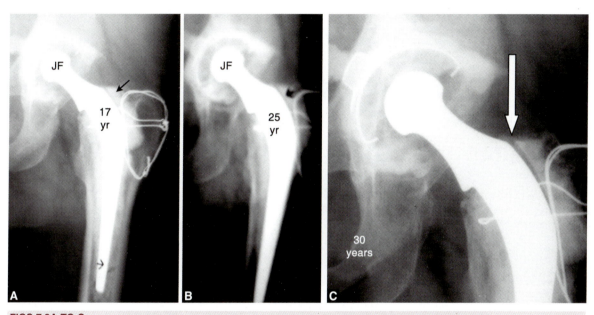

FIGS 7.2A TO C

(A) Radiograph obtained 17 years after surgery performed in a 56-year-old woman for the care of osteoarthritis. (B and C) Radiographs taken 25 and 30 years after surgery respectively. Notice the presence of a metal/cement radiolucent line on Zone 7 that did not progress with time

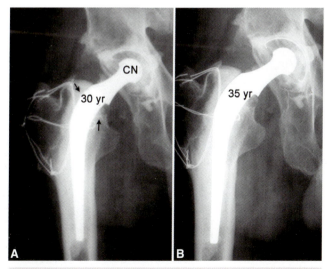

FIGS 7.3A AND B

(A) Radiograph obtained 30 years after surgery performed in a man of 39 years of age for the care of idiopathic osteoarthritis. He is 6f. 3in. tall and has remained very active. (B) Radiograph obtained 35 years postoperatively. Notice that the metal/cement radiolucent line on zone 7 did not progress. There is a healthy mild hypertrophy of the cortex distally

day, I cannot speak of my "learning curve" without experiencing an uncomfortable feeling.

We have conducted comparative studies of our experiences with the Charnley total hip and the Titanium (STH) prosthesis. The following are tables that demonstrate that in virtually all parameters the Charnley arthroplasty performs better than the STH prosthesis (Figs 7.21A to F).

Currently, it appears that some noncemented porous-covered prostheses are performing very well. My own personal experience with them over the past 20 years has been most gratifying. Hopefully some day an investigator will study the results obtained with these prostheses and compare them the cemented Charnley arthroplasty. I suspect that the Charnley prosthesis will withstand the comparison very well even though the newer implants will win the day.

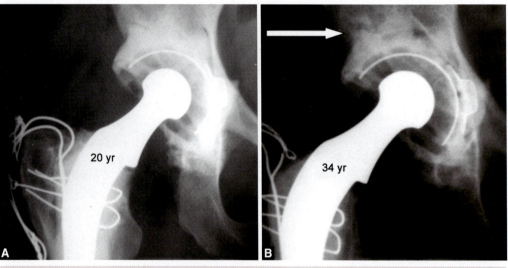

FIGS 7.4A AND B
Radiographs obtained 20 and 34 years postoperatively in a man 40-year-old at the time of surgery. Notice the lack of progression of the bone/cement radiolucent line in the acetabulum, and the minimal wear

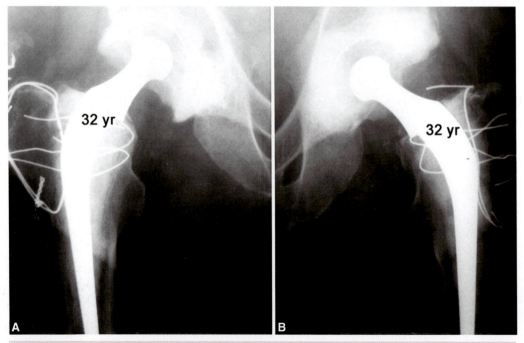

FIGS 7.5A AND B
Radiographs of bilateral Charnley arthroplasties obtained 32 years postoperatively. Notice the broken trochanteric wires, the rather imperfect cementing technique but also the absence of wear or lysis

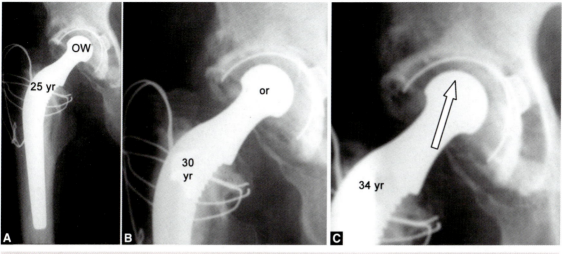

FIGS 7.6A TO C

Radiographs of Charnley arthroplasty performed in a very active tennis player: 25, 30 and 34 years after surgery. Notice the wear of the polyethylene socket

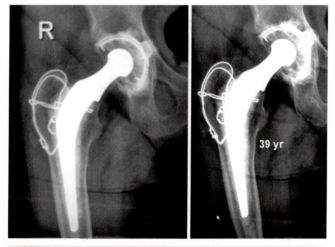

FIG. 7.7

Radiograph of the hips of a woman, who at the age of 39 years had a Charnley arthroplasty for the care of post-traumatic avascular necrosis of the right femoral head

Section 1

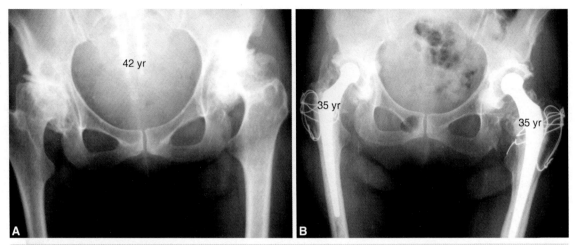

FIGS 7.8A AND B

(A) Bilateral osteoarthritis in a 42-year-old woman. (B) Radiographs obtained 35 years after surgery. Patient has remained active and asymptomatic. Notice the absence of measurable wear

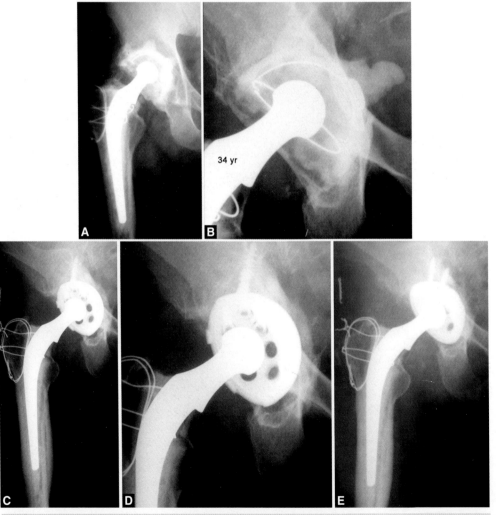

FIGS 7.9A TO E

(A) Radiograph of Charnley arthroplasty performed in a 36-year-old woman for the treatment of post-traumatic arthritis. This film was taken 25 years post-surgery. There was no evidence of impending failure. (B) Radiograph taken 34 years post-surgery. The acetabular cup has migrated into the acetabulum and it is loose. (C and D) The arthroplasty was revised with a noncemented porous acetabulum. However, I mistakenly placed the cup in a too vertical position while attempting to obtain complete coverage of the metallic cup. (E) The arthroplasty was revised again and the socket placed in a more horizontal position

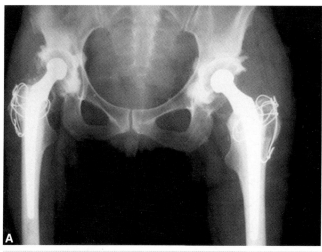
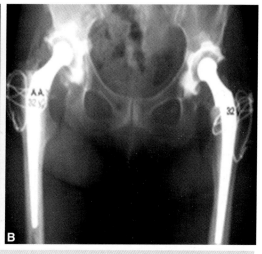

FIGS 7.10A AND B

(A) Early postoperative radiograph of bilateral Charnley arthroplasties. (B) Radiograph taken 32 years postsurgery. Patient has remained asymptomatic but her activities have decreased as her age advances

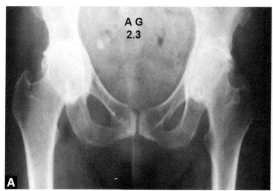
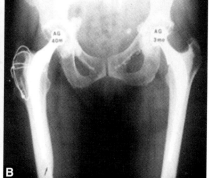
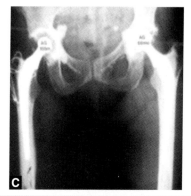

FIGS 7.11A TO C

Radiograph of osteoarthritis of both hips. The right hip was replaced with Charnley prosthesis, and the left with a titanium allow femoral component. Radiograph illustrating the frequently seen distal hypertrophy when a stiff implant is used. This in itself is a good sign providing proximal stress shielding does not appear proximally

Section 1

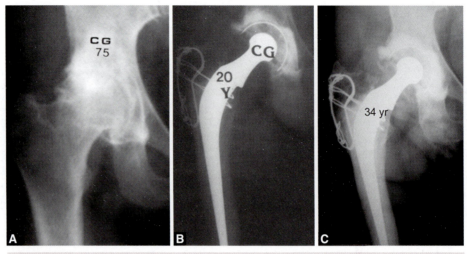

FIGS 7.12A TO C

(A) Radiograph of osteoarthritis in 34-year-old woman. (B) Radiograph obtained 20 years later. There appears to be no evidence of measurable wear, lysis or radiolucent lines. (C) Radiograph taken 34 years after surgery

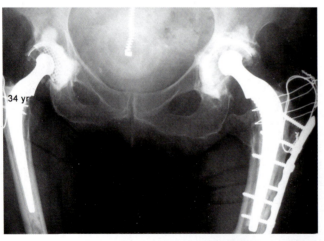

FIG. 7.13

Radiograph of bilateral Charnley arthroplasties 34 years after surgery. Patient was 45-year-old at the time of surgery. She had sustained a fracture of the left femur a year earlier, which was stabilized with a plate

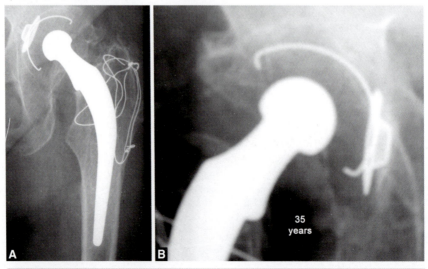

FIGS 7.14A AND B

Radiographs of Charnley arthroplasty obtained 35 years after surgery. Notice the absence of barium in the cement and the absence of wear in the polyethylene acetabulum

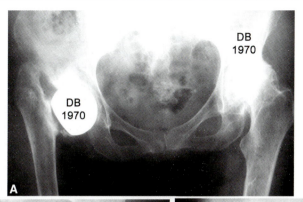

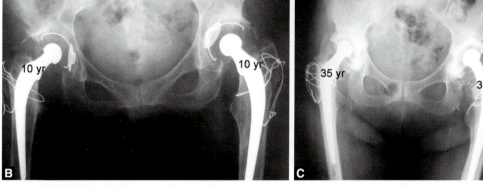

FIGS 7.15A TO C

(A) Radiograph of arthritic hips of a 45-year-old woman. The right hip had been replaced with a mold arthroplasty, which allegedly failed within 5 years. (B) Radiograph taken 10 years after bilateral Charnley arthroplasties. (C) Radiograph 35 years after surgery. The right femur had sustained a fracture which was treated with plate

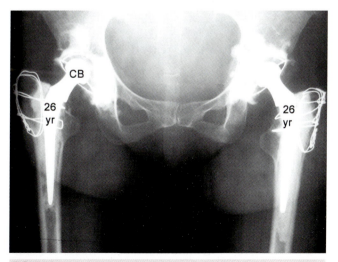

FIG. 7.16

Radiographs of Charnley arthroplasties obtained 26 years postsurgery. Patient was 18-year-old at the time of surgery and suffered from rheumatoid arthritis. She was lost to follow-up following these films

Section 1

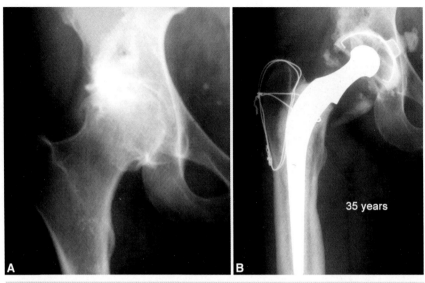

FIGS 7.17A AND B

(A) Radiograph of osteoarthritic hip of a 40-year-old woman. (B) Radiograph obtained 35 years postoperatively. The radiograph illustrates the desirable feature of a cemented arthroplasty: (1) Complete coverage of the acetabular component. (2) 45 degree orientation of the acetabular cup. (3) Proper placement to the trochanter. (4) Neutral attitude of the femoral component. (5) Filling of the canal by the stem in more than 50 percent of its diameter

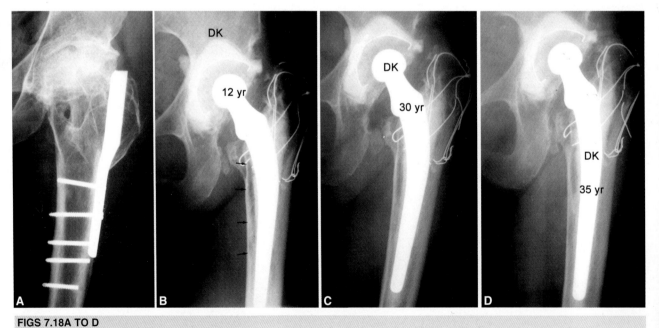

FIGS 7.18A TO D

(A) Radiograph of osteoarthritic hip following osteotomy of the femur in the car of congenital. (B to D) Radiographs obtained 12, 30 and 35 years postsurgery

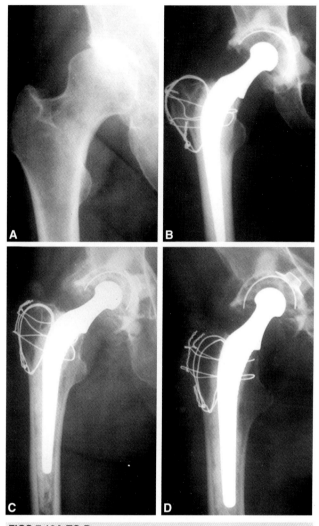

FIGS 7.19A TO D

(A) Osteoarthritic hip of a 52-year-old woman. (B) Postoperative radiograph showing the appropriate wiring of the trochanter. (C and D) Radiographs depicting the gradual fragmentation of the wires at 20 and 32 years postoperatively. Notice the absence of measurable wear or lysis

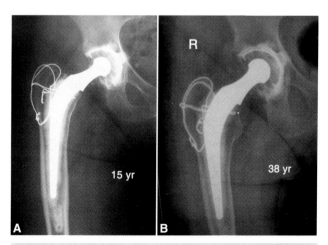

FIGS 7.20A AND B

(A) Radiograph of Charnley arthroplasty obtained 15 years after surgery. (B) Radiograph taken 38 years postsurgery

Section 1

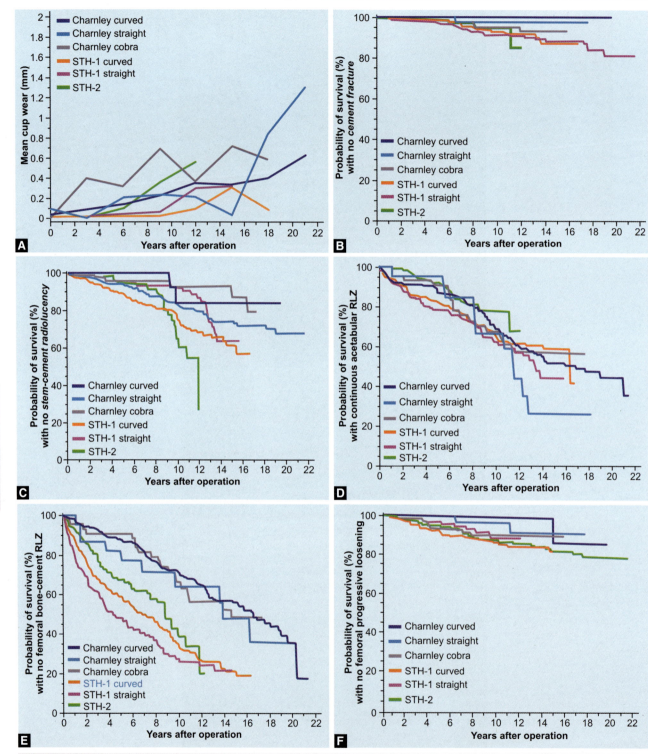

FIGS 7.21A TO F

Survivorship analysis of comparing the results obtained with Charnley total hip arthroplasties with those I obtained using a titanium totally cemented prosthesis (STH). Though the clinical and radiological results had indicated minimal differences between the two implants when they were analyzed after a 6 years follow-up, significant differences became evident over the ensuing years. In virtually all parameters the Charnley prosthesis performed better

*References**

46, 51, 55, 57, 61, 70, 76, 104, 113, 117

* References provided at the end of the book after annexures.

8

Broken Wires and Nonunion of the Greater Trochanter

I suspect that one of the main reasons for the loss of interest in the Charnley arthroplasty was the frequent failure of fixation of the osteotomized greater trochanter. Had Charnley given up on his firm adherence to the concept of osteotomy, the popularity of his implant and overall technique and philosophy would still be more widely popular. However, that was not possible. Charnley believed until the end of his life that the trochanter issue was a most important technical detail in his operation and the area he enjoyed the most. Solving the problems associated with the osteotomized trochanter was the challenge he really wanted to resolve.

Charnley had studied carefully every conceivable aspect of total hip arthroplasty, and the effect of trochanteric osteotomy was to him a seminal one. The transfer of the trochanter distally and anteriorly was, according to him, the best way to ensure a sound increase in the length of the lateral lever arm of the hip. He had recognized that the medial lever arm of the hip was significantly longer than the lateral one. Balancing this discrepancy could be accomplished by deepening of the acetabulum and implanting a small diameter prosthetic head, in that manner shortening the medial lever arm. The transfer of the trochanter distally and anteriorly would lengthen the lateral arm. He had data to prove his point, however, perhaps not strong enough to justify the addition surgery and the gaining of minor reductions of stresses on the joint itself.

After my return from his institution in England in the Spring of 1970, we conducted studies hoping to find additional data to support Charnley's views. Unfortunately, our findings indicated that the transfer of the osteotomized trochanter contributed in only a minor way to the reduction of stresses.

In the meantime the orthopedic community continued to experience frustration with the technical difficulties encountered in the fixation of the trochanter and the frequent breakage of the fixating wires. Nonunion of the trochanter became a common complication, and the esthetic component (radiologically) created by the broken wires became a significant one. The breakage of the wires and the occasional nonunion of the trochanter were not in themselves serious problems since the broken wires not always produce pain, and the nonunited bone seldom produces a detectable weakness of the abductor musculature.

It is true, however, that intact or broken wires on occasion produced a trochanteric bursitis that if not responsive to local injections, requiring their removal. We had learned early during our personal experiences that wires frequently break no matter how they are fastened or how strong they are. And that once a wire breaks at one level, it usually continues to break into smaller fragments. *This is due to the fact that the constant motion of the hip in many directions and the contraction of surrounding muscles place bending stresses on the wires with a resulting continued fragmentation of the metallic implants.* A clear comparison can be made with any wire that one bends repeatedly; it warms up every time it is bent until it finally breaks.

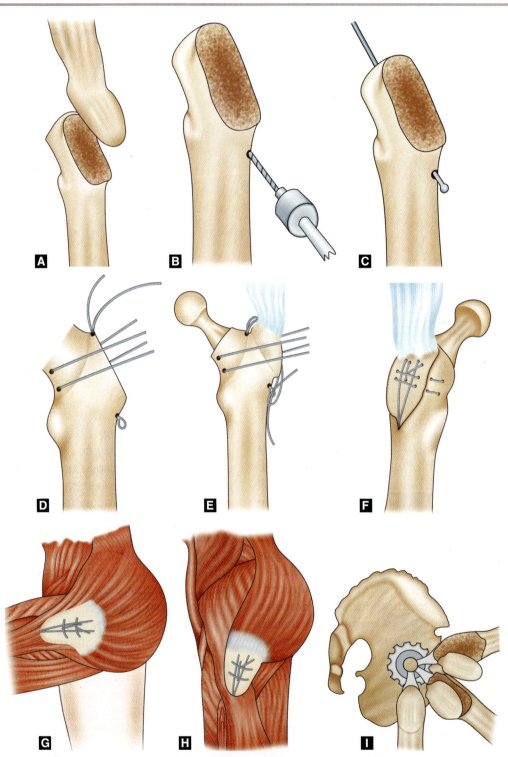

FIGS 8.1A TO I
Schematic drawings of the consecutive steps taken in the reattachment of the osteotomized greater trochanter, beginning with the placement of a wire laterally and wrapped temporarily over the proximal femur. Next is the placement of the 2 horizontal. The trochanter is then transferred distally and anteriorly under tension. The wires are then fastened as tightly as possible. Illustration of the correct and incorrect placement of the trochanter

Section 1

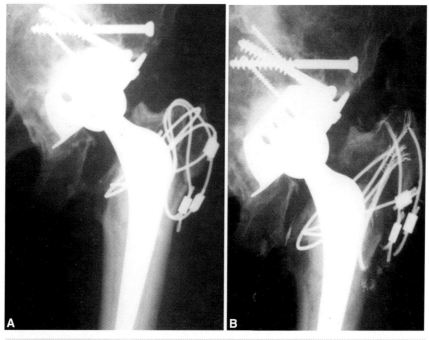

FIGS 8.2A AND B
(A) Postoperative radiograph showing the reattachment of the trochanter using filiform wires.
(B) The wires broke into smaller pieces. Their migration into the metal/plastic interface is possible

We developed our own technique of wiring in the early 1970s (Figs 8.1A to I). It is likely that the prognosis improved but did not completely prevent wire breaking.

Others advocated filiform wires (Figs 8.2 and 8.3), while yet others developed plates and hooks hoping to reduce complications (Figs 8.4A to E). No technique has proven completely successful. *The filiform wires, in my opinion, create other problems, perhaps of a greater importance.* Because this wire is composed of multiple thinner strands of metal, when it breaks and continues to break into smaller fragments, the small fragments spread themselves through a wide area. The possibility of the small fragments migrating into the joint space is a real one. The resulting third-body wear phenomenon then created will generate plastic and metal debris with the resulting lysis of the femur and or acetabulum.

The nonunion of the osteotomized trochanter, as I indicated early, does not preclude normal function without apparent weakness of the gluteus musculature (Figs 8.5A to C). I am sure, however, that if critical measures of strength are taken, some weakness will be found. In addition, *a significantly displaced trochanter results in an increase of rotation of the hip that may result in dislocation of the hip when extreme degrees of rotation are introduced* (Fig. 8.6).

Several times I have noticed that patients with nonunited trochanters walk with the limb in external rotation. To some people this is unpleasant (Figs 8.7 to 8.13).

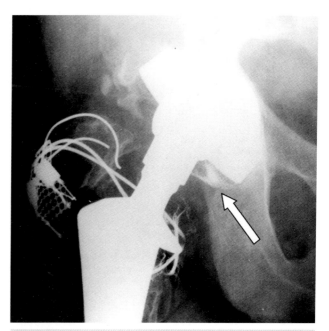

FIG. 8.3
Filiform wires used to stabilize the greater trochanter. The wires fractured and traveled proximally and distally. They might create a third-body wear process

Section 1

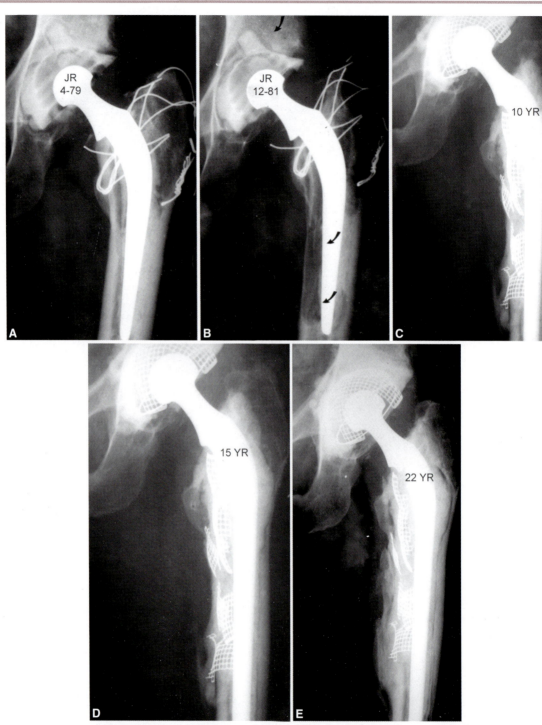

FIGS 8.4A TO E

(A) Radiograph of cemented prosthesis showing early evidence of loosening and lysis. (B) Two years later there was significant amount of femoral lysis and loosening of both components. Notice the additional broken wires. (C) Radiograph illustrating the postrevision arthroplasty 10 years later. Bone graft had been placed under the wire mesh. (D and E) Radiographs taken 15 and 22 years postrevision. The width of the radiolucent lines has not increased and the degree of wear is minimal

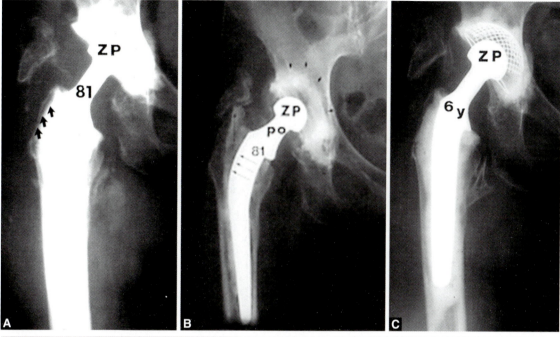

FIGS 8.5A TO C

(A) A failed arthroplasty revised in 1981. The greater trochanter was ununited. (B) At the time of the revision I elected to leave the trochanter unattached. A radiograph taken 6 years postoperatively shows the ununited trochanter. (C) Twenty years later the patients is asymptomatic and the hip is stable

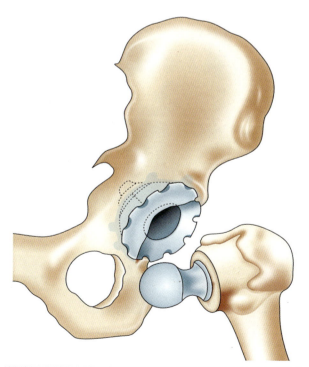

FIG. 8.6

The additional external rotation of the hip resulting from a nonunited greater trochanter might result in an anterior dislocation

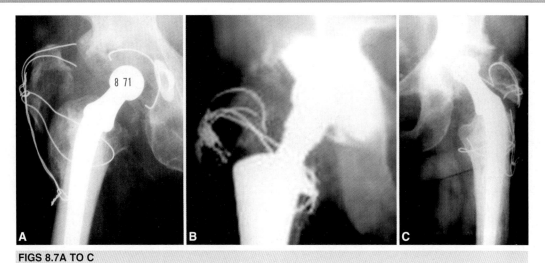

FIGS 8.7A TO C

Three representative examples of nonunited greater trochanters that were stabilized with three different techniques

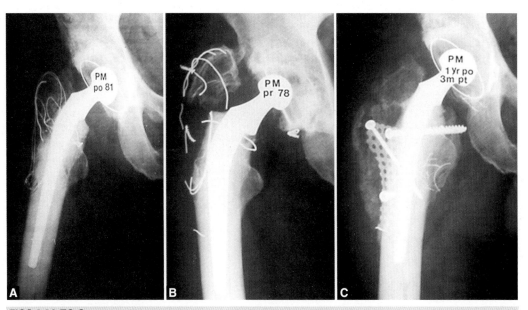

FIGS 8.8A TO C

(A) A nonunited trochanter wired in place at the time of revision arthroplasty. (B) The wires broke and the trochanter displaced superiorly. (C) Radiographs taken after a third procedure to obtain union. A wire mesh and screws were used. The trochanter slipped away from under the wire-mesh

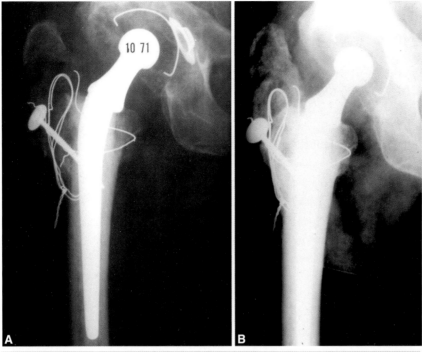

FIGS 8.9A AND B

(A) Radiograph of nonunited greater trochanter after a second attempt to obtain union. Notice that the trochanter "slipped" under the wires and migrated superiorly. (B) Three years later the trochanter remained ununited. Nature's attempt to achieve union resulted in heterotopic bone forming in the area

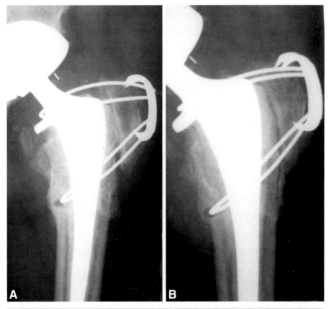

FIGS 8.10A AND B

After four attempts to achieve union, a strong fibrous union took place following the use of a staple and wires

Section 1

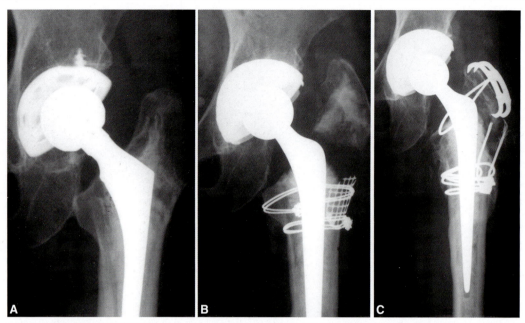

FIGS 8.11A TO C

(A) Radiograph of hybrid arthroplasty experiencing wear of the polyethylene liner. (B) A revision was allegedly carried out at another institution, during which a nondisplaced fracture of the femur was created. Wires were used to prevent displacement of the fragments. Within a few weeks the wires fractured and the trochanter displaced superiorly. (C) Allegedly because continued discomfort, the trochanter was stabilized with a staple and wires. The nonunion persisted and the wires broke

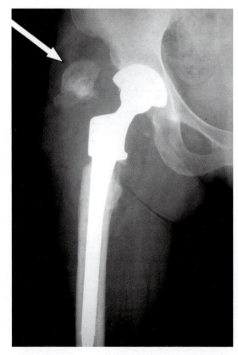

FIG. 8.12

Revision arthroplasty that required significant gain of length left the ununited trochanter separated from the femur in a major way. Attempts to reattach the trochanter under these circumstance almost inevitable results in a continued nonunion. In order to prevent dislocation, in the event there is great residual instability, it is best to use a self-constrained acetabular component. Methods designed to provide stability relying on sections of iliotibial band have been reported by others, however, the results have been mixed

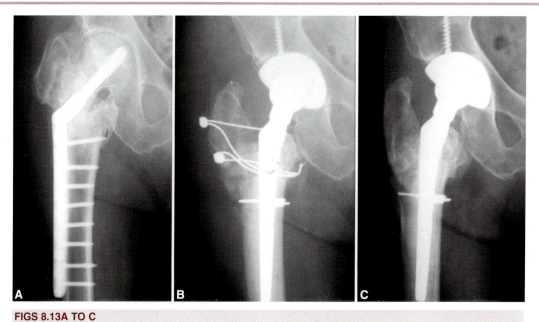

FIGS 8.13A TO C

(A) Failed fixation of subtrochanteric fracture. (B) A total hip replacement was performed and the trochanter was stabilized with wires. (C) The trochanter healed and the wires were removed

9

Metal-backed Cemented Acetabula

Some time in the early 1980's, the concept of reinforcement of cemented acetabular fixation with a metallic mesh component gained some popularity. The idea had come from finite analysis studies that suggested that the distribution of stresses around the acetabular component of a cemented arthroplasty was improved in that manner. I never embraced the concept and continued to adhere to Charnley's teaching, and to the fact that up to that time I was quite satisfied with the results I was obtaining with the traditional method of cement stabilization.

Time has shown that the appearance of radiolucent lines between the acetabular bone and the column of cement is not necessarily the product of abnormal distribution of mechanical stresses but more likely the presence of debris, and the resulting chemical and histological changes. In any event, the concept of the metal-backed cemented acetabulum gained immediate acceptance in the surgical community in the late 1970's and early 1980's.

I had become suspicious of the value of the innovation and of possible harmful effects of the reinforced cup, when we found that at another institution a large number of implanted femoral-cemented titanium prostheses with metal-backed components experienced early failure accompanied with significant metallosis. Up to that time we had not found evidence of metallosis in seventeen consecutive acetabular components that we had retrieved from patients who had cemented titanium femoral replacements. These prostheses had been inserted without metal-backed acetabula. However, when the same titanium prosthesis was used with metal-back acetabula, metallosis and early failures were frequently demonstrated. Careful analysis of the removed specimens was conducted in our laboratories at the Orthopedic Hospital of Los Angeles. *Harry McKellop demonstrated that the cement around the polyethylene socket fragmented and generated debris that also carried metal from the plasma-sprayed cup. The fall of these fragments in the plastic-metal articulation produced a third-body wear phenomenon.*

The finding of this phenomenon with titanium prostheses can be explained on the grounds that titanium is a relatively softer material when compared with harder ones, such as stainless steel or cobalt-chrome alloys.

Surgeons in the Los Angeles area who had used the metal-backed-acetabula also experienced the same problems. Their radiographs depicting the complications were made available to us. This opportunity made possible to us to conclude that the metal-backed component create cement and metal debris that eventually find their way into the joint, initiating then a third-body wear process and the resulting bone lysis in the femur and acetabulum (Figs 9.1A to C).

I am not aware of any reports dealing with a similar complication using different metals. I suspect however, that the problem occurred with cobalt-chrome and stainless steel because virtually overnight the popularity of the technique ended. This may not be a good example

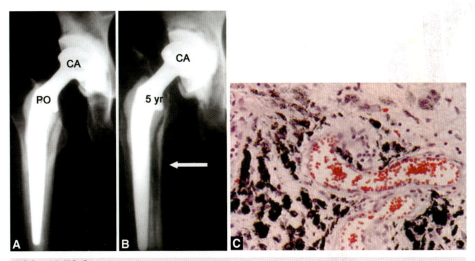

FIGS 9.1A TO C

(A) Postoperative radiograph of cemented titanium arthroplasty reinforced with a metal-backed acetabulum. (B) Radiograph obtained five years later demonstrating loosening of both components and lysis in the femur and acetabulum. (C) Microscopic slide of capsular tissues obtained during revision surgery demonstrating the presence of metal in them

to illustrate the unfortunate fact that, much too often, implants and techniques that ultimately fail when introduced into the general orthopedic community show a high rate of complications, neither the developers nor the manufactures publicly acknowledge the problem. The products continue to be sold, if not locally, at least in developing countries. Surgeons, as a rule, continue to use the techniques or implants until it is accidentally learned that bad results were recognized months, if not years earlier.

I had a personal experience along this line. A number of years ago I encountered a high incidence of failures with a noncemented prosthesis. We prepared a report on the subject and sent it for publications to one of our popular journals. The main reason for the rejection of the paper was that "the prosthesis we had used was no longer being sold, since it had been replaced with the Model II". I expressed my unhappiness with the editor's decision by asking him, "If 5 years down the road someone were to report the complication rate with the Model II being higher than Model I, would that paper be rejected because Model III had replaced Model II?".

I informed the editor that the Model I implant was no longer sold in North America, but was strongly marketed south of the border as an implant that could be used as a cemented as well as an uncemented prosthesis. C'est la vie

References*

39, 56, 72

* References provided at the end of the book after annexures.

Section 1

10

The Posterior Surgical Approach

Despite the fact that the lateral approach to the hip was the one used almost exclusively for total hip surgery for a number of years after the Charnley arthroplasty was introduced in the United States, this approach is currently rarely used. I personally used the lateral transtrochanteric approach exclusively for five consecutive years, following the few months I spent at Charnley's institution in Wrightington, England, in the spring of 1970. More recently, Joel Matta began to use a modified anterior approach top the hip with very good results. His approach is a modification of the Heuter's approach, which is truly an anterior, not an anterolateral approach, as the Charnley's approach is..

I vividly recall the following anecdotal experience: In 1975, I stopped using Charnley's transtrochanteric approach and began to use a posterior approach without trochanteric osteotomy. I also began to use titanium and abandoned the stainless steel implants. After a couple of years of experience with the new system I wrote to Sir John informing him of my departure from his technique. He wrote back a most interesting letter, which began with thanks for my keeping him informed of my change. He said that he was not surprised to hear the news, which he interpreted as a sign of the enthusiasm of youth. After criticizing my use of titanium, and making a few other points, he ended his letter saying that I had missed my call: "You do not have the mentality of an orthopedic surgeon.. By approaching the hip from behind, you have shown that you have the mentality of a gynecologist". Several years after his death, I discussed that letter with his widow, Lady Gill,

who informed me that he had shown her the letter before he mailed it to me, and he had been concerned over my change of direction.

Most orthopedic surgeons today use either a posterior approach or a modified anterolateral one. Routine osteotomy of the greater trochanter is reserved by some exclusively for complicated revision arthroplasties for operations that require major gain in length to the extremity, such as in the case of a congenitally dislocated hip with significant shortening of the limb.

The posterior approach makes possible replacement arthroplasty in virtually all instances. The exposure to all bony and soft tissue structures is very good. The danger of vascular or nerve injury is minimal by simply adhering to guidelines (Figs 10.1A to C).

It has been fairly well documented that the posterior approach to the hip, which requires internal rotation of the hip and its flexion during the insertion of the femoral component, is less likely to have an adverse effect on the major vessels, leading to the initiation of thromboembolic disease. The anterior approach to the hip, on the other hand, requires external rotation and flexion of the hip. In this instance the vessels experience a greater kinking, likely to initiate the damage that leads to thromboembolic disease. My own experience has supported the concept that the posterior approach is safer than the anterior one in this regard (See *Thromboembolic Disease*).

For the performance of total hip surgery through the posterior approach, the patient should lie on his side

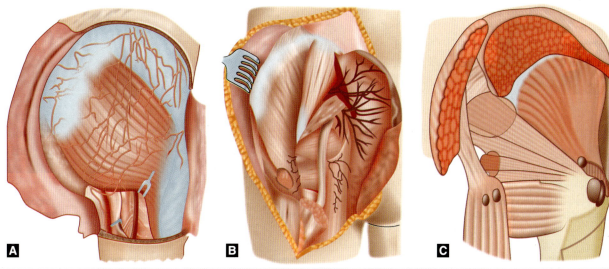

FIGS 10.1A TO C

(A) Illustration of the gluteus maximus muscle, which is not transected during surgery. At most its attachment to the iliotibial band is sectioned and later repaired upon completion of surgery. (B) Illustration of the relationship between the sciatic nerve and the small rotators of the hip and the piriformis muscle. (C) Illustration of the posterior aspect of the hip showing the gluteus medius and small; rotators of the hip

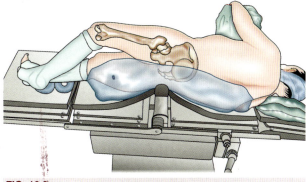

FIG. 10.2

The patient lies on the sound side and is held in place with either a suction bag or with other simple methods of stabilization

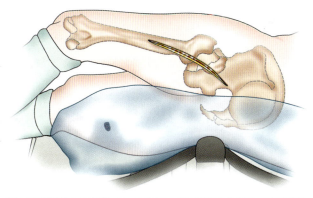

FIG. 10.3

The surgical incision is made in an almost totally vertical direction slightly behind the greater trochanter, extending from above the greater trochanter to the proximal third of the femoral shaft. Its length must be determined on the basis of the patient's degree of adipose tissues, the presence or absence of contractures, shortening of the extremity or rotational deformities. What is important is not the length of the incision but the making of the surgical intervention free of preventable technical problems. After all, wounds heal from side-to-side, not from end-to-end

with the hip uppermost. In order to ensure that a true lateral position is maintained throughout the entire surgical procedure, some type of system must be used, either in the form of a deflated "beam bag' or metallic supports. In this instance a beam-bag is illustrated (Fig. 10.2).

The following illustrations (Figs 10.3 to 10.13) depict the posterior surgical approach and the important surgical details to be observed. Though the drawings emphasize the cemented technique, the same other details are applicable to the noncemented arthroplasty. In general, a noncemented hip arthroplasty is easier to perform, though surgical precision is also essential.

Adequate exposure of all structures is an indispensable prerequisite (Figs 10.4 to 10.18).

Otherwise, a number of complications can occur. Through a too small an incision, exposure of the acetabulum may not be possible, resulting in poor orientation of the prosthetic component. Contractures, particularly those associated with limitation of internal rotation, makes the exposure of the neck of the femur extremely difficult if not impossible. Attempts to forcefully rotate the leg could result in a fracture of the femoral neck or shaft. The same is true for the insertion

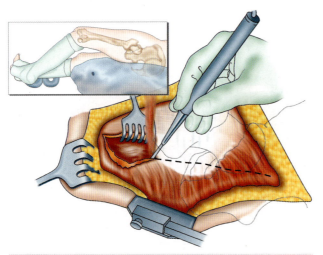

FIG. 10.4

The iliotibial band is incised generously along the axis of the femur

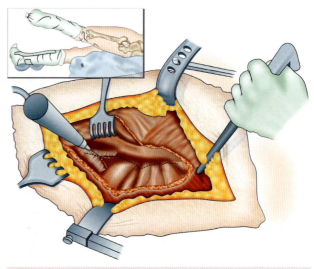

FIG. 10.5

Retraction of the incised iliotibial band reveals the small rotators of the hip and the insertion of the gluteus maximus on the shaft of the femur. There is no need to sever this muscle unless there is significant limitation of motion of the hip or a previous surgery that has resulted in inelastic scarring which prevents adequate exposure of the deep structures

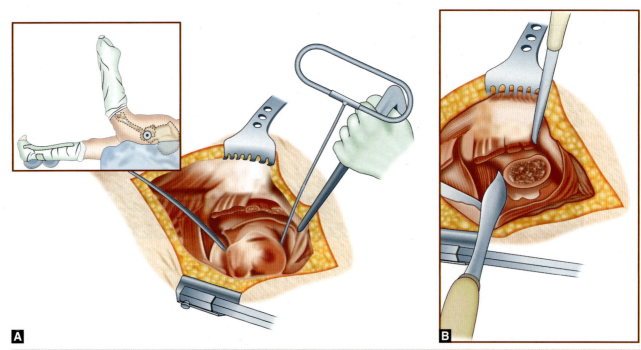

A

B

FIGS 10.6A AND B

(A) Once the capsule is exposed, it is incised along the long axis of the femoral shaft. Then the hip is dislocated by means of flexion, adduction and internal rotation of the leg. I do not hesitate to remove the entire posterior capsule if the dislocation is difficult. The head of the femur is removed either with a Gigli saw or with an electrical saw. (B) Once the head is excised the remaining neck of the femur is exposed

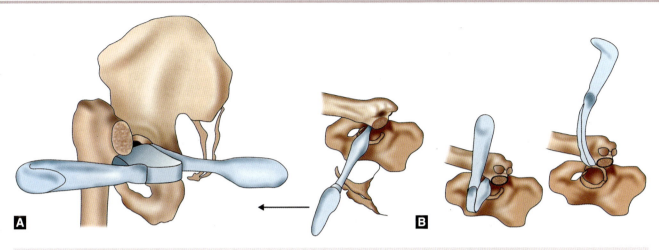

FIGS 10.7A AND B

(A) The acetabulum is exposed by inserting a retractor over the anterior wall of the acetabulum. Care must be exercised to avoid injury to vessels and nerves inside the inner pelvis. (B) Illustration of the maneuver that is carried out to expose the acetabulum

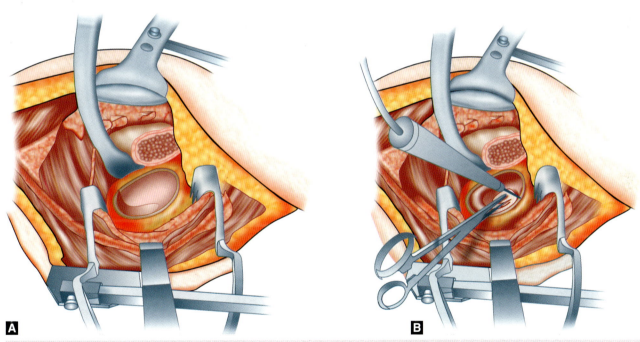

FIGS 10.8A AND B

(A) Once the posterior capsule has been separated or removed, the exposure of the acetabulum is very satisfactory. At this time major osteophytes are removed with the aid of a rongeur. Despite the fact that removal of the osteophytes might increase bleeding, it is better to remove them, not only in order to facilitate the surgery, but also to prevent impingement of the femoral neck against them, leading to dislocation. (B) Remnants of the ligamentum teres are removed

Section 1

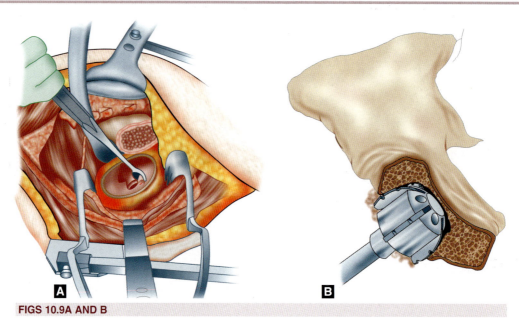

FIGS 10.9A AND B

(A) With the aid of a curette, additional soft tissues are excised. (B) The acetabulum is reamed until its depth is deemed appropriate to accommodate the acetabulum component. This is more easily done with power tools while exercising caution to avoid excessive penetration into the bony pelvis

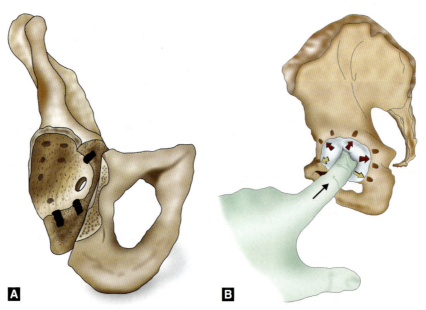

FIGS 10.10A AND B

(A) Several holes are made on the surface of the acetabulum, into which the acrylic cement is later injected. This step is obviously unnecessary if a noncemented implant is used. Up to this point the surgical technique is the same. (B) The acrylic cement is firmly pushed into the holes and throughout the entire surface of the acetabulum

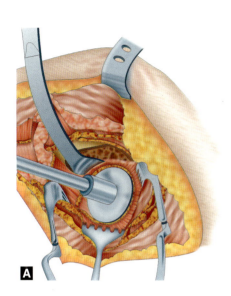

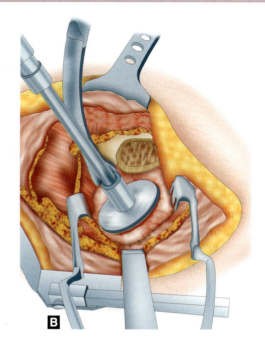

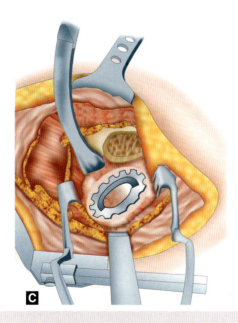

FIGS 10.11A TO C

(A and B) Care must be exercise to avoid placement of the acetabular component in improper positions of exaggerated anteversion or retroversion. Usually between 10 and 15 degrees of anteversion are desirable. This applies to cemented as well as non-cemented arthroplasties. A 45 degrees angle of inclination in relation of the horizontal is also desirable. There are instruments to assist the surgeon in obtaining the best alignment of the component. (C) The plastic acetabular component is then placed over the still polymerizing cement and held into position until the cement has hardened completely

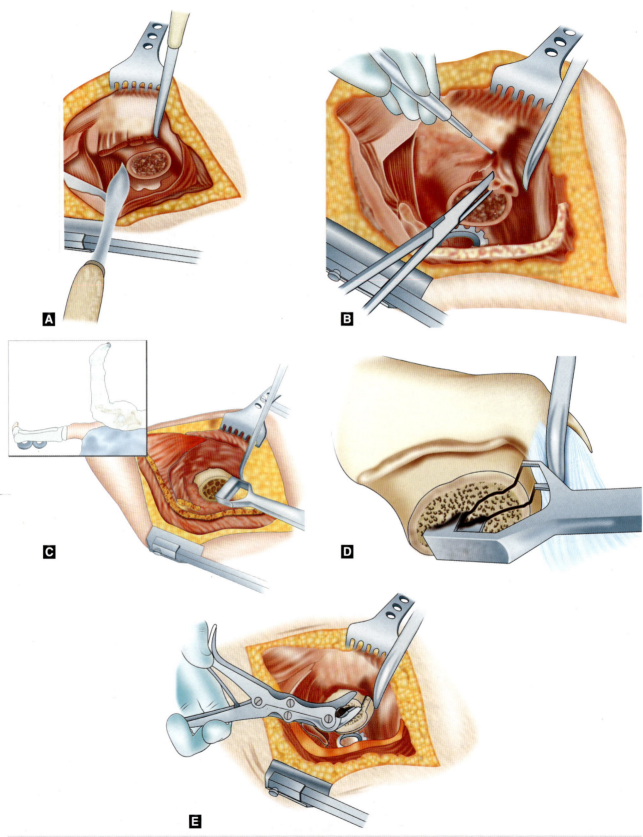

FIGS 10.12A TO E

(A) The sectioned femoral neck is once again exposed. (B) Remnants of soft tissues from its most lateral aspect are excised. (C) With the aid of a "cookie- cutter" a wedge of bone is removed form the lateral aspect of the neck. (D) Closer view of the excised bony wedge. (E) Residual bone that may interfere with the insertion of the prosthesis is removed with the aid of a rongeur

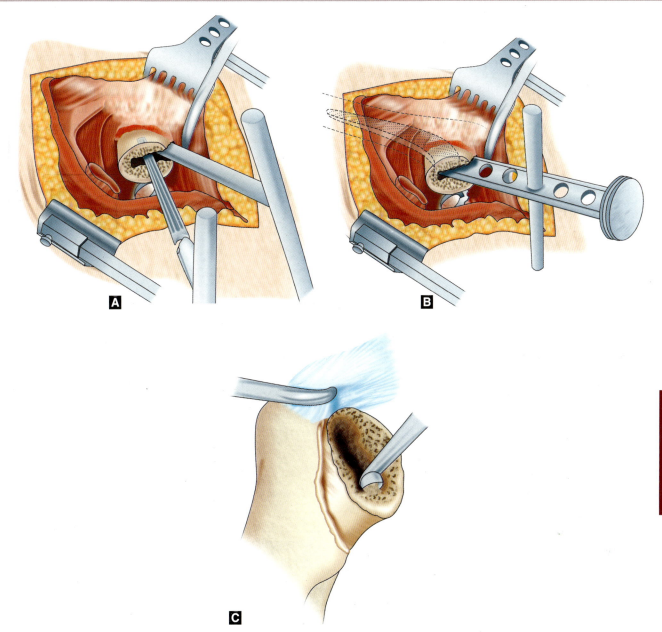

FIGS 10.13A TO C
The medullary canal is opened with a moderately blunt instrument to avoid perforation of the femoral cortex. A Moore rasp is then inserted in the medullary canal emphasizing the firmly rasping of the lateral surface

of the femoral component, which is often necessary when severe shortening of the extremity needs correction. Lengthening of the leg places tension on the surrounding nerves. *In order to lessen the tension on them the semi-rigid tissue must be released.*

The removal of the head is not always easy, particularly if the Ligamentous Teres is intact as in the case of an acute fracture of the femoral head or in the early stages of avascular necrosis. *Fortunately, in most instances of osteoarthritis or rheumatoid arthritis this*

ligament is severely degenerated and mechanically weakened.

If the removal of the head becomes difficult despite deliberate rotation and levering it against the rim of the acetabulum, it is best to split the head with an osteotome and then remove the fragments separately. This maneuver is often necessary in instances where the femoral head is severely enlarged, as in the case of arthrosis secondary to Perthes disease. The same is true when the surgical incision is small, which

Section 1

compromises the exposure of the various soft and bony tissues in the area.

When a noncemented prosthesis is used, the steps thus far described are the same. However, subsequent steps require additional rasping and reaming of the medullary canal to ascertain that the fit of the implant against the cortical wall of the femur is as perfectas possible. Radiographs (Figs 10.14 to 10.18) of multiple noncemented arthroplasties are shown throughout the text.

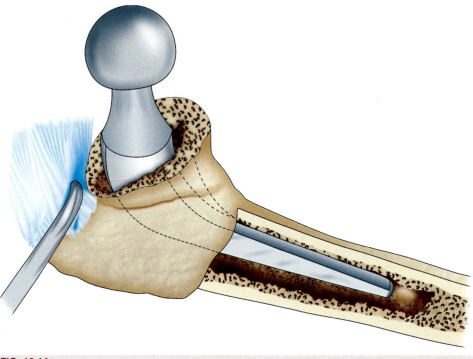

FIG. 10.14

Prior to the insertion of the cement into the canal a trial placement of the prosthesis should be done to ascertain its neutral position

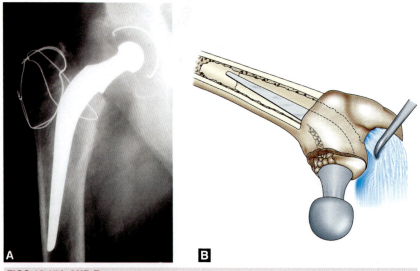

FIGS 10.15A AND B

The varus position of the prosthesis that should be carefully avoided

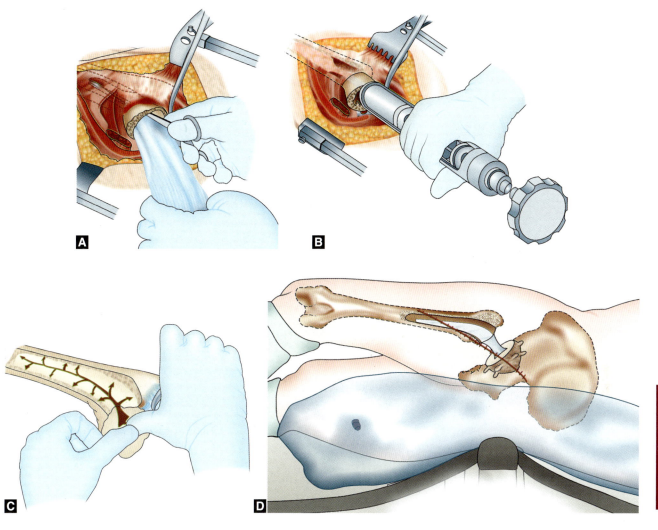

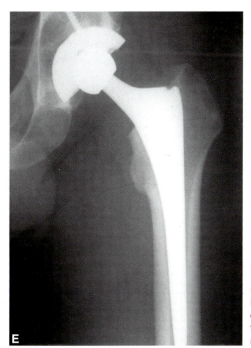

FIGS 10.16A TO E

(A) The medullary canal is dried prior to the insertion of the cement. (B) The cement is injected into the medullary canal. (C) Once the syringe has been emptied, the cement is further pressurized with the surgeon's thumbs. (D) Upon completion of the procedure the femoral component should be in a neutral attitude. (E) When a noncemented stem is used its fit in the canal must be as precise as possible

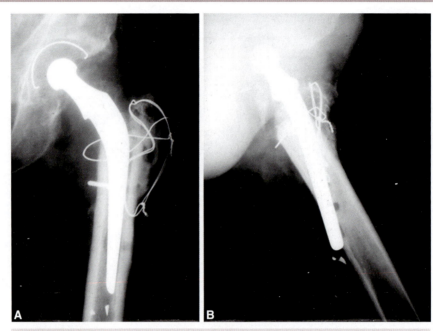

FIGS 10.17A AND B

(A) An anteroposterior radiograph suggests good placement of the components. (B) The lateral radiograph depicts the perforation of the medullary canal and the exit of the stem through the cortex

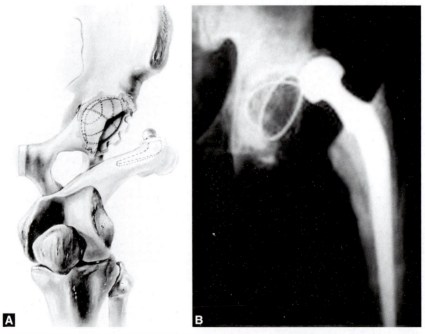

FIGS 10.18A AND B

(A) Drawing of a posterior dislocation of a total hip arthroplasty demonstrating how flexion of the hip, accompanied with adduction and internal rotation, produce the complication. (B) Radiograph of a superior dislocation of a total hip arthroplasty. One single view of the hip cannot clearly tell the direction of the dislocation in the anteroposterior plane. However, posterior dislocations usually produce an internal rotation of the extremity, while an anterior dislocation produces an external rotation of the leg

*References**

21, 82

───────────

* References provided at the end of the book after annexures.

11

Leg-Length Discrepancy

Millions of people have walked this earth for millions of years with one lower extremity shorter than the other without ever having noticed the difference. Tailors are familiar with this pattern, and therefore, when fitting customers for new pants they check both sleeves. Minor discrepancies are not associated with late sequella, such as arthritis of the spine or adjacent joints as some borderline quacks want us to believe. Asymmetry is very common in other parts of the body as well: one eye smaller, one nostril wider, one testicle longer, one breast lower are frequently observed.

Upon finding out after completion of an uncomplicated total hip arthroplasty that the operated extremity is longer than the normal one, can create an unhappy scenario that may become a nightmare to the surgeon. For reasons not clearly understood, patients who have this experience are, often, deeply concerned over the limp the sudden discrepancy produces. *A situation where a residual additional shortening of less than one centimeter results from surgery, is rarely a problem, as far as the patient is concerned.* They seem to get used to the change within a very short time. However, if the leg is made longer than the opposite leg, it is likely that the patient will complain for a long period of time. It is my experience, that most of them eventually forget the "problem" and cease to complain. It is unfortunate that there are surgeons who contribute to making the situation of a "longer leg" a problem, and in doing so provoke litigation against the surgeon who performed the operation.

As I indicated earlier, patients usually get used to the greater length of the operated extremity. To assuage their initial concern, the prescription of a lift in the shoe in the shorter leg can be prescribed.

One can confirm the nature of mild length discrepancy in the length of an extremity by placing a lift in one of the shoes and walk around with the lift for a couple of days. The chances are that at the end of the second or third day the difference in length is less noticeable. Wear the lift for a couple of weeks and the discrepancy might be forgotten.

A number of suggestions have been advanced regarding the most effective means to ensure that at the end of surgery both lower extremities are of the same length. The simplest and most commonly used one is the placement during surgery of two Steinman pins as reference points: one in the iliac crest and the other in the proximal femur. The distance between them is recorded prior to the dislocation of the hip, and the Figures 11.1A and B is kept in mind while selecting the most appropriate length of the prosthetic head/neck component.

This simple method works well in most instances. However, to rely entirely on it may lead to unexpected disappointments. Sometimes, a flexion contracture may go unrecognized, resulting in increasing unnecessarily the length of the operated extremity.

It should be kept in mind also that on occasion the patient may have, prior to surgery, one leg longer than the other secondary to a fracture of the tibia or femur sustained earlier in life, or a paralytic disease that left one extremity shorter than the other. Therefore, the surgeon should not rely entirely on the figures obtained from measuring on X-rays plates the distance between the two points in the pelvis and the femur.

When an adduction contracture is present and its presence has not been of a very longstanding nature, it is not unlikely to see a spontaneous correction of the

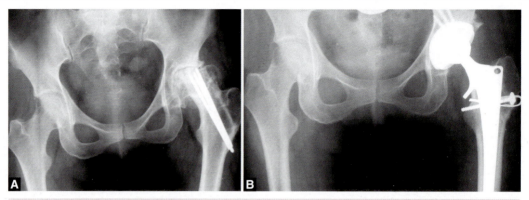

FIGS 11.1A AND B

Radiograph of pelvic obliquity secondary to surgically treated slipped capital epiphysis. (A) If the obliquity is not considered in determining the true discrepancy of the lower extremities, it is likely that a total joint replacement will result in a much the obliquity spontaneously improves. (B) Radiograph obtained one year after surgery demonstrating a significant spontaneous improvement of the pelvic obliquity

deformity over the ensuing months. Some adduction deformities, secondary to trauma, that affected the sacroiliac joints, never improve. This fact must be kept in mind at the time of surgery.

Patients who have associated structural scoliosis often hope that their gait will be improved following replacement of their arthritic hip. Though often some benefit is achieved in this regard, there is no reliable method to predict its effectiveness.

I suspect the best way to ascertain that the appropriate ultimate length of the operated obtained is to use the various techniques: the discrepancy suggested by the preoperative films, the distance between the 2 pins, the clinical measurement of the length of the two extremities prior to surgery, and the assessment of contractures, pelvic obliquity and related spinal deformities.

Many surgeons pay a great deal of attention to the "shucking" produce from manual traction of the extremity for the selection of the appropriate neck length. I also use the method but pay relatively little attention to its findings. Not that I completely ignore them because major separation between the socket and the prosthetic head may lead to later dislocation, but because this phenomenon is influenced by several factors. If we were to insert longer and longer prosthetic necks in order to eliminate all "shucking", there will be a legion of patients walking around with their operated legs longer than necessary.

Even though the appropriate length of the neck has been selected, some "shucking" may still be present in some patients with very elastic tissues. With patient with less elastic tissues subjected to even stronger traction, will show no separation between the acetabular and femoral components.

Another factor that heavily influences the separation between the acetabulum and prosthetic head is the extent of soft tissue striping carried out by the surgeon. Those who like to perform the surgery through a small incision are less likely to see major "shucking". Others, including myself, who prefer a wide exposure of the hip joint and, frequently, surgical severance of the insertion of the gluteus maximus from the shaft of the femur, as well as posterior capsulectomy, observe a greater "shucking" during traction. Moderate "shucking" is not a problem since scarring and tightening of the tissue is inevitable; resulting in a satisfactory tightening of the tissues.

I have treated several patients experiencing painful symptoms when attempting to flex the hip following total hip surgery. A diagnosis of iliopsoas tendonitis was made and treated with local infiltration of hydrocortisone and Novocain. In a couple of instances, as much as 12 months elapsed before permanent improvement was obtained. Once, I had a patient who experienced severe groin pain on the 4th postoperative pain as she attempted to flex the hip, trying to get out of bed. At first I suspected a dislocation, however, clinical and radiological examination rule it out. It was not until a few days later that the presence of a fracture of the lesser trochanter was recognized. It is likely that the lesser trochanter was incompletely fractured at the time of surgery, and that sudden contracture of the iliopsoas muscle a few days later completed the fracture (Figs 11.2A to D).

It is of historical interest to note that Austin Moore deliberately osteotomized the lesser trochanter whenever he performed his endoprosthetic replacement in osteoarthritic patients. He felt that this "inconsequential" step was beneficial and never considered it as a possible cause

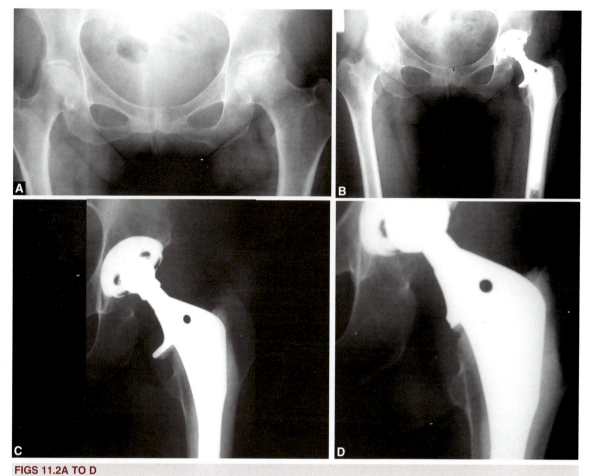

FIGS 11.2A TO D

(A) Preoperative radiograph of the pelvis of a sixty-four-year-old woman suffering from osteoarthritis of the left hip. (B) The condition had been treated at another institution using a hybrid arthroplasty. The operated left leg ended up being longer than the right leg to a degree that troubled the patient in a significant degree. She refused to accept a period of waiting hoping that the limp she was experiencing would become less noticeable. Another reason for the refusal to accept my recommendation was the fact that the pain was more severe during active flexion of the hip, suggesting iliopsoas tendonitis produced by a long prosthetic collar. (C) Radiograph of the long collar, which I suspected was responsible for the iliopsoas tendonitis. (D) Postoperative radiographs showing the shortened prosthetic neck, which was accomplished by replacing the neck-head component with a shorter one

of dislocation or of permanent weakness of hip flexion. The temporary weakness improved over a short period of time (See *Dislocation in Total Hip Surgery*).

In the presence of hip pathology, women, because of the usually wider pelvis are more likely to experience a greater limp than men with narrower pelvis. The same is true for those people who have a valgus femoral neck, compared to those with varus femoral necks. These facts, supported by data that was originally generated in France, explain why people of the same height but of opposite gender, and who demonstrate identical radiological changes, females demonstrate a greater limp. People affected with paralytic diseases, like poliomyelitis, prove the point: the females limp more than their male counterparts.

It may be appropriate to introduce at this time a somewhat related piece of information. It has been long-believed that there is significant difference in the TKA between men and women. That thus is true because women are more likely to have valgus knees, while men most likely have varus knees. I recently read a very well documented article indicating that the etiology of this is premise is incorrect. The authors demonstrated that the difference disappears when comparisons are made between people of the same height. That is, for example, women and men measuring eight feet tall show similar TKA.

12

Hip Dislocation, Dislocated Total Hips and Acetabular Containment

The introduction of CT scans and MRIs in orthopedic diagnosis has had incalculable benefits.

Long before such sophisticated machines became popular, I had the opportunity to work with Doctor Herman Epstein, from Los Angeles, for nearly 13 years. He conducted long-term follow-up studies of many indigent patients at the USC-LACH, often at his own expense. This made it possible for him to make observations of great importance. He came to the conclusion that all traumatic dislocations should be surgically managed because he found out that, in many instances, small free pieces of bone and cartilage were floating in the joint, eventually producing late degenerative arthritis. Today, the MRI or CT scans show them with certainty (Fig. 12.1).

It used to be customary to prevent early weight-bearing following reduction of traumatic posterior hip dislocations. The reasons for such a practice never made any sense to me. First of all, re-dislocation of posterior dislocations is very unlikely unless extreme degrees of flexion associate with internal rotation are introduced. Secondly, the intact articular surfaces do not require precautions against weight-bearing. Thirdly, curtailing weight-bearing should not have any influence on the condition of the important vessels, which in the event they were initially severed, would lead to avascular necrosis.

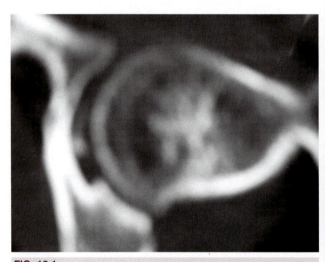

FIG. 12.1

Illustration of small bony fragment at the bottom of the acetabulum following a traumatic dislocation of the hip

This was my reasoning, even during my residency, when traction in bed for a period of six weeks was the recommended method of treatment. My approach to the issue has been radically modified with time. I have seen patients following close reduction of dislocated hips develop osteoarthritis at a later date, without avascular necrosis. In these cases, is it possible that the initial injury could have crushed the articular cartilage and damaged it irreparably at that time? Or that bony fragments in the joint went unrecognized? Methods to determine the condition of the cartilage with the use of MRI and CT scan are in their infancy. In the near future, I hope such techniques will be available and my question will be answered.

Although we would like to be free of dislocations in total hip surgery, it appears that we will be confronting them from time-to-time, particularly in the case of revision arthroplasty. Much has been said about its etiology, prevention and treatment but no last word has yet been written on the subject.

I don't think it serves any purpose to rehash what has been said many times before about the importance of proper orientation of the acetabulum during total hip surgery. *In my opinion, malposition of the acetabulum is not the common cause.* For a dislocation to occur, the malposition must be significant since the hip may be stable even in the presence of a socket anchored without anteversion. A socket in a few degrees of retroversion does not always necessarily result in dislocation when the surgery was performed through a posterior approach. We demonstrated this quite well using an artificially created hip that allowed us to study various attitudes of the acetabulum. It is universally accepted that the inclination of the acetabular component should ideally be that of 45 degrees, and the socket should be well contained under the bony roof. Our studies, definitely indicated that the inclination of the socket does not need to be very precise. A few degrees of greater or lesser inclination are not necessarily harmful. Under artificial mechanical simulators we demonstrated this. What the studies did make clear is that containment is much more important. When comparing nearly 900 total hip arthroplasties with a maximum follow-up of 17 years, the incidence of acetabular loosening was significantly greater when the socket was not well contained. The sockets that were placed with an inclination of 50 degrees did better than those placed more transversely. The amount of wear was the same in both groups; and such was also true for the rate of dislocation.

It must be kept in mind that all these prosthetic replacement were cemented. In such a case, it is possible that the transverse nature of the socket location makes possible a titter-tatter mechanical environment less likely to be present when the cup is in a more vertical position. Placing the acetabulum in the allegedly preferred 45 degrees inclination is oftentimes impossible if the bony socket is shallow and cannot be deepened further without breaking into the inner pelvis. *The surgeon is then forced to place the socket in a vertical position in order to achieve coverage, which is more important.*

It is likely that the observations and conclusion we drew from cemented socket do not apply to porous implants, and that complete converge is less essential. *It has been documented from observations of post-mortem specimens that stability of the socket may be very good even if the porous surface demonstrates only a small area of bone ingrowth.*

I suspect that most dislocations are the product of soft tissue imbalance. A prosthetic replacement that shortens the extremity too much leaves major soft tissue instability. This does not mean that all total hip replacements that end-up with a shorter leg eventually dislocate, since scaring down of the tissues can provide the necessary tethering that ensures stability. The clicking about which some patients complain during the first few weeks following surgery and its eventual disappearance testifies to that effect.

It is a common practice to "shuck" the hip joint prior to selecting the best possible femoral neck length. Though I do pay attention to the findings from such maneuver, I do not rely too heavily on my findings (See *Length Discrepancy*). Often, one is able to obtain significance separation between the prosthetic head and the artificial socket in the presence of the desired length of the extremity, due to unusually high degree of elasticity of the capsular tissues. Other times the same phenomenon can be seen when major stripping of soft tissues from the surrounding bony structures was necessary.

Attempts are being made by some to develop navigation systems that will "guarantee" the proper insertion of a noncemented femoral component. The proposed systems require additional surgical time for the fulfillment of technical detains and the reading of computerized data. I think such as effort is an unnecessary one. The proper placement of the femoral component has been standardized and made simple and predictable. With rasps of various sizes the corresponding appropriate permanent prosthesis can be selected in such a manner that the so-called "ideal" relationship with the femoral cortex and the wall of the implant can be obtained. I have said, "so-called ideal relationship" because I am not sure that such a perfect relationship throughout the entire canal is necessary. I have seen hundreds, if not thousands of clinically and radiologically "perfect" results in patients whose femoral stems did not meet the specified criteria for a good technique (See Chapter 19: *Factors that Determine Success in Total Hip Surgery*). That the system "ensures" the most accurate determination of leg-length is also misleading. It assumes that the single feature to be considered in restoring length is the distance between the lesser trochanter and a line that transects both ischial tuberosities. Though this measurement is very useful and should be considered in all instances, it ignores the fact that in many instances the cause of dislocation is soft tissue instability, rather than length discrepancy. *One might read from these measurements a certain degree of shortening or shortening of the operated extremity without realizing that the diseased limb, or the normal opposite one, had suffered a fracture in early life, resulting in either overgrowth or undergrowth that the X-rays of the hips fail to identify.* It also ignores the fact that a pelvic obliquity often gives misleading readings resulting in significant difference in the length of the extremities once the procedure is completed (See *Leg-length Discrepancy*).

I worry about the role that making a leg too long plays in the etiology of dislocation. *This is particularly true in patients with tight hamstrings.* I discovered this while performing surgery in an individual with significantly tight hamstrings. I deliberately inserted a temporary implant with an excessively long neck. When the hip was reduced and the hip ranged, the stability of the joint was good as long as the knee was kept in flexion. However, when I flexed the hip to approximately 80 degrees and then extended the knee, the hip dislocated posteriorly. The tight, inelastic hamstring created the pathological situation. Applying a brace postoperatively under those circumstances is likely to result in subsequent dislocations particularly if a commonly, ill-conceived brace that limits flexion, is applied.

Hip dislocation braces that limit flexion of the hip do, in my opinion, more harm than good. When a patient, fit with a brace that limits flexion beyond 75 degrees, sits down, the normal hip, which easily reaches 90 degrees of flexion, forces the operated hip to dislocate posteriorly. *Hip dislocation braces should not limit flexion of the hip; simply adduction and internal rotation.* Failure to adhere to this design explains why so many surgeons have grown dissatisfied with the use of braces for the prevention of recurrent dislocation of artificial hips.

Braces to prevent dislocation that cover too much of the pelvis and thigh are not necessary. *All the hip-dislocation brace needs to do is to ensure that the hip cannot be adducted and internally rotated.* That can be accomplished with a very light appliance that simply needs a thin pelvic band and a small, adjustable thigh band. The brace I have used in the recent past creates those limitations very effectively. It is designed to permit normal ambulation with an economic narrow gait but forces the hip to abduct as the patient assumes the sitting position (Figs 12.2A to E).

It is important to recognize that most dislocations of total hip arthroplasties occur not during activities requiring extreme degrees of motion but during the process of sitting down or getting up from a bed or chair. Usually, when a patient holds the knee in extension (as it is often mistakenly recommended) and then proceeds to sit down the hip is adducted and internally rotated. The dislocation ensues. If the hip and knee are flexed from the beginning of the process of sitting down or getting up, a dislocation is not likely to occur. The overwhelming majority of these dislocations have acceptable coverage and orientation of the acetabulum. Needless to say, the presence of a very large osteophyte could precipitate the dislocation, but this is very rare, since its presence would have been recognized at the time of surgery when the stability of the hip was tested.

Repeated dislocation of total hip prostheses frequently end-up needing surgery. Many times the procedure is helpful and the dislocations stop because the hip is "tightened" and the newly stripped soft tissues have a new chance to scar down in a tighter fashion. Self-constrained sockets that retain the head in place and prevent dislocations are in vogue at this time and early results seem satisfactory. We should remember, however, that Emile Letournel, in the 1970's developed a similar socket only to find at a later date that the rate of polyethylene wear was too high (See *Self-constrained Acetabular Components*).

Patients with very thin or very muscular thighs are more prone to dislocate their total hips. In a couple of instances I have seen patients who twenty five years after surgery dislocated a total hip implant, while carrying out activities that they had regularly performed over the years without any problem. The only detectable finding was a significant loss of weight that was clearly visible on their thinner thighs. Wear of the polyethylene was not a factor in these particular cases.

Sciatic palsy following traumatic dislocation of a normal hip is common. However, this neurological complication is very rare in the case of dislocation of a total hip arthroplasty. I have never seen such a problem. I assume that most dislocation of prostheses

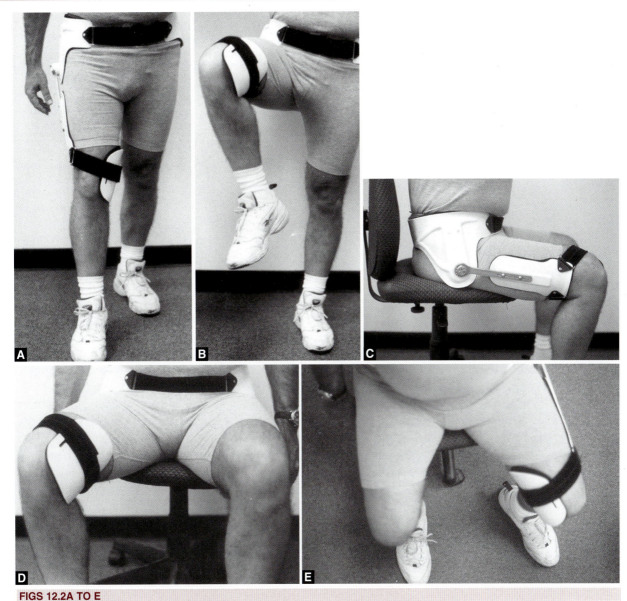

FIGS 12.2A TO E

Photographs illustrating a specially designed hip-dislocation brace. The brace prevents adduction and rotation of the hip. *The pelvic joint is constructed in such a manner that during ambulation the leg swings in a normal fashion, however, during flexion of the hip, the hip abducts and externally rotates*

occur in the absence of major trauma. *In the case of traumatic dislocation of previously normal hips, when a sciatic palsy develops, it is very likely that the palsy is limited to the peroneal component of the sciatic nerve.* Many surgeons mistakenly assume that the nerve is traumatized at the level of the hip in order to explain the resulting pathological picture. However, this is rarely the case, since the neurological pathology takes place below the knee, not at the level of the hip joint. As the hip dislocates superiorly, the nerve is stretched, but since the posterior tibial component runs in a straight direction from the hip to the foot, the stretching is easily tolerated; on the other hand, the peroneal component of the nerve is relatively fixed around the neck of the fibula, experiencing greater stretching when the hip dislocates. This is easily supported by the fact that manual pressure over the nerve behind the fibula produces pain.

References*

33, 40, 57

Section 1

_____

* References provided at the end of the book after annexures.

13

Self-constrained Acetabular Components

The introduction of the self-constraint acetabulum became a major contribution to total hip surgery. Thus far there appears to be no major downside for the use of the appliance, and I anticipate its use will become wider with the passing of time. Emile Letournel, from Paris, designed a self-constrained acetabulum some 30 years ago but its use was abandoned within a few years. Excessive wear of polyethylene was seen with frequency. It appears that the design of the implant was incorrect since abutment of surfaces occurred within normal motion of the hip. This abutment created damage to the plastic material and therefore the production of plastic debris.

I suspect those major drawbacks of the original implant have been overcome. My experiences, though limited, have been rewarding. I have not as yet seen a complication traceable to the implant. However, not enough time has elapsed to justify its use in every instance when instability of the hip is detected in primary surgery. In the case of revision surgery when major instability is detected, I do not hesitate to use the implant at that time (Figs 13.1A to C).

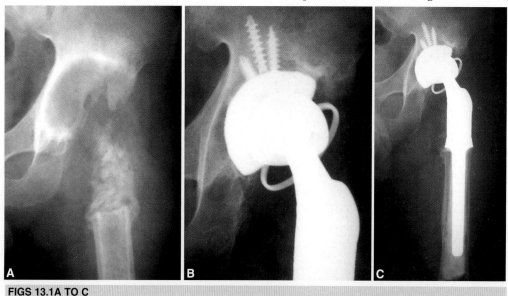

FIGS 13.1A TO C

(A) Radiograph obtained after removal of an alleged infected total hip arthroplasty that left the patient with a very short extremity. At the time of the revision surgery, the trial prosthesis demonstrated significant instability. (B) A self-constrained acetabulum was used to render the hip stable. (C) Radiograph of the femur and implant

There have been some reports of dislocation of the acetabular component. This is easily understood, as one considers the fact that when a conventional total hip reaches an extreme degree of motion, and an additional stress come into the picture, such as an unexpected force tending to increase that degree of motion, the joint dislocates. A similar mechanical situation in the case of a constrained implant, would result in loss of fixation of the screws from the acetabulum. An osteoporotic pelvic bone, makes this eventuality a more likely one.

In addition, sudden, excessive forces being resisted by the stable component, such as a fall, can produce a fracture of the femur from the great rotary forces to which the bone is then subjected.

My satisfaction with the self-constrained acetabulum (Figs 13.2A to F) has been so great that I have suggested the possibility of using it in all elderly patients with displaced fractures of the femoral neck (See Primary Total Hip Replacement for Fractures of the Femoral Neck in the Elderly). I base this view on the fact that in this age

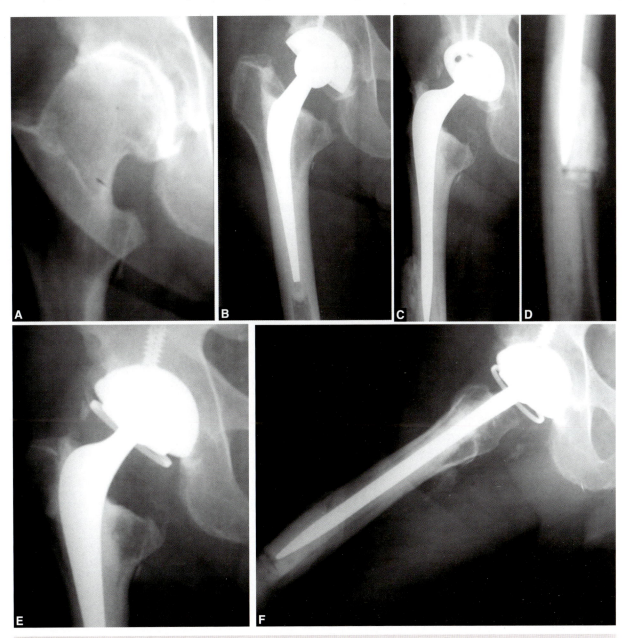

FIGS 13.2A TO F

(A) Radiograph of osteoarthritic hip in a man 60-year-old. (B) I replaced the hip with a noncemented prosthesis. (C and D) The patient dislocated his hip 2 weeks after surgery and was treated at another institution. The surgeon chose to revise the components and in the process perforated the femur. (E and F) Allegedly the hip dislocated again. He then implanted a self-constrained acetabulum

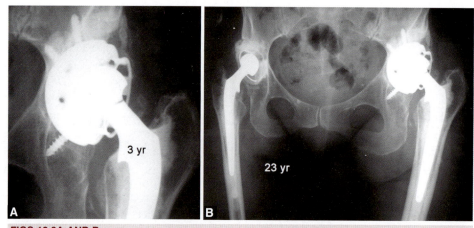

FIGS 13.3A AND B

Radiographs of a self-constrained acetabulum in the left hip that was used in order to create stability with a vertically placed acetabular component. The X-ray on the (A) also shows the titanium arthroplasty performed 23 years earlier. (B) Another surgeon replaced the hip with a cemented prosthesis...

category the endoprosthesis is associated with a high incidence of dislocation. In addition, immediate full weightbearing ambulation has been discouraged for reasons I do not clearly understand. Therefore, if those fractures that have a notoriously bad prognosis when treated by means of internal fixation were to receive a noncemented or cemented total hip arthroplasty with a self-constrained acetabulum, there would not be a need to curtail immediate weight-bearing ambulation without precautions against dislocation (Figs 13.3A and B).

This theoretical approach will not be practical at this time, primarily because of the unreasonable cost of the surgical implants. If industry were to manufacture reasonably inexpensive prosthesis, I suspect much would be gained. With the currently popular treatments of internal fixation or primary endoprostheses the cost of care is very significant. Many of these elderly patients, because of the limitations and problems just outlined, require nursing home care and extensive rehabilitation, the propose approach would eliminate such needs.

14

Minimally Invasive Total Hip Arthroplasty

The performance of surgery through smaller incisions, using in some instances new instrumentation, has gained interest in the treatment of a multitude of conditions, ranging from gallbladder or inguinal hernias repair, aortic aneurysms and disk removal. There should be no doubt that the advances these new techniques brought forward have benefited countless people. The morbidity associated with some of the surgeries performed through traditional long incisions has been dramatically reduced. It is likely that the advent of these techniques were inspired by the success that knee arthroscopy has had in the last few decades.

More recently, the idea of performing total hip surgery through smaller incisions has captivated the orthopedic community with a degree of polarization not frequently observed. Several surgical approaches that make possible the performance of the arthroplasty have been advocated.

When first brought forward, any revolutionary concept that seriously challenges tradition generates controversy. It is within our nature to grow comfortable performing surgery in the manner in which we have previously executed it. We witnessed this reaction when arthroscopy was first introduced in the armamentarium of the orthopedist. Its acceptance required a relatively long period of time. We had grown accustomed to making long incisions that allowed the inspection of the joint in a very satisfactory manner. The idea of inspecting and treating damaged menisci or cruciate ligaments through a lens appeared irrational. That view was held by most orthopedist for some time. However,

it is history. Once orthopedists learned how to handle the instrumentation appropriately, the thought of returning to open surgery was unthinkable.

It is possible that the same course of events will follow minimally invasive total hip surgery. However, I have reservations. Unless obvious benefits become readily apparent; the performance of the procedure is made relatively simple and the associated morbidity is reduced, most surgeons will be unwilling to experiment with the new toy.

The idea of performing hip arthroplasty through a small incision is not new. In the mid-1970's I visited Buenos Aires, where I had the opportunity to see Doctor Fermin Garcia perform total hip replacements through what he called a mini-incision. Indeed it was an incision much shorter than the one I had learned from Sir John Charnley. I did not think Doctor Garcia was having difficulties carrying out the procedure. I was impressed.

He gave me a movie depicting the procedure, which I replayed upon my return home. Then, I replaced a hip using his technique. It was obviously a departure from the way I had performed total hip surgery for the past 8 years. Nothing went wrong and the patient did well. I admit, however, that the exposure of the acetabulum and proximal femur was not as good as the one I had become accustomed to. I elected not to use the mini-incision again. I had not gained anything from the experience, despite the fact that it is likely that the patient had lost a little bit less blood. So what, I said, she will rebuild it in no time. The rehabilitation of the patient was not modified. I do not know if the degree of pain she experienced was less that it would have been otherwise. Pain is difficult to measure. Some people go through major surgery and leave the hospital a few days later having required a minimal amount of analgesics. Others, with less serious or longer surgery cry with pain in degrees we do not comprehend. Furthermore, the psychological make up of the individual and the anticipation of pain make a great deal of difference. To spend sleepless nights trying to unravel that mystery does not pay.

A few years earlier I had seen Maurice Muller perform hip arthroplasties using an incision that was as long as the distance from his 5th finger to his thumb. Even though I never liked his anterior approach to the hip, because I felt the exposure of the femur was not as good as the one provided by a posterior approach, he did a wonderful job and made it look like a simple procedure. He was an artist.

During my younger academic days I devoted a great deal of time to the study of amputation surgery and prosthetics. I was deeply impressed with the great difference that seemed to exist in the reaction of different people to the news that they had to lose a limb. The differences were mainly along ethnic lines. Those of Northern European ancestry, as a rule, accepted the event relatively well and without external evidence of great grief or emotion. Those of African descent also accepted the loss of the limb pretty much the same way, but did not seem able to hide the fear of the amputation. For those with Mediterranean ancestry, particularly Latin Americans, the event was a major one. Crying and moaning was the rule. Relatives came to the hospital to console the grieving patient, asked many questions and wanted to know every single step that would take place before and after the surgery.

The same is probably true for hip surgery. The amount of pain and the length of disability are influenced by the ethnic and racial factors surrounding the individual. I have discharged from the hospital a relatively small number of patients as early as three or four days following total hip surgery. They were able to carry out most activities of daily living and had graduated to one crutch or cane before leaving the hospital. The incisions were of the length I had used for the past 35 years. The mini-incisions do not have the exclusivity on early hospital discharge.

A few years ago I was asked by a prestigious journal to review a paper submitted to them dealing with the subject at hand. The following are excerpts of my letter. "I doubt these alleged advantages the "minimally invasive procedure" have been documented.

a. *Less surgical dissection:* This "advantage" applies only to the skin and iliotibial band, not to the capsular tissues and bone. The capsule is incised or excised in the same manner with all known techniques, and the neck of the femur osteotomized also in an identical fashion. That being the case, one wonders what is the real "advantage" of reducing the "dissection" of the skin (other than perhaps less pain), since the skin heals from side-to-side and not from end-to-end. With these "easy cases" the performance of surgery takes longer when exposure is more limited. The author pays no attention to the fact that hip replacement performed through a very small incision compromises the surgeon's ability to obtain good exposure of essential features. The procedure therefore is more difficult and more likely to be associated with complications.

b. *Reduced blood loss:* The advocates of the 'new technique' (it is not) indicate that the arthroplasties is easy to perform by conventional methods and are the primary indications for the minimally invasive procedure. It must be recognized that in such instances, the performance of the arthroplasty by conventional means is associated with minimal bleeding, often without the need for transfusion. Therefore, what is the "real" advantage of the "minimally invasive" technique in regard to "bleeding"? Though, it is very likely that the amount of bleeding from the severed soft tissues is less with smaller incisions, what meaningful difference a few more cubic centimeters of blood loss makes in the short or long-term outcome? Is it possible that the greater trauma inflicted on the forcefully retracted soft tissues, necessary when a small incision is used, may be more important than the additional amount of blood loss?

c. *Less postoperative pain:* It is logical to assume that the amount of pain from a smaller incision should be associated with less pain. The literature has not as yet discussed the methodology used to determine the degree of postoperative pain. Were the conclusions drawn from the number of injections of narcotics or ingestion of analgesics received by the patients? How many patients have participated in prospective studies? Were the patients operated through the new technique compared with a similar group of patients who had the arthroplasties performed with traditional techniques? Has the placebo effect been evaluated? To the best of my knowledge none of those things have been done. Furthermore, one must be aware that many hip arthroplasties are performed under epidural anesthesia, which often is maintained for 24 hours, and therefore pain is not a problem. Ambulation of patients anesthetized either with epidural or general anesthesia is begun on the first postoperative day, many of them requiring minimal amount of narcotics or analgesics. However, there are times when patients experience unexpected degrees of pain. It has to do with the personality of the individuals. The same, I am sure, is true regardless of the surgical technique used. As with the previous item, what is the meaningful "advantage" gained from the minimal reduction of pain, which is easily treated with simple medications?

d. *A shorter hospitalization:* A glance at the history of total hip arthroplasty shows that the length of hospitalization has gradually decreased. It began with four (4) weeks and currently averages five (5) days. Not all patients are discharged from the hospital and immediately returned home. Many factors come into the picture: the patients' age (most hip arthroplasty patients are elderly); their overall general condition; associated pathology; presence or absence of relatives at home willing to assist the recently operated relative; and many others. A period of observation during the first few days after surgery are used to monitor medical and orthopedic related matters: taking measures to prevent dislocation; bladder and pulmonary complications, teaching transfer activities; examining the extremities for impending thromboembolic disease; and many others. Ignoring the advantages that these measures offer, only for the sake of shortening hospitalization by a couple of days is difficult to justify.

e. *Early non-assisted ambulation:* This is an attractive feature, which can be achieved not only with small surgical incisions but also with longer ones. However, the orthopedic community has not been able to settle the issue concerning the desirability of immediate full-weightbearing following surgery. The issue was discussed in reference to cemented arthroplasties, and has been raised again with non-cemented prostheses. Marketing the technique based on the merits of immediate weight bearing ambulation may not be appropriate.

The author uses references to Christensen's work to support his or her views. I question the analogies presented, i.e. the telephone, photocopy machines, personal computers. The same applies to some medical developments such as angioplasty, laparoscopic cholecystectomy. These medical related innovations were introduced to the medical community after extensive evaluation of clinical results. Data was presented to peer-review journals and eventually the procedures became popular. This is not the case yet with "minimally invasive arthroplasty".

"I have concluded that there is no data in the literature to strongly suggest that the method of minimally invasive total hip replacement" has proven safe and effective. Publications in non-peer review journals and presentations at several meetings during the last years have been highly anecdotal, and so is this paper. The issue at this time has been emotionally charged and the incidence of complications with the technique has been virtually ignored.

"Publication of this article would, in my opinion, be interpreted by many as an endorsement of an unproven technique. Without sufficient follow-up and clear documentation and peer review of results, publications of papers of this nature often do more harm than good. The history of our discipline is rich with such examples: ballerinas carrying out athletic pirouettes a few weeks after hip replacement surgery, or professional football players falling to the ground under the force of his opponents, who nonetheless found themselves within a short period of time having their artificial joints surgically revised. Isoelastic prostheses, carbon composite implants, surface replacement arthroplasties were marketed and widely used before they were appropriately tested. Soon they were abandoned, but not before much harm was done. If the "minimally invasive technique" is eventually proven efficacious, then its dissemination through the literature will be justified. Based on the above arguments, I suggest this paper not be published at this time. There is ample time for additional experiences with the technique, which might make the technique universally accepted."

I admit that the above criticism of the "new technique" was perhaps prematurely harsh. Since, then I have read reports from reputable surgeons who appear to have documented their experiences appropriately. In addition, I suspect that something beneficial has already come out of the interest generated by the subject. It has made us realize that the long incisions that we traditionally used are not always necessary. I benefited from that lesson, and began to make smaller ones, without going to the extremes recommended by some.

One thing that the technique has accomplished is to demonstrate the power of effective marketing.

*Reference**

103

* Reference provided at the end of the book after annexures.

15

The Effect of Age in Total Hip Surgery

It is generally believed that the age of the patient has much to do with the way in which the implant and surrounding bone perform over a long period of time. Instinctively, we all share that view. However, experiences have not always supported that perception. I have seen patients with cemented total hip implants who had surgery in their twenties, thirties or early forties (Figs 15.1 to 15.3), who after 37 years after surgery showed no clinical or radiological changes to suggest impending failure. Some of those implants looked as good as they did the day after surgery. On a number of occasions these patients lived very active lives and

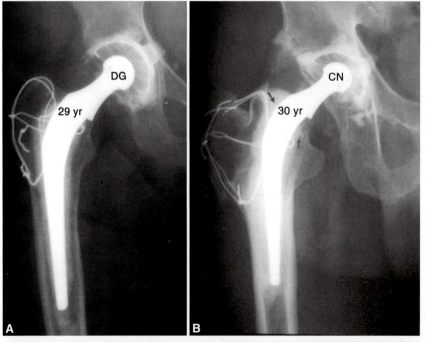

FIGS 15.1A AND B

Two different patients: (A) Radiograph obtained 29 years postsurgery, originally performed for the treatment of rheumatoid arthritis in a 19 years of girl. (B) Radiograph taken 30 years after surgery performed in an active osteoarthritic man 38 years of age

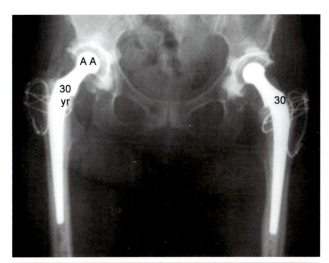

FIG. 15.2

Thirty-year-old bilateral total hip Charnley arthroplasties performed for the treatment of osteoarthritis in a 35-year-old woman

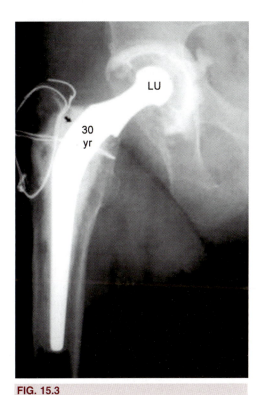

FIG. 15.3

Thirty-year-old Charnley arthroplasty performed in a 40-year-old woman for the treatment of osteoarthritis

were heavy and tall. Other older patients, light in weight and who lived rather sedentary lives demonstrated signs of failure in a short period of time.

The long-term survival I am referring to deals with cemented arthroplasties. They are the only ones with which I can claim to have had the opportunity to follow for such long periods of time. Experiences with

noncemented prostheses is much shorter, therefore we do not know whether they will provide equal or better results. There is suggestive evidence that some of now-popular noncemented implants will last as long if not longer than cemented Charnley arthroplasties. I sincerely hope that will be case. *However, we must remain cautious, and remember that we have been repeatedly disappointed by the short-life span of prostheses we were marketed to be the final solution to all problems.* To complicate matters is the fact that hip replacement has become a big business, not only to the surgeons but to the manufacturing industry of surgical implants. It is unfortunate that at the time of this writing it is being said that with "modern" implants there is no need for patients to avoid any strenuous exercises. Indulging in all kind of sports is OK because the artificial joints will last them the rest of their lives. I think we are playing with fire, and the chickens will some day come back to roost. The data at this time is still weak and to make such recommendations is probably inappropriate and unprofessional.

As a result of the exaggerated commercialization of medicine, it has become increasingly difficult to find honest reports regarding the true findings from follow-up studies. Too much data is fabricated to protect individuals who cannot tolerate even the thought that their results are not as good as they expected them to be. Their publications, therefore, are not creditable.

I have personal anecdotal experiences to support my views. On a recent occasion I heard a very well-known hip surgeon, who carries the title of professor and chairman of orthopedics at a major medical school, report an almost complete absence of complications in a group of 18,000 total hip replacements performed at his institution within a given period of time. He emphasized a near-perfect system of follow-up where all patients' progress was monitor with great accuracy. What he did not know was that at I was providing follow-up care to two of his patients. I had asked them during their initial visit to my office about their experiences with their surgeon and further communications with him. Both had responded in the same manner: "I was very well impressed with my surgeon when I first met him. He is charming" When I asked about postoperative contacts, they replied, "He is too busy, I never saw him after surgery. His residents and therapists took care of me". Concerning post-surgical discharge from the hospital their comments were, "I never heard again from him or from his assistants".

To imply that this is a universal practice would be very unfair, because there are many surgeons who honestly report on their experiences. However, others do not. This is why I tell residents in training to be extremely careful about taking for granted the veracity of whatever information they read. *Accepting as truth only a small percentage of the data is the wisest approach.*

What is the explanation for such apparently inconsistent results? Much speculation has surrounded the issue and no clear-cut conclusions have been reached. *Many of my best total hip arthroplasties, among the thousands I have performed over the years, were cemented Stainless Steel Charnley replacements performed with the crude thumb-packed cementing techniques of the early 1970's.* Those implants were cemented on both sides of the joint; no metal-backed acetabula were used; no irrigation, pressurization or plugging of the canal was done; the polyethylene material was probably of a better quality, and the sterilization process less damaging to the plastic material.

I also suspect that our infatuation with bigger and stronger prostheses has also been responsible for the higher rate of complications. This came to my mind in a clear way a few weeks ago when I heard a presentation dealing with prosthetic replacement of the femur and tibia in children suffering from malignant tumors. The presenting surgeon during his discussion of complications indicated that future improvements should be made concerning the strength of the implants. The statement was made despite the fact that none of the prostheses he had used had broken. The failures he reported had been of the osseous structures; not of the implants.

I commented on his presentation by saying that *stronger prostheses will increase the number of complications, since, as a rule, stronger prostheses are stiffer and therefore more likely to increase the difference in the modulus of elasticity of the bone versus that of the implant.* Such an increased difference worsens the stress shielding that leads to bone weakening in some areas and hypertrophy in other areas (See *Titanium Total Hip Prostheses*).

We have reviewed our clinical material (Figs 15.4A to D) several times over the past years and have carefully looked at the issue of age in relation to success or failure of cemented total hip prostheses. We found that, in general, older patients experience a lower number of radiological changes with the passage of time. *Women have a higher incidence of bone-cement radiolucent lines on the acetabular side. I have long suspected that older women may have a more "flexible" pelvic bone that because of its lower modulus of elasticity in comparison to that of the prosthetic component, deforms to a greater degree during weight bearing. This repeated deformation probably leads to later loosening.*

We identified that age, per se, is not the reason for the difference between the two groups. The disease for which the operation had been performed is the most important finding. Patients with avascular necrosis have the worst radiological results. It happens, however, that most patients with avascular necrosis are younger. *If the group of patients with avascular necrosis is removed from our entire series the difference in performance between the young and the old disappears.*

On the other hand, it is only fair to admit that this is true only if the two groups are followed for the same period of time. It is likely that young people with total hip implants, if they live to an old age, will have a higher incidence of complications. John Charnley, who rarely made a wrong observation or prediction, categorically stated that no total hip implant would last thirty years in an athletic individual. I guess that to some extent he was wrong but his warning should be remembered as our enthusiasm with the operation increases. He was thinking at that time that wear would be the ultimate problem that made total hip implants failed. Perhaps, the problem of wear will some day soon be solved. If and when that happens we will be able to finally say that prosthetic replacement of the hip is truly a long-lasting procedure.

Longer follow-up with noncemented prostheses have indicated a high rate of success. It is likely that these implants will eclipse others methods of fixation for a long time to come.

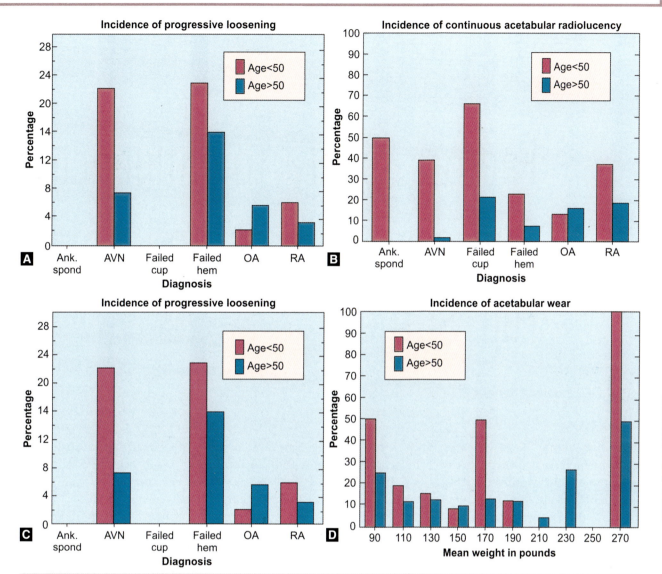

FIGS 15.4A TO D

If the patients who undergo prosthetic replacement for the care of AVN are deleted, the performance of the implants becomes very similar. Surgery for AVN seems to render the worst results

*References**

58, 59, 70, 104, 117

Section 1

* References provided at the end of the book after annexures.

16

Factors Likely to Influence Success in Cemented Total Hip Surgery

A great deal has been written about total hip replacement. If we were to believe everything we read we would be utterly confused. Almost everybody has "excellent" results according to the thousands of publications. Every new prosthesis is marketed as "new and improved"—as in the case of toothpaste or soap—as the product of extensive research. If that were true, one could choose any of the nearly 350 different prostheses in the market and count on having perfect results.

The fact remains that complications occur with any and all implants and that very little research goes into the design of many of the modifications. In actuality, the difference between various implants is minimal and represents only minor changes in shape, length, width, angle or texture.

New implants appear in the market on a frequent basis simply because the competition between the manufacturers is fierce. Each company has to protect its turf to keep ahead of the pack. The president of a major manufacturing company told me once that as soon as they released a new implant they are already working on its modification which would be released the following year. This pattern has been tempered somewhat in recent years after industry realized it was too expensive.

Several years ago, I moderated a panel dealing with total hip arthroplasty. A very well-known surgeon flashed slides on the screen showing a virtual absence of complications with his "own" prosthesis. His list of the complications had only zeros before them. Three years later I had the opportunity to moderate a panel, where the above-mentioned surgeon was one of the speakers. This time he was describing his newer prosthesis and telling the audience about the absence of complications. As expected, zeros appeared regarding complications. I took advantage of the situation and asked the distinguished surgeon, what reasons he had for having modified his earlier implant, since he had not had complications with it. I changed the subject before he had a change to answer the question. I did not want to embarrass him. In retrospect, I should have.

I do not intent to go into a lengthy discussion regarding the many factors that influence the behavior of total hip implants. I will limit my comments to cemented arthroplasty based on a review of my own experiences. My results support the views of others. I will not discuss noncemented implants because I have not critically reviewed my own experiences with them. Their follow-up is relatively short, having a maximum of approximately 20 years.

Recent European literature is reporting possible advantages with cemented implants, something that has shocked the American orthopedic community, since in the United States we have grown accustomed to believe on the superiority of the noncemented ones. These reports call for a new assessment of the issue at hand.

1. *The metal* of the prosthetic head. *Titanium is the wrong material to use.* Stainless steel or cobalt chrome is better. I feel titanium alloys, as we know them today, are too soft and likely to be scratched, resulting in the release of metal debris that eventually produce bone lysis. Titanium alloys have powerful toxic metals such as aluminum and vanadium. *It is well known that when total hip fails, the urine and blood show the presence of those metals at the same ratio present in the alloy.* Other popular alloys, such as those primarily composed of cobalt and chromium, also contain toxic metals. However, since the composite does not scratch easily, it is less likely to release particles. To date we have no evidence that serious clinical problems have been associated with those metals in patients with total hip implants. However, a totally complacent attitude about this fact cannot be justified, based on data presented by people like *Patrick Case, from Bristol University, who has identified chromosomal abnormality in areas of metallosis.*

It may be argued that the problems I encountered were exclusively due to the use of titanium alloy heads, and that the results would have been better if I had used prosthetic heads made of cobalt-chrome or ceramics. I agree with that premise, however, a cemented stem, if it becomes loose at the stem-cement interface, can generate metal debris as it is scratched from its repeated motion against the cement. Furthermore, I also suspect the same can occur with noncemented prostheses that become loose in the medullary canal. This is not a very likely probability because the cortical bone is softer than the metal. However, metal debris can fall into the medullary canal, arising from friction between the screws fixing the acetabular cup and the holes in the cup. Likewise, debris can be produced by corrosion at the level of the modular components (See *The Titanium Experience*).

2. The *type of socket* remains debatable. My own experiences comparing totally cemented prostheses with *hybrid ones, indicated a better performance of the noncemented ones, as far as the acetabular side was concerned, but inferior regarding the femoral side.* I must admit, once again, that the worse results were likely to be to the fact that I had used monoblock titanium alloy femoral components. Others, however, using Cobalt-Chrome implants have had similar experiences (See *Hybrid Total Hips*)

3. The *attitude of the acetabular cup* has been traditionally believed to be ideal when it measures 45 degrees of inclination. When we reviews our result it was discovered that in a number of instances I had inadvertently cemented acetabula with a higher degree of inclination. However, those hips behaved as well as the more transversely placed ones. Furthermore, we suspect that the more vertical cup has an advantage over the more transverse one, as it seems to be subjected to lesser "teeter totters" weight bearing stresses (See *Acetabular Orientation*).

4. *The socket should be fully covered with bone. Coverage is more important than orientation. It is better to place a socket in 55 degrees of inclination than to have it incompletely covered with bone.*

5. A few degrees of *anteversion* have always been recommended. This stands to reason, but a neutral attitude is not always bad. It is difficult to dislocate a hip prosthesis that has a socket in neutral. Dislocation has a variety of etiologies, many of which are far more important than the lack of full anteversion (See *Dislocation of Hip Prostheses*).

6. The *orientation of the femoral component* is relatively important. *The best attitude of the implant is in few degrees of valgus.* Varus produces a higher incidence of radiological complications. However, I am convinced that varus is bad only if it decreases significantly the thickness of the medial-proximal column of cement. If the canal is wide, a few degrees of varus still permit the presence of a wide medial column of cement (Fig. 16.1).

7. The *thickness of the cement* at the "calcar" level *is best if it is between 2 and 5 millimeters.* Too little cement probably fragments and initiates the production of harmful debris. A column of cement greater than 10 millimeters also appears to be associated with a higher incidence of radiological complications (Figs 16.2A and B).

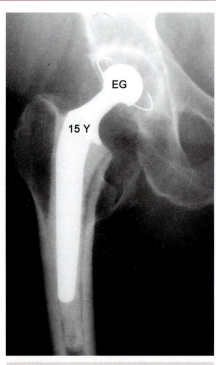

FIG. 16.1

Titanium alloy cemented prosthesis inserted in a varus position. A thick column of cement at the level of the calcar seems to ensure long-term stability

8. The stem should fill more than 50 percent of the medullary canal. Careful review of our experiences confirmed the validity of the argument (Fig. 16.3).

9. A distal *plug* may be desirable. I say, "May be desirable", because I am not convinced it makes biological sense. It is rather naïve to claim that pressurization of the cement is not possible without a plug. It may not be as great without it but there is no data to suggest that maximum pressurization is ideal (See *Pressurization*). Some of my best results were obtained with the original Charnley prostheses when the cement was driven into the canal under thumb pressure. I admit that aesthetically the plugged canal "looks better" and that revision surgery is easier when the cement mass does not extent too far below the tip of the prosthesis. *The possibility exists that polyethylene debris may pool above the plug and create lysis of the bone. Without the plug it should be able to seep beyond that point and be free of compressing stresses.*

10. The *age* of the patient, up to this point, is important. Younger patients are more likely to experience complications. However, our data

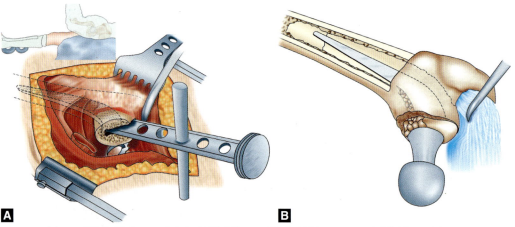

FIGS 16.2A AND B

In order to obtain a thick column of cement medially, at the level of the calcar, the lateral aspect of the femur must be forcefully rasped

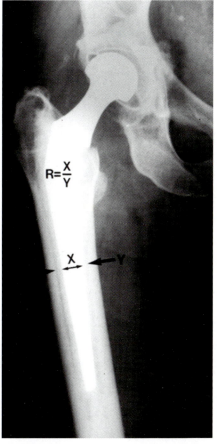

FIG. 16.3

The *diameter of the stem* should not be either too large or too small. *It appears that at seven centimeters below the calcar more than 50 percent of the canal should be filled with the stem*

showed that the risk of femoral component loosening was similar in young and old patients. *The risk of socket loosening is higher in younger patients and the risk of acetabular loosening is higher in female patients.*

11. *The disease for which the operation is performed is of the greatest importance.* Patients with avascular necrosis do not do as well as those with osteoarthritis. The fact that avascular necrosis is usually a condition of the young helps to explain why most people believe that young patients are more likely to experience failure of their total hip implants. If from the overall series one eliminates the patients with AVN, the results indicate that the difference between the young and the old are not as significant.

12. The column of cement should extend below the tip end of the prosthesis.

References*

34, 37, 39, 55, 56, 58, 59, 66, 70, 72, 76, 91, 104, 113

Section 1

---

* References provided at the end of the book after annexures.

17

The Effects of Material and Prosthetic Design

Ever since total hip replacement became popular in the early 1970s, a number of modifications have been made to the original Charnley prosthesis. It was an expected and logical development. Not only was the Charnley implant a patented product, but the desire to improve on his design was a powerful human impulse.

It is likely that emphasis on making changes within such a relatively short period of time may have slowed down the progress that could have been made if the research community had concentrated in addressing wear, which was the crucial issue that John Charnley had emphatically identified as the one that needed the greatest attention. Instead of zeroing in on improving the wear properties of polyethylene, the new prostheses simply dealt with the size of the head, the shape and length of the neck, the geometry of the stem, the properties of the cement, and similar important but not fundamental issues.

The mistaken belief that acrylic cement was responsible for the development of bone lysis gave birth to the noncemented prosthesis, and it was assumed that with biological fixation of the components the problem would be eliminated. That hope did not crystallize. Quite the contrary. The first noncemented prostheses demonstrated a higher incidence of lysis. It was not until additional major improvements were made that lysis was brought under control, though not completely eliminated. It appears that healthy modifications to the stability of modular components, the shape and depth of the

screws into the acetabular cup, the size of the porous surface, and other details were responsible for the improved results.

The material of the implants, their size and shape represented a topic of great interest to many members of our laboratories over which I presided, first at the University of Miami, and later at the University of Southern California. *We developed and used the first titanium alloy prosthesis to be clinically tested in the United States.* The initial results with the implant appeared to be as good if not better than those we had obtained with the stainless steel Charnley implant. *However, with greater experience we came to the conclusion that the titanium alloy implant was not a good one.* Its greater softness made the material subject to scratching from freed acrylic cement particles or from metallic ones released from other structures (See *Titanium Prostheses*).

During a period of nearly three decades I used 6 different designs of cemented total hips: 3 different Charnley implants (curved Charnley, Straight–narrow Charnley, a heavy cobra Charnley and the curved STH, the straight-narrow STH, and the STH2. The radiological performance of these implants was analyzed by Edward Ebramzadeh in our laboratories a USC and subsequently published in the literature. The six prostheses had distinct mechanical properties due to differences in shape and/or material. For example, the straight-narrow Charnley stem was more rigid than the identically shaped titanium alloy straight-narrow STH stem, because the modulus of

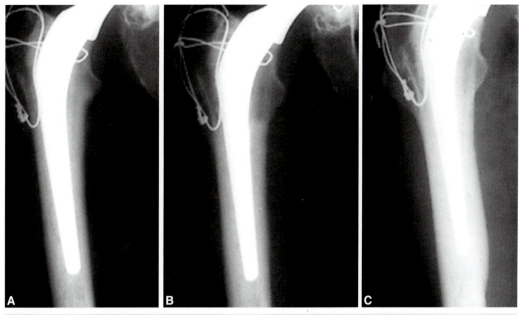

FIGS 17.1A TO C

Composite illustration of radiographs of a Charnley arthroplasty demonstrating the frequently seen hypertrophy of the distal femur resulting from the high stiffness of the femoral component. The process took 16 years to reach the present hypertrophy

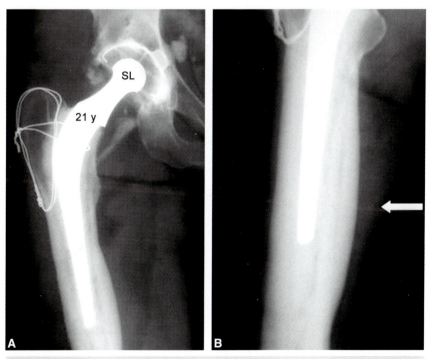

FIGS 17.2A AND B

Radiographs showing the distal hypertrophy of the femur in a Charnley prosthesis. To this degree, this phenomenon is a salutary one

elasticity of stainless steel is twice that of titanium alloy. Likewise, the curved Charnley stem was twice as rigid as the curved STH stem. The stainless steel Charnley cobra stem was the most rigid of all six femoral stem designs, due to the additional dorsal flanges and larger dimensions as well as the modulus of elasticity of its material, stainless steel.

Radiographs (Figs 17.1 and 17.2) obtained over the years indicated that the more rigid stainless steel femoral stems were at lower risk of developing bone-

Section 1

cement radiolucent lines than the titanium femoral stems. Nonetheless, the Charnley cobra stem, which was the most rigid, was not at the lowest risk of developing bone-cement radiolucent lines.

Only one cement fracture and no progressive loosening was observed with the Charnley cobra stems, the most rigid of the stems in the study. The risk of cement fracture and progressive loosening was lower with curved Charnley than the curved STH stems. *However, most radiolucent lines at the cement/stem interfaces were not progressive, and many remained stable for long periods of time, consistent with an observation made in our laboratories by Zhen Lu and his associates: that small amount of debonding can be associated with an actual decrease in peak stresses within the cement and at the interfaces.*

Our studies clearly demonstrated that titanium alloy, in the presence of third body metal or cement particles, can experience significant surface damage resulting in accelerated metal and polyethylene wear, excessive osteolysis, and subsequent loosening of the components. In subsequent studies of titanium alloy femoral components, retrieved in revision surgery, severe wear was observed when a metal-backed acetabular cup- plasma sprayed- had been implanted (See *Retrieved Titanium Prostheses*).

It was also demonstrated that the STH 2 prosthesis was associated with the greatest risk of developing wear, as well as the greatest risk of developing lysis in the adjacent femur. *The risk of lysis was greater with all titanium alloy implants, regardless of the shape of the stems.*

The information gathered from this and other studies conducted in our laboratories have given strong evidence that titanium alloys heads are not acceptable as weight bearing surfaces. I suspect that the disadvantages of titanium can be extended to all prostheses made of this material. We suspect this problem, because the softness of the alloy, which is subject to scratching, applies also to the stem, which if loose may be scratched by the surrounding cement or particles of metal arising from the acetabular component, the Morse taper, the screw-hole junction, or the porous surface in the acetabular or femoral components.

Without any supporting evidence, I suspect some of the problems we have identified with cemented titanium stems apply to noncemented implants. Loosening of the stem associated in the presence of metal debris arising from modular femoral components, screws fixing the cup or porous acetabular components might result in lysis of the femur or acetabulum.

As I have indicated in previous chapters, our apparent obsession with bigger and stronger prostheses has created more problems than solutions. Bigger prostheses are usually stiffer, creating in that manner abnormal concentrations of stresses along the surrounding bony structures that compromise their quality.

Recent work with Tantalum as the substrate metal suggests further improvements. Longer follow-up studies are necessary. Ceramics are offering good results, however, occasional fractures of the material and "squeaking" continue to be of concern.

References*

48, 51, 54, 65, 72, 76, 104

18

Bilateral Simultaneous Versus Staged Total Hips

The most appropriate way to deal with the arthritic hip when the condition is bilateral has been a source of concern ever since total hip arthroplasty entered the armamentarium of the orthopedic surgeon. I have also been interested in the subject for quite some time. Despite the fact that we have reviewed my experiences, I still have reservations regarding the best approach to this situation.

Bilateral hip disease that necessitates total hip replacement is not uncommon. Some of these patients are severely disabled with pain, deformities and contractures. Appropriate surgical management and rehabilitation in these patients are oftentimes challenging requiring careful planning.

Doctor Anukul K Goswami, from England, who worked with me as a fellow, reviewed my data hoping to identify as clearly as possible the clinical results and to determine indications for simultaneous THA, and to document the incidence of complications occurring during and after simultaneous bilateral THA.

The incidence of thromboembolic phenomenon in patients who were operated on both hips (Figs 18.1 to 18.4) within one year period was also compared with the simultaneous group. The database that was evaluated consisted of 1473 patients with 2400 THA surgery who underwent hip replacement during a period of 25 years. Two hundred sixty-nine (18.3%) patients had bilateral hip surgery out of 1473 patients. Thirty-four (2.3%) patients had bilateral one-stage operation, 35 (2.4%) in 4 weeks and 83 (5.6%) between 6 weeks and 12 months. 269 patients had bilateral

surgery, of which 34 patients had bilateral simultaneous hip surgery. Thirty-six patients had surgery within 4 weeks on each hip. Thirty-five out of these 36 had surgery in a single hospitalization period. Another 83 patients were operated between 4 weeks and one year. The results of simultaneous hip surgery were compared with the group of patients consisting of 36 patients who were operated on both the hips within 4 weeks period. Thirty-five of the 36 patients who had surgery within 4 weeks of surgery had been operated in a single hospitalization phase.

I had carried out the procedures to accommodate preconceived notions. *Bilateral flexion-and adduction contractures of the hips, associated with limb length disparity was, in my opinion, the principal indication of the single stage bilateral procedure.* I had come to the conclusion that unilateral hip replacement successfully eliminated the flexion contracture, but the patient's ability to maintain the gained motion was often lost due to the fact that during the sitting position the contracted opposite hip continued to determine the degree to which the operated hip was allowed to flex.

We found out that delaying surgery in the second hip by four weeks or less, significantly increased the anesthesia time, need for blood replacement, length of hospitalization and days for rehabilitation. *There was an increase in the incidence of thromboembolic complications following bilateral total hip arthroplasty when done within 6 weeks.* The risk of thromboembolic complications following one stage bilateral hip surgery was significantly less when compared to those who were

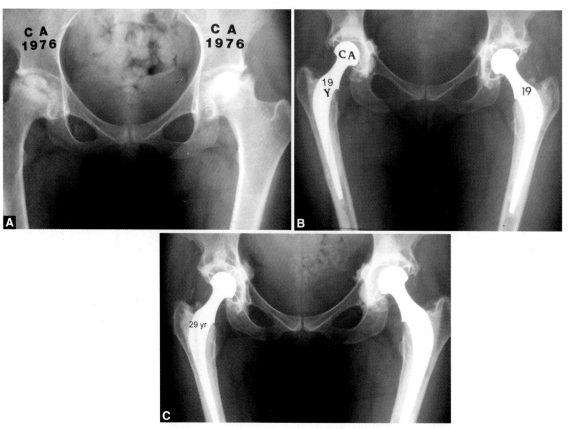

FIGS 18.1A TO C

(A) Avascular necrosis of the femoral heads in a 17-year-old girl with lupus. (B) Radiograph of bilateral simultaneous cemented titanium alloy total hip arthroplasties obtained 19 years postoperatively. (C) Radiograph obtained 29 years postoperatively. Patient has remained active and has two grown-up children

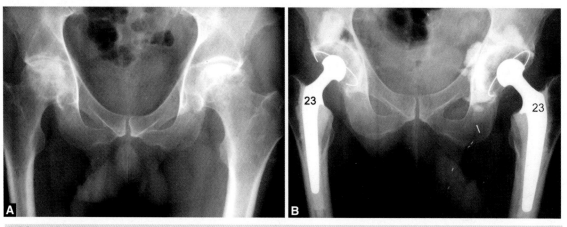

FIGS 18.2A AND B

(A) Idiopathic bilateral avascular necrosis of the femoral heads in 50-year-old surgeon. (B) Both hips were replaced simultaneously. Radiographs obtained 23 years postoperatively. The physician has remained active and asymptomatic

operated in two stages in 6 weeks. If carefully planned, bilateral single-stage arthroplasty seems preferable to bilateral two stage procedures.

Currently, *I do not hesitate to perform adductor tenotomy prior to making the surgical incision to expose the hip joint.* It facilitates in many instances the performance of the procedure. Bilateral adductor tenotomy and soft tissue release around the hip was done in four cases in the simultaneous group as against two in the group where the surgery was done in four

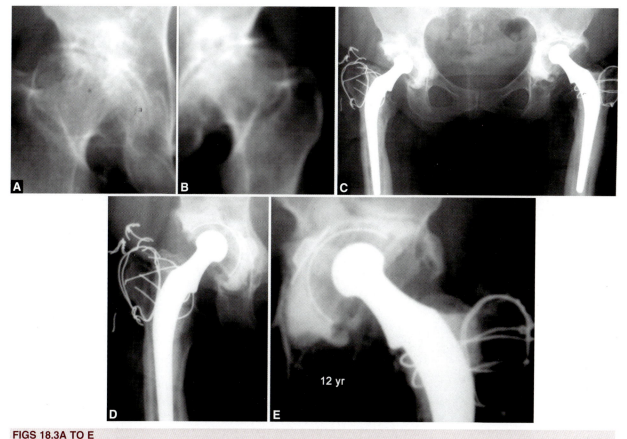

FIGS 18.3A TO E

(A and B) Bilateral hip osteoarthritis in a 65-year-old woman. (C) Radiograph obtained 10 years post-bilateral Charnley arthroplasty. Notice bilateral wear and signs of loosening of the left hip. (D and E) Radiographs taken 12 years after surgery showing the degree of wear and the widening of the bone cement radiolucent line in the acetabulum. The patient was minimally symptomatic and died 2 years later

weeks. Following surgery, the improvement in pain, range of motion, and deformity was satisfactory in both groups. However, one patient, who had bilateral procedure within 13 days, dislocated both her hips during the hospitalization phase. She had a long convalescent period in a rehabilitation center. During her stay in the rehabilitation center she also fractured her femur in a fall. This complication was successfully treated conservatively.

Hospitalization period and days to rehabilitate was significantly higher in patients who had surgery in two stages. (60% increase in hospitalization period, 83% for rehabilitation period (p<0.1). Postoperative dislocation occurred with one patient in each group. Both of these occurred within the hospitalization period.

There were no deaths secondary to pulmonary embolism in the two groups. However, the incidence of deep vein thrombosis and nonfatal pulmonary embolism was higher in patients who had one stage surgery when compared to the group where surgery was done on both hips within 4 weeks. The difference

was not found to be statistically significant. To identify the risk of developing thromboembolic complication following two-stage bilateral hip operations, data was gathered on patients who had been operated within one year. Statistical analysis indicated a significant risk of developing thromboembolic phenomenon if both hips were operated within six weeks. The incidence and risk of thromboembolic phenomenon following bilateral hip surgery done after 6 weeks was similar to the patients who had unilateral surgery. Spinal and epidural anesthesia significantly reduce the risk of thromboembolic complications following hip replacement surgery. With a significantly higher number of patients operated under epidural anesthesia (11 out of 34) in patients with bilateral single stage surgery when compared to the group of patients who were operated within 6 weeks (2 out of 37), the precise implication of lowered incidence of thromboembolic complications in the simultaneous group is unclear.

There is an increased risk of thromboembolic complications following two-staged bilateral hip

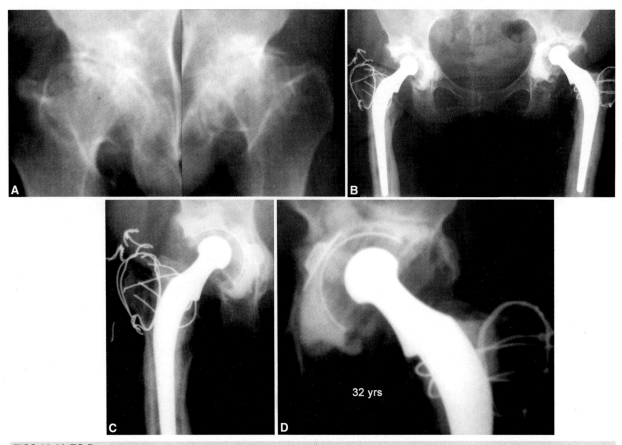

FIGS 18.4A TO D

(A) Radiograph of bilateral osteoarthritic hips in a 59-year-old woman. (B) Radiograph of right hip obtained 10 years postoperatively. (C and D) Radiograph of both hips taken 32 years postoperatively. Notice relatively mild wear of the right acetabulum, as well as the more severe wear of the left acetabulum. A radiolucent line is visible at the bone-cement interface on the left

surgery performed within six weeks when compared to a single stage procedure. Patients with bilateral severe hip disease with flexion-adduction contractures and hip pain, is preferably managed with bilateral single stage surgery. This significantly reduces the postoperative morbidity, and allows early mobilization and rehabilitation. There is also significant reduction in hospitalization period with attendant reduction in costs of inhospital care. If for any reason the one stage operation is not be possible, the second stage operation should be deferred until at least after 6 to 8 weeks. Careful selection of patients for bilateral one stage surgery is preferred over surgery done in 6 weeks (See *Thromboembolic Disease*).

The incidence of revision surgery was similar in both groups. In the simultaneous procedure group eight hips were revised in six patients within the average follow-up period of 8.9 years. In the two stage procedure group eight hips were revised in five patients in an average follow up period of 12.2 years.

The hospitalization period was also significantly increased in patients who are operated in two stages within 4 weeks. The increased cost of inhospital is further inflated by additional cost of rehabilitation services, and costs related to management of post-operative morbidity.

The anesthesia time was found to be significantly increased in patients who had operation within 4 weeks, while the time taken for operation on both hips remained the same. The need for blood replacement was found to be significantly higher in patients who had operation in two stages. There were no fatalities and none had any deep infection.

*Reference**

113

_____

* Reference provided at the end of the book after annexures.

19

The Titanium Total Hip Experience

I hold the dubious distinction of having conceived and used the first titanium total hip prosthesis in the United States. At that time I was unaware that Pierre Boutin, from Pau, France had just begun to use an implant made of the same titanium alloy (aluminum 10, venadium 4). He, however, used ceramic heads rather than the monoblock titanium implants I used. *I wished I had known about Boutin's work, and followed his approach. It would have saved me the inferior results I obtained with the monoblock titanium implant.*

The idea of using titanium occurred to me when I saw a couple of my patients who had experienced fractures of stainless steel Charnley prostheses I had inserted a few years earlier. Similar complications were being reported in the literature in various parts of the world. We also had already noticed the presence of resorption of the femoral calcar and suspected this was due to stress shielding of the proximal femur. The parallel frequency of distal femoral hypertrophy could also be explained by the greater concentration of stresses distally being created by the stiff stainless steel. It was not until years later that we learned that the benign bone resorption may have also been created by plastic debris arising from the polyethylene acetabulum.

By the mid 1970s I had some knowledge about the mechanical properties of titanium because of my interest in fracture healing. *We had documented through clinical and laboratory studies that diaphyseal fractures managed without rigid immobilization healed faster than those treated with rigid fixation. We speculated that motion*

at the fracture site brings about stresses at the fracture site that encouraged osteogenesis. Zimmer Manufacturing Company had recently conducted clinical and laboratory research with an intramedullary femoral nail made of a titanium allow. The concept fascinated me, as I suspected the lower modulus of elasticity of the nail would allow greater stresses at the fracture site and motion at that level. These features should expedite healing, creating a stronger callus. We used the nail a few times, but its production was shortly afterwards discontinued, allegedly because of the increased cost of the material.

After the brief experience with the new nail, it occurred to me that using titanium alloy prostheses, designed to have a lower modulus of elasticity that the ones made of stainless steel or cobalt-chrome alloys, could eliminate the resorption of the cortex we had observed with stiffer metals. With those thoughts in mind, I approached engineers at Zimmer. I suspect thy already had thought about using titanium for prostheses since the reception of my comments were enthusiastically and rapidly embraced.

Working with Zimmer's engineers we designed a total hip titanium alloy prosthesis that resembled the Charnley implant. The size of the head, however, was 28 millimeters in diameter; the Charnley, 22 millimeters. The offset of the titanium implant was also 4 degrees lower than the Charnley prosthesis (Fig. 19.1). Extensive laboratory studies (Figs 19.2A to D) were conducted regarding the mechanical and wear properties of the new implant and were found to be very good. Locally, at the University of Miami,

Hip Surgery

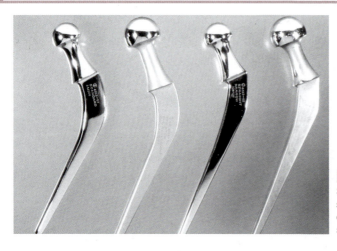

FIG. 19.1

Schematic drawing of the STH prosthesis and its relationship with the surrounding structures. Photograph illustrating the similarities and difference between the stainless steel Charnley prostheses (polished surfaces) and the titanium alloy prostheses (mat surfaces)

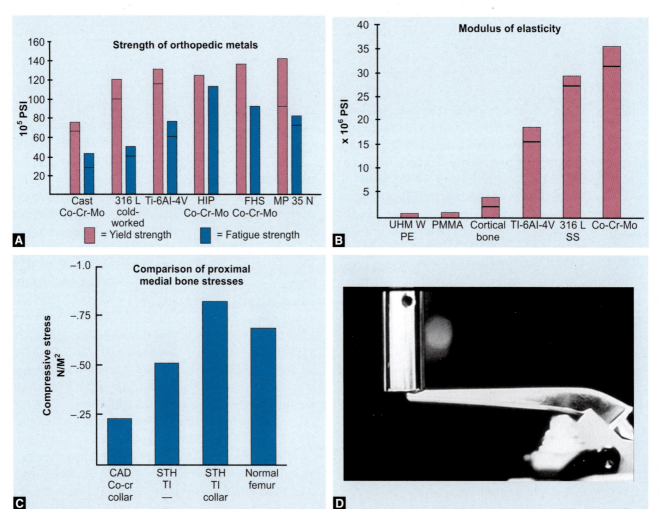

FIGS 19.2A TO D

(A to C) Barographs depicting the laboratory findings indicating the different mechanical properties of the STH implant versus others. (D) The bending stresses to which the implants were subjected to determine some of their mechanical properties

Loren L. Latta, PhD, director of research for the orthopedic department, conducted the initial testing of the prototype implant.

Indeed, the titanium prosthesis transferred stresses in a more desirable manner throughout the entire proximal femur and wear against polyethylene appeared to be even superior to stainless steel and cobalt chrome alloys (Figs 19.3A to D).

Years later, after I moved to the University of Southern California, Ian Clarke, PhD and Harry McKellop PhD, at different time directors of orthopedic research at the new department, (located at The Orthopedic Hospital, and affiliate of the University) corroborated the initial results: polyethylene against titanium heads, under clean conditions, *wears as well if not better than stainless steel or cobalt-chrome alloys (Fig. 19.4).*

However, Rostoker, a distinguished engineer from Chicago, did indicate, that even though the wear properties of the material were good under laboratory conditions, its wear behavior was unpredictable. In the early 1970's the engineers at Zimmer could not explain this phenomenon and decided to ignore it. Years later,

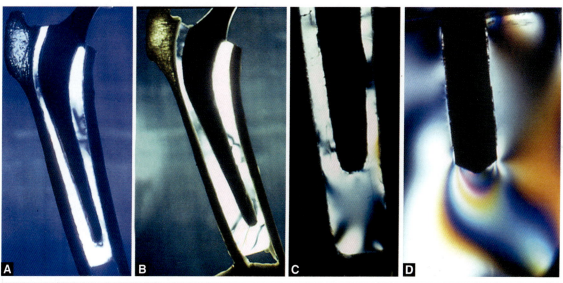

FIGS 19.3A TO D

Illustration of test determining stress distribution

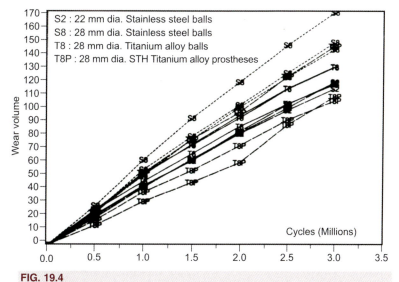

FIG. 19.4

Data concerning the wear of polyethylene against different metals. This example indicates that under the wear testing machine *titanium alloy implants of 28 mm in diameter wear very well.* This work was done by Harry McKellop, PhD

Section 1

Rostoker's observation proved to be prophetic. We should have been more cautious and pay closer attention to his observation. It would have saved us a lot of grief.

We consulted with others in the United States, such as Patrick Laing, from Pittsburgh, who had earlier published his work on titanium alloys. To the best of my knowledge, he had not worked with total hip prostheses.

Our initial clinical experiences with the new implant that the manufactures had elected to call the STH Prosthesis (Strength-titanium-prosthesis) were very encouraging. Simultaneously I had abandoned the use of the lateral approach to the hip and the trochanteric osteotomy that Charnley's recommended.

Grateful to Charnley for his teachings and friendship I contacted him and informed him that I was no longer using his implant, osteotomizing the greater trochanter or using the lateral approach, and had moved to a titanium implant, and was approaching the joint through a posterior approach.

My letter prompted a very interesting response. After thanking me for providing him with information about my change in philosophy and technique, he proceeded to say that I had never really learned how to perform his operation correctly; that using a "flexible" metal was a big mistake; and ventured to add that I had missed my call. He wrote, *"You do not have the mentality of an orthopedist, but that of a gynecologist"*. My approaching the hip from behind had proved his point. Our relationship was slightly strained. Obviously, he resented my leaving his fold. After all we had developed a very good personal relationship and I had invited him on several occasions to lecture at various meetings sponsored by the Academy and the University of Miami.

A few years later when I reported my results with the STH prosthesis before the International Hip Society in Bern, Switzerland, I titled my presentation "A Gynecologists approach to Total Hip Surgery" and dedicated the presentation to Charnley, who was in the audience. We both had been founding members of the Society, which at that time had only twenty members. The audience, after learning the genesis of the title of my talk, enjoyed the levity. My relationship with Charnley went back to normal. A couple years later the Queen of England knighted him.

Our original publication relating to the first six years of follow-up with the new implant, indicated that the overall

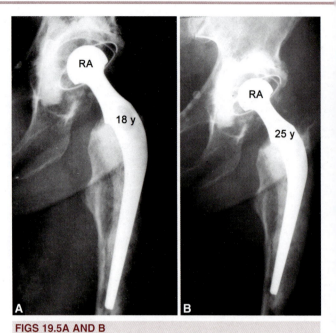

FIGS 19.5A AND B

Radiograph of STH prosthesis 18 and 25 years postoperatively, inserted in an acromegalic patient. Similarly, many other patients have shown excellent result for periods currently approaching the 30 years mark as the following radiographs demonstrate

behavior of the titanium prosthesis was comparable, if not slightly better, than the Charnley stainless steel implant. Unfortunately, subsequent longer follow-up began to reveal a higher incidence of radiological changes with the STH prostheses. The revision rate was also higher. Eventually, I abandoned its use all together. The fact remains that many monoblock titanium prostheses have performed extremely well over a relatively long period of time. A very active acromegalic patient (Figs 19.5A and B) functioned without any clinical problems for over 27 years. His X-rays have shown a thin metal-cement radiolucent line on zone 1 for over twenty-five years without signs of progression (Figs 19.6 A to C).

Suspecting that perhaps the thin stem of the initial STH prosthesis was creating too much stress on the column of cement due to its greater elasticity, the implant was modified to have different diameters and stem-neck angle (Figs 19.7A to D).

This modification did not prove to have been a good one. When our material was reviewed later it was found out that the complication rate with the new implant (STH 2) was higher. Obviously the cause of greater failure was eluding us (Figs 19.8A to D).

It appears that titanium, as an articulated surface against polyethylene sockets is very good, but only under "clean" conditions. That is, if no third bodies are present between the metallic head and the plastic acetabulum. Any material

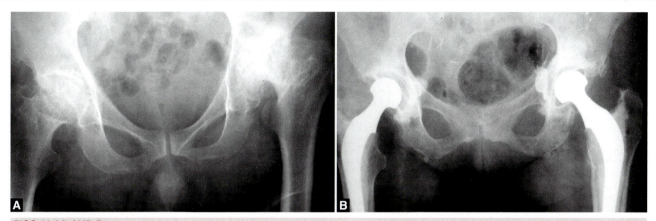

FIGS 19.6A AND B

(A) Preoperative radiograph of bilateral hip osteoarthritis of an active patient suffering from osteoarthritis. (B) Radiographs obtained 18 and 26 years after surgery

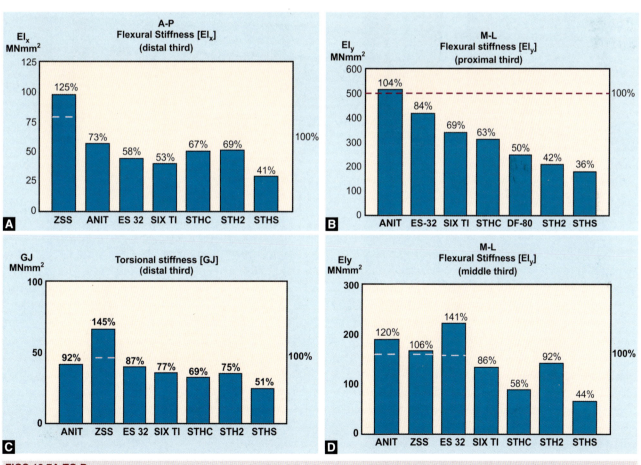

FIGS 19.7A TO D

Barograph illustrating the modulus of elasticity of various femoral stems with different geometry and or metal. This data clearly shows that the stiffness of an implant does not entirely depend on the material used, since a prosthesis made of a titanium alloy (lower modulus) can be made of a stiffer than one made of an alloy with a higher modulus (cobalt-chrome) simply by modifying its geometry

Section 1

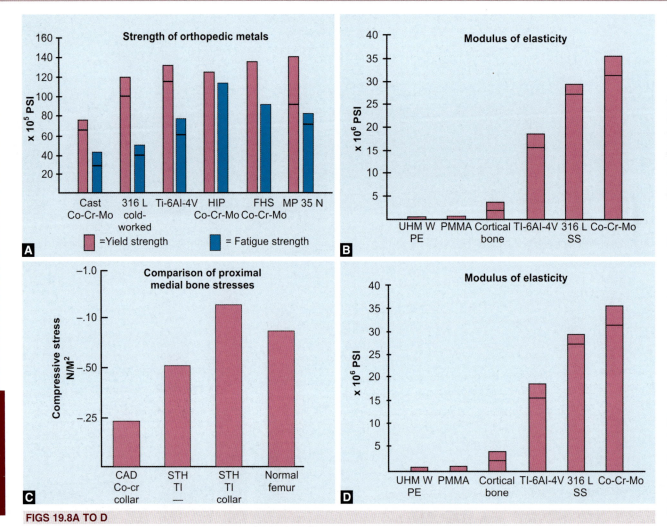

FIGS 19.8A TO D

Barographs of various tests conducted prior to the fabrication of the original titanium hip prostheses

capable of scratching the relatively "soft" alloy, if interposed between the two surfaces can initiate a third body wear process. I first became aware of the problems others were having with titanium prostheses from reading of anecdotal reports of massive metallosis encountered in isolated instances. Claims were immediately made that the wear properties of titanium were poor and the original work of Rostoker was cited.

The hospital for special surgery, in New York, had developed a titanium alloy total hip prosthesis that was strongly marketed by Zimmer. Some time in the late 1980's I was informed by the director of research at Zimmer that the surgeons at that hospital were seeing early failures with their titanium implant, associated with severe metallosis. Accompanied by him I traveled to New York where we had an opportunity to confirm the findings of serious early failures and the associated presence of metal debris. This took place in the presence of the local surgeons and pathologists.

I was flabbergasted at the magnitude of their failures and returned home puzzled by them. I could not explain them. Their implant was made by the same manufacturer, using the same material. The geometry was the only difference between their prosthesis and ours. It was hard to believe that mild geometrical differences in the stem (Figs 19.9A and B) would explain the problem.

I was particularly troubled because at that very same moment we were in the process of submitting for publication a manuscript reporting on *17 surgically retrieved STH prostheses that had not shown any evidence of metallosis, either under the naked eye or under the microscope.* Trying to explain the differences became extremely difficult. We then elected to withhold submission of the paper awaiting a local review of our findings.

The new review did not indicate anything contrary to the original findings. It was at the moment that I

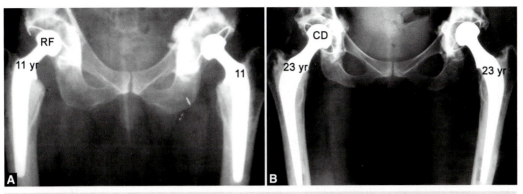

FIGS 19.9A AND B

(A) Radiograph of the original titanium alloy prostheses (STH) with narrow stems taken 23 years postoperatively.
(B) Radiograph of the modified STH prosthesis with a wider stem taken 11 years postoperatively. In neither instance there was evidence of wear, signs or loosening or lysis

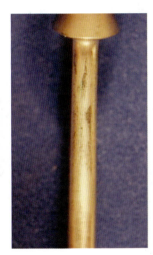

FIG. 19.10

Photo of failed loose titanium prosthesis demonstrating the burnishing of the stem, probably secondary to motion of the stem against the acrylic cement

recalled that the X-rays of the failed implants I had seen in New York had their acetabular components cemented with metal-backed polyethylene cups. Ours did not. It dawn on us then that this could be an explanatory factor. Simultaneously, Frank Schiller, a local Los Angeles orthopedist who had used a few STH prostheses informed me of his bad experiences with our implant and the presence of metallosis recognized at the time of revision surgery. His failed implants had been stabilized with metal-backed acetabula (Fig. 19.10).

We obtained his removed specimens and studied them in the laboratory. Harry McKellop did the work and reported the strong probability that very small pieces of metal and cement may have fallen from the cemented metal-backed sockets into the joint, precipitating a rapid and aggressive third body wear process (Figs 19.11A to C).

Once, when I was about to cement the acetabular cup, I noticed that the implant the nurse was handing me was a metal-backed one. She proceeded to inform me that the vendor of the implants had generously replaced the "old cups" with newer ones, which were "much better". It was the only metal-backed cup I ever used. Within a couple of years it failed and at surgery we demonstrated metallosis. (See *Metal-backed Acetabular Cups*)

Harry McKellop observed, measured and correlated the degree of dulling of the heads with burnishing of the stem we had revised, and concluded that there was *a direct correlation between the degree of burnishing of the stem— a reflection of motion between the stem and the cement—and the dulling of the heads—a proof of wear. There was no direct correlation, however, in regards to the length of implantation* (Figs 19.12A to C). Failed prosthesis that had been in place for long periods of time often demonstrated less dulling and burnishing, that in more recently implanted components. This indicated the possibility of a late, sudden presence of a third body capable of initiating the wear process. It probably came from the stem as it moved against the column of acrylic cement.

The fact that the surface of the metallic heads of retrieved failed implants that had been removed with an intact mantle of cement, and where the failure had obviously taken place at the bone-cement interface, did not show dulling of the head, further supported the initial hypothesis (See *Retrieved Titanium Prostheses*).

Corrosion from modular components, motion between the plastic liner and the metal cup, and poor wear properties of the polyethylene are the most popular explanations for lysis with noncemented prostheses. Regardless as to what theory is eventually

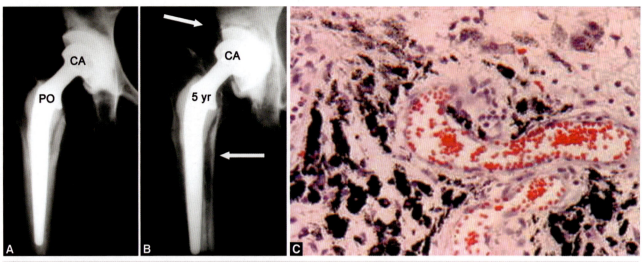

FIGS 19.11A TO C

(A and B) Radiographs of an STH titanium prosthesis obtained shortly after surgery, and five years later. Notice the loosening of the prosthetic components and the significant lysis of the femur. (C) Histological slide of capsule around the stem. Notice the metal in the tissues. The metal-backed cemented acetabulum showed this lytic complication with great frequency, probably secondary of loose particles of meal and cement coming from the acetabulum and seeping into the medullary canal and over the metal shell

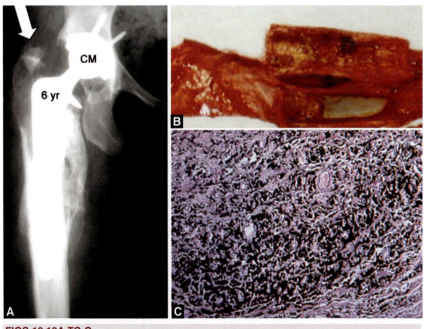

FIGS 19.12A TO C

(A) Radiograph of cobalt-chrome prosthesis demonstrating lysis in the greater trochanter and proximal femur produced by metal debris. (B) Appearance of the window made in the femur. Notice the dart staining due to metal debris. (C) Histological slide of tissues from the area showing severe metallosis

proven most accurate, the fact remains that motion between the metallic stem and the cortical bone of the femur might be sufficient to generate metal debris. If it travels to the joint in sufficient amounts it may initiate polyethylene wear and the resulting lysis. I have seen instances (Figs 19.13 to 19.21) where histological evidence indicated lysis produced by metal with complete absence of polyethylene debris (See *Lysis*).

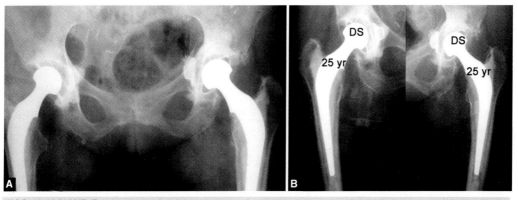

FIGS 19.13A AND B

(A) Osteoarthritic hips replaced simultaneously with cemented STH titanium alloy implants. (B) Radiographs obtained 25 years postoperatively. Notice the minimal wear and the absence of lysis or radiolucent lines

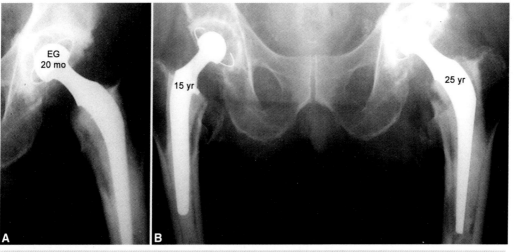

FIGS 19.14A AND B

(A) Radiograph of a 20-month-old titanium alloy (STH) prosthesis in a heavy and active pilot 46 years old at the time of surgery. (B) Radiograph obtained 25 years after surgery to the left hip, and 15 years after surgery to the right hip. The patient expired shortly afterwards

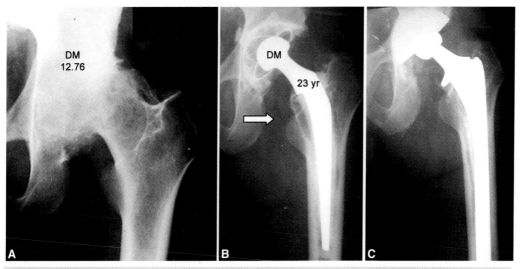

FIGS 19.15A TO C

(A) Radiograph of the arthritic hip of a 44-year-old man. (B) Twenty-three years after surgery the hip was asymptomatic, but lysis had become apparent. (C) Twelve months later the hip was revised with a noncemented implant. Radiograph obtained 3 years later

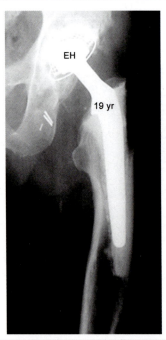

FIG. 19.16

Radiograph of cemented STH titanium prosthesis obtained 19 years after surgery performed in a 67-year-old man. The patient had sustained a fracture of the femur 25 earlier. Notice the thick column of cement separating the stem from the proximal femoral cortex. It appears that if a thick column of cement is preserved at that level the incidence of loosening is less when compared with those instances where the column of cement, (as a result of the varus attitude) is too thin or nonexistent

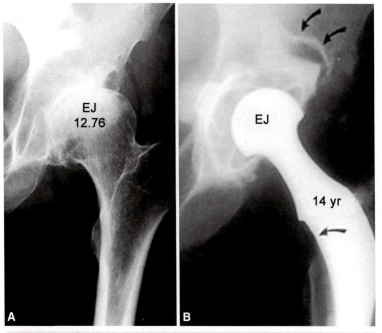

FIGS 19.17A AND B

(A) Radiograph of arthritic hip in a 43-year-old woman, secondary to hip dysplasia. (B) Radiograph obtained 14 years after surgery. Notice the lytic lesion in the acetabulum and the minimal wear of the polyethylene liner

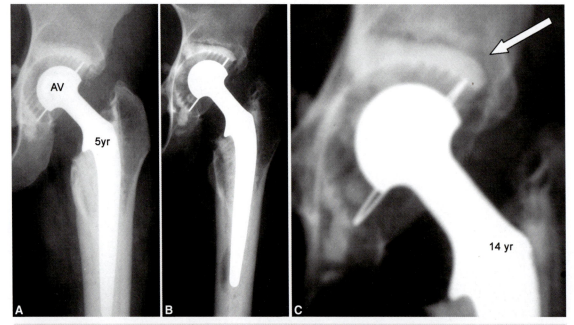

FIGS 19.18A TO C

(A) Radiograph obtained 5 years post-titanium total hip replacement. There is no evidence of wear or lysis. (B and C) Radiographs taken 14 years after surgery demonstrating loosening of the acetabulum, and early loosening and lysis on the femoral side

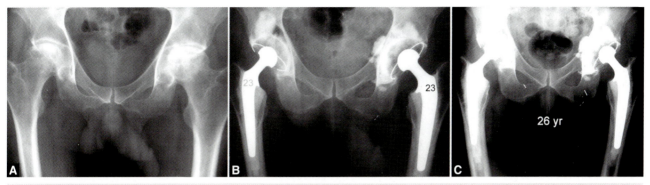

FIGS 19.19A TO C

(A) Radiograph of bilateral avascular necrosis of the hips in a 45-year-old physician. (B) Radiograph taken 23 years postoperatively. The hips were replaced with cemented STH-2 implants. (C) Radiograph taken 26 years postoperatively. Acetabular wear is apparent in the left hip. The patient has remained asymptomatic

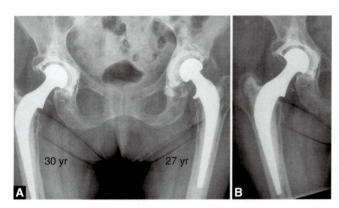

FIGS 19.20A AND B

(A) Radiograph of an STH arthroplasty (right) obtained 30 years post-surgery performed in a 55-year-old rheumatoid arthritic patient. The left hip was replaced 3 years later with a different type of implant. Notice the preserved bone/cement relationship in the right hip, but a clear radiolucent line on the left hip. (B) Closer view of the STH arthroplasty

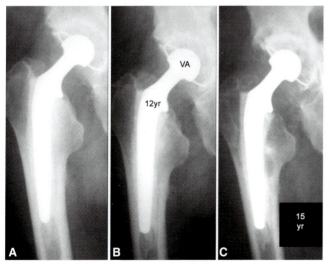

FIGS 19.21A TO C

(A) Postoperative radiograph of the arthritic hip of a 67-year-old osteoarthritic man (B) Radiograph taken 12 years postoperatively. Notice the mild wear and no absence of lysis, or loosening. (C) Radiograph obtained 15 years postoperatively demonstrating lysis of femur and loosening of the acetabulum

*References**

21, 22, 23, 24, 25, 26, 28, 30, 32, 34, 36, 37, 38, 39, 43, 46, 48, 50, 56, 58, 59, 66, 70, 72, 76, 103, 110

Section 1

_____

* References provided at the end of the book after annexures.

20

Retrieved Titanium Implants

I have discussed in previous chapter our experience with a titanium 6-4 alloy hip prosthesis, and *have concluded that this material is not a good one to use as an articulating metal against UHMW polyethylene.* We had developed the titanium alloy in anticipation that is lower modulus of elasticity, when compared with Cobalt-Chromo and Stainless Steel, would provide a more physiological distribution of stresses throughout the femur, preventing in that manner the stress shielding that stiffer metals create. Loren L Latta, PhD, Director of Research in our Department at the University of Miami conducted the earlier investigations.

The initial clinical experiences when studied six years after the onset of the study, indicated that the radiological and clinical results were comparable to those obtained with the Charnley arthroplasty. However, observation of data that extended beyond the first six years began to cast doubt on the appropriateness of using titanium. *The incidence of complications, particularly that of loosening and lysis was greater than the one observed with other materials.*

Easy explanations for the adverse effects were not available. A great deal of confusion surrounded the issue, particularly due to the fact that laboratory investigations, conducted prior to the clinical use of the prosthesis, had shown that the titanium alloy produced lower wear of the polyethylene than stainless steel. Further studies conducted by Ian Clarke, Harry McKellop and their associates in our laboratories at the University of Southern California (Orthopedic Hospital of Los Angeles) had strongly encouraged the continuation of the project. *It was later demonstrated that the excellent performance of titanium against polyethylene existed only in an absolutely clean environment.* The presence of a contaminant, such as particles of cement or metal, created a scratching of the relatively soft titanium, which in turn produced plastic debris that eventually traveled to the bone/cement interface creating lysis.

A number of interesting observations were made by the investigators, which ultimately established clear foundations for the understanding of the behavior of titanium and other metals as a weight bearing components. Some of the most important data came from the study of implants that had been removed form the body after experiencing loosening. Similarly, valuable information came from the analysis of radiographs of patients who had experience revision of the acetabular component, and required revision of socket, while leaving intact the titanium femoral stem.

Severe, self-perpetuating abrasive-corrosive wear of the titanium alloy could be initiated by the entrapment of third-body particles between the metal and polymer, some times with particles of acrylic cement, and always with metallic particles, as from porous coated prostheses. The micro-scratching (dulling) commonly observed on the bearing surfaces of retrieved titanium alloy components appeared to be primarily due to entrapment of third-body acrylic and/or metallic particles that were initially generated by fretting of loosened prostheses, for example, at the stem-cement interface. Nitrogen hardening of the titanium surfaces, e.g. by diffusion or ion-implanting, provided additional protection against cement particles, but did not prevent severe abrasion by entrapped metallic particles.

Under clean conditions, the mean wear rate of the polyethylene pins was least against the conventional titanium alloy disks, intermediate against the stainless steel disks and greatest against the nitrated titanium alloy disks, averaging 0.20, 0.08 and 0.27 cubic millimeters per million cycles, respectively. In general, such pin-on-disk tests have produced volumetric wear rates much about an order of magnitude lower than is typical of hip simulator tests, and of retrieved implants. The relative wear rates, and the incidence of runaway wear, provide insight into the likely behavior of the materials *in vivo*.

The STH hip prosthesis consisted of a one-piece titanium alloy femoral components inserted with acrylic cement, articulating against a one-piece, all polyethylene acetabular cup, also inserted with cement. The wear of the STH prosthesis *in vivo* was assessed through examination of tissues and implants that were recovered during twenty revision surgeries in seventeen patients. The hips were revised after an average of 63 months (range= 12 to 134 months), for aseptic loosening of the femoral component in eight cases, of the acetabular component in one case, and of both components in eight cases. One prosthesis was revised to correct recurrent dislocation, one due to infection and one was revised to remove a fracture plate on the proximal femur.

Samples of capsular tissues obtained at surgery were processed by routine techniques. The extent of the histological reactions and the amount of polymeric or metallic debris were graded on the semi-quantitative scale developed by Mirra for his study of revised stainless steel and cobalt-chrome alloy prostheses. Those STH femoral components and acetabular cups that were removed from the patients were examined in the laboratory for evidence of wear.

At revision, none of the 20 STH titanium alloy prostheses exhibited signs of severe metallic wear, and there was no discoloration of the adjacent tissues. The ratings for the extent of histological response, for the incidence of giant cells and for polyethylene debris were comparable to those reported by Mirra for failed stainless steel and chrome-cobalt prostheses. In contrast, the tissues from the titanium alloy STH prostheses showed a higher incidence of acrylic debris than Mirra reported, but a lower incidence of acute and chronic inflammation. This was consistent with the fact that the TH prostheses were removed primarily for aseptic loosening, which typically involves fragmentation of the cement mantle, whereas the hips in Mirra's study were revised primarily for infection, which would be accompanied by an inflammatory response.

Isolated particles of metal were found in tissues from only two of the STH hips, a lower incidence than was reported by Mirra for stainless steel or cobalt-chrome components. While it is possible that some titanium particles were overlooked in the tissue samples, or that titanium particles may have been located in areas of the capsule that were not collected during the revision surgeries.

The contact area of the balls on ten of the 13 retrieved STH femoral component exhibited visibly dull patches, consisting of a dense pattern of fine scratches. In addition, the surfaces the stems of the STH stems components, which originally had a matted finish, often exhibited bright burnishing areas, presumably caused by fretting against the surrounding acrylic cement mantle (Figs 20.1A to E). The fact that very few metallic particles were observe in the peri-prosthetic tissues under light microscopy suggested that, if titanium alloy wear debris was generated by ball dulling and/or stem burnishing, this was probably in the submicron range.

The extent of ball dulling appeared to be related to the extent of stem burnishing. This is, when the femoral components were first place in rank order according to the amount of dulling on the femoral head, and than according to the amount of burnishing of the stem, the rank orders for the two forms of wear were found to be strongly correlated. In contrast, neither ball-dulling nor stem-burnishing was significantly correlated with the duration of use of the prostheses. Furthermore, the two stems that were removed with nearly intact cement mantles (that were later broken away in the laboratory) showed little or no burnishing of the stem, nor dulling of the ball. Taken together, these observations strongly suggest that both the dulling of the balls and the burnishing of the stems occurred primarily after the prostheses were substantially loose, rather than gradually over the lifespan of a well-fixed implant (Figs 20.2A to C).

I first became aware of problems with titanium alloy prostheses when the director of research at Zimmer, the company that made the STH, called me on the

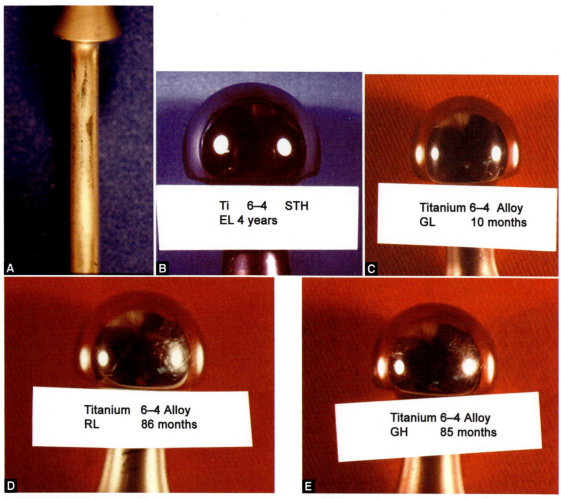

FIGS 20.1A TO E

Photograph of a retrieved cemented titanium stem demonstrating the typical burnishing produce by the movement of the loose implant against the acrylic cement

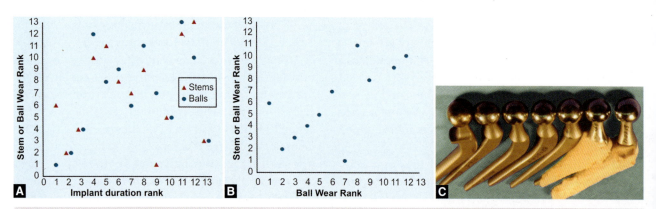

FIGS 20.2A TO C

(A) Illustration of the lack of correlation between degree of head dulling and prosthetic stem burnishing suggesting that those abnormal changes are not produced as a result of a gradual response to metal/polyethylene contact, rather by some type of sudden third-body wear phenomenon. (B) Illustration of the direct correlation between dulling of the prosthetic stem and the burnishing of the prosthetic head. (C) Photo of 7 retrieved titanium prostheses. Notice the dulling of the prosthetic heads, except for the last two on the right, which came loose at the cement/bone interface, but remained fixed to the cement mantle. This picture strongly demonstrates the fact that a loose stem at the prosthetic/cement interface scratches the metal, generating a debris that eventually travels to the articulation

phone to tell me that the staff at the Hospital for Special Surgery, in New York, was experiencing severe complications with their own titanium alloy implants. They had allegedly recovered several implants associated with massive wear that developed over a very short period of time. The two of us met with the surgeons, pathologist and researchers at the Hospital for Special Surgery where we were shown a number of their complicated cases. They had developed their own titanium alloy implant a few years after we developed ours. I was indeed shocked to see the nature and severity of their complications.

At first I could not understand why they should have complications, which up to that time we had not witnessed. Their prosthesis was manufactured by the same company and its design though different from ours could not explain the problems. When my visit to New York took place we were ready to submit to the Journal of Bone and Joint Surgery our findings form the revision of the twenty STH titanium prostheses, I made reference in an earlier paragraph. The report, as I stated before, reported the absence of metallosis in the tissues surrounding the prostheses.

Upon my return to Miami I discussed my experience with Harry McKellop, PhD, Director of our laboratories at USC/Orthopedic Hospital of Los Angeles. McKellop was already a well-known investigator whose contributions to wear properties of materials used in surgery were universally accepted. He took very seriously the problems I had seen in New York and initiated further studies in an attempt to elucidate what at that time appeared to be inexplicable. His findings and conclusions I have discussed above.

The first clue to the explanation of our results versus those of the New York group was my recollection that the failed implants I was shown during my visit had a metal-backed acetabular reinforcement. We had never used the acetabular reinforcement. McKellop addressed that issue and concluded that particles of metal and cement from the acetabular interface had fallen into the joint initiating a rapid third-body wear process (Figs 20.3A to E).

During the process of studying the problem in great earnest, an orthopedic surgeon from Los Angeles informed me that he had used the STH prosthesis a few time with very undesirable results. He had encountered loosening within a few years after implantation. He gave me the films of one of his patients (Figs 20.4A and B) demonstrating loosening and lysis five years after surgery. As I suspected he had used the metal-backed reinforcement I had seen in New York.

Amongst the many studies prompted by McKellop's findings was the review of a few patients (Figs 20.5 and 20.6) on whom I had revised failed acetabular

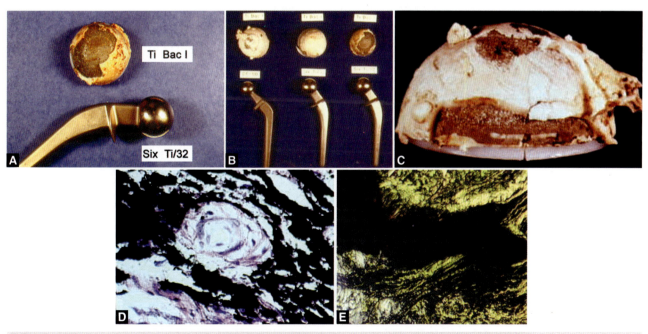

FIGS 20.3A TO E

(A to C) Photographs of cemented titanium implants using metal-backed acetabula. The fragmentation of the cement is readily recognized. It is very likely that small particles of cement, probably accompanied with metal particles coming from the plasma sprayed metal, travel into the joint initiating a third-body wear process. (D and E) Microscopic sections illustrating the metal staining of failed titanium implants associated with metal-backed acetabula

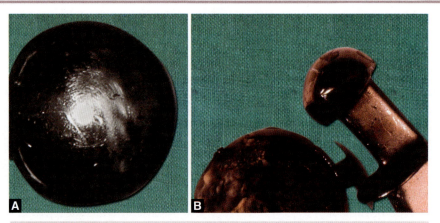

FIGS 20.4A AND B

Photo of a blackened and worn out titanium prosthetic head obtained from a failed arthroplasty where a metal-backed cemented acetabulum was used

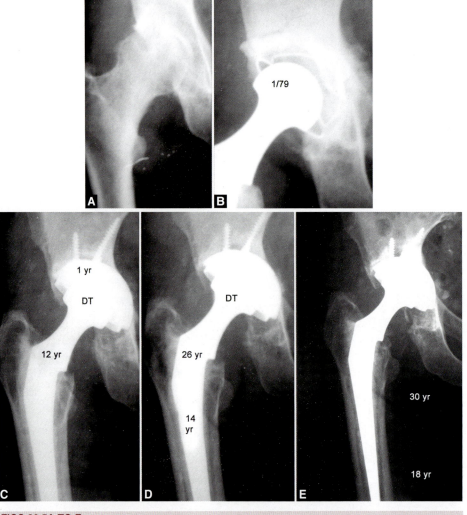

FIGS 20.5A TO E

(A) Radiograph of arthritic hip in a 54-year-old woman. (B) Radiograph obtained 2 years postoperatively. A titanium STH prosthesis was used. Notice the wear of the polyethylene 2 years postoperatively. (C and D) Radiographs obtained 12 and 26 years after surgery, and 12 and 14 years after revision of the acetabular component. (E) Radiograph obtained 30 years after the initial surgery, and 18 years since the revision procedure. Notice the apparent lack of measurable wear of the polyethylene

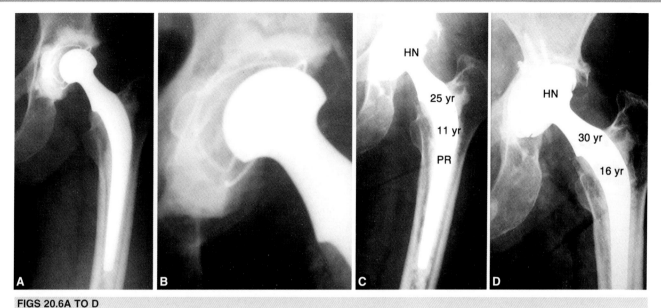

FIGS 20.6A TO D

(A) Radiograph of titanium STH prosthesis in a 57-year-old woman 2 years after surgery. (B) Radiograph obtained 10 years after surgery. Notice the loosening of the acetabular component and the wear of the polyethylene liner. (C) Radiograph obtained 25 years after surgery, and 11 years after revision of the acetabular component. (D) Radiograph taken 30 years after surgery, and 16 years after revision of the acetabular component. Notice the apparent absence of wear of the polyethylene liner

components with STH femoral components. The acetabula had become loose and required revision. Upon finding the femoral components intact I elected not to revise them. The cemented plastic components were replaced with porous components. I have been able to follow 2 of the 5 patients for more than ten years, and have documented the fact that measurable wear of the polyethylene liners had not taken place. This observation supports McKellop's findings that the titanium head is polished over the years in such a manner that its wear properties are improved (See *Metal-backed Acetabula*).

The superior/medial migration of noncemented acetabular component into the pelvic bone should not be explained entirely on a mechanical basis. It is very likely that this phenomenon can be due to polyethylene or metal debris deposited over the convexity of the metallic socket, resulting in softening of the cancellous bone permitting its migration.

*References**

34, 42, 48, 56, 66, 72, 73, 91

* References provided at the end of the book after annexures.

Section 1

21

Acetabular Grafts

There are those who believe that bone grafting of the shallow acetabulum is frequently necessary. I do not think so. This does not mean that the shallow acetabulum should never be grafted, for indeed there are times when the grafting is absolutely necessary. In many instances (Figs 21.1 to 21.3) is possible, however, to obtain good containment of the artificial acetabular component without resorting to grafting.

If the original shallow acetabulum present in the case of completely dislocated congenital hips the need for grafting is more common. In those instances when the acetabulum is only moderately shallow as a result of hip dysplasia, its deepening usually suffices. An acetabular component that does not have complete bony coverage is not necessarily vulnerable, if the acetabular replacement is of the noncemented type. On the other hand, cemented acetabular components require complete coverage. I have come to the realization that in many instances, when a graft was used in a effort to provide full coverage of the porous shell, only a very small portion of it provided support to the artificial socket.

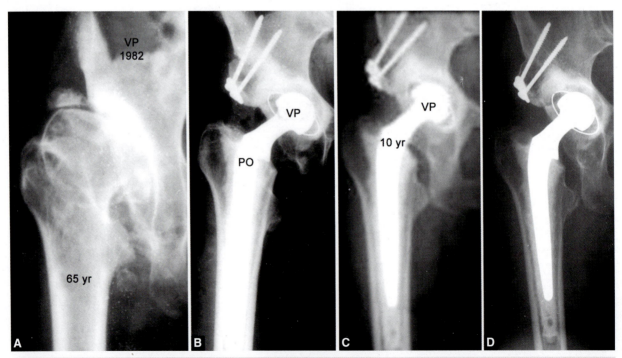

FIGS 21.1A TO D

(A) Radiograph of osteoarthritic hip secondary to congenital hip dysplasia. (B) The total hip arthroplasty was reinforced with a bone graft. In retrospect it appears the graft was unnecessary since the depth of the acetabulum provided sufficient coverage of the plastic socket. (C) Radiograph obtained ten years later. (D) Radiograph taken 23 years after surgery

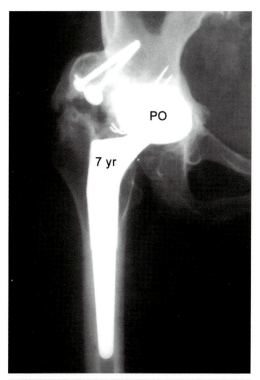

FIG. 21.2

Radiograph of a total hip arthroplasty, probably performed for the care of congenital hip dysplasia. A graft was used by her surgeon hoping to provide a deeper socket. *Obviously the graft was unnecessary*

Militating against bone grafting of the acetabulum is the fact that large grafts may undergo late resorption or collapse. Progressive revascularization and remodeling of the dead bone may prompt the late collapse, since the new bone does not yet have the mechanical properties necessary to withstand the powerful forces to which the acetabulum is subjected. If no revascularization occurs, the cumulative stresses on the nonviable bone may result in its collapse. There are those, like Rene Marti, from the Netherlands, who holds opposite views and has reported very convincingly that full incorporation of the graft eventually takes place (Figs 21.4A to C).

The placement of cancellous bone to fill large defects has been proven to be effective when used with the technique of "impaction" developed by professor Thomas Sloof, from the Netherlands. However, I am rather skeptical about the routine use of cancellous graft whenever a defect is found. *I doubt the value of adding a second interface to the system.* I suspect the technique of packing may not be fully indicated when using porous acetabula. *To expect the "dead" bone graft to grow into the porosity of the metallic cup may be wishful thinking.* The remaining normal bone on the deficient acetabulum is more likely to achieve growth into the porous surface (Figs 21.5 and 21.6) (See *Acetabular Augmentation and Bone Impaction*).

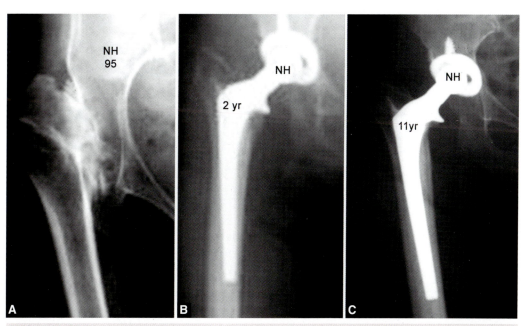

FIGS 21.3A TO C

(A) Radiograph of sequella of a congenitally dislocated hip. (B) Despite the shallowness of the acetabulum it was possible to obtain very satisfactory coverage of the porous cup, without the need of a graft. The surgery was performed without trochanteric osteotomy, which is usually the case. (C) Radiograph obtained 11 years post-operatively. The patient has remained unhappy because the gained length resulted in her inability to done her shoes as easily as she had done it before surgery

Section 1

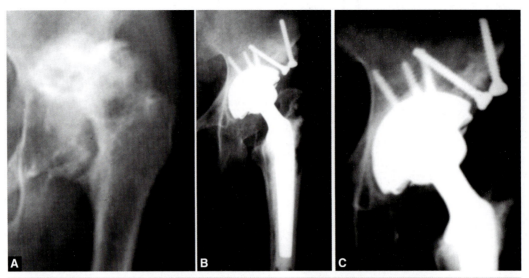

FIGS 21.4A TO C

(A) Radiograph of an arthritic hip following a fracture dislocation of the acetabulum. The acetabular component was placed at the level of the original acetabulum requiring a bone graft to the superolateral acetabulum. (B and C) Radiographs taken after surgery 10 and 15 years postoperatively. The 15 years radiograph suggests mild resorption of the graft

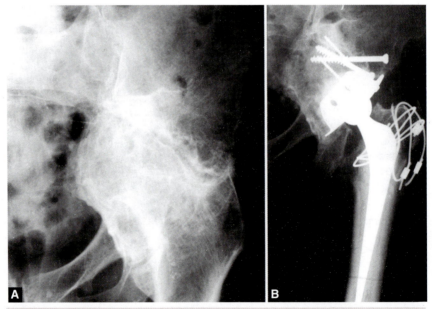

FIGS 21.5A AND B

(A) Radiograph of an old fracture/central dislocation of the hip. (B) The femoral head was used as an acetabular graft. I have found that large medial defects such as those encountered following an ununited fracture of the medial wall of the pelvis can be managed well by transfixing the femoral head to the surrounding pelvic bone. Under those circumstances the acetabular cup should be cemented

In earlier days I frequently used cement to build a deficient acetabulum (Figs 21.7A and B).

Once, I elected to leave in place a well-fixed cemented acetabular component and simply replaced the femoral component. The polyethylene socket was in a protrusio situation. I cemented a new plastic socket on top of the old, one after drilling several holes into the polyethylene cup and packing more cement (Figs 21.8 to 21.10).

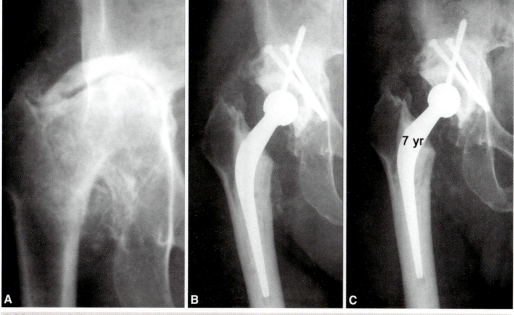

FIGS 21.6A TO C

(A) Radiograph of old fracture dislocation of the acetabulum. (B) The femoral head was left in place and secured with metallic screws. (C) Radiograph obtained 7 years after surgery. There is not radiological evidence at this time of incorporation of the graft into the normal pelvic bone. The patient expired from unrelated causes a few months after this film was obtained. He was asymptomatic

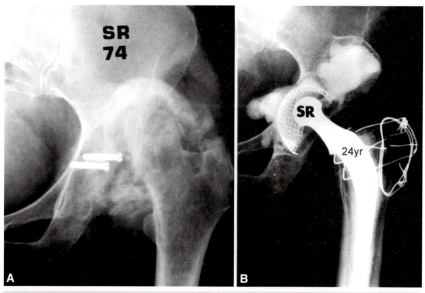

FIGS 21.7A AND B

(A) Old chronically dislocated hip. (B) Charnley prosthesis inserted after filling the acetabular defect with acrylic cement. Twenty-four years after surgery the patient was asymptomatic

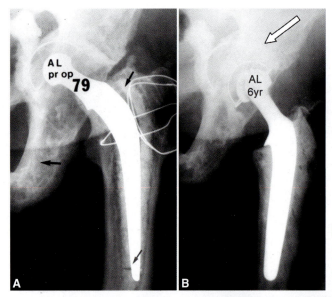

FIGS 21.8A AND B

(A) Failed cemented femoral component on a patient with Paget's disease. (B) During revision surgery the acetabular cup was left in place. *A new plastic acetabular implant was cemented over the old one and the femoral component was revised*

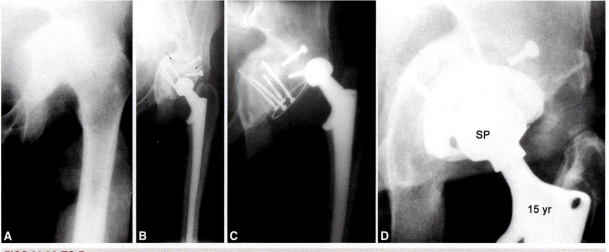

FIGS 21.9A TO D

(A) Posttraumatic osteoarthritis. (B) The femoral head was left in place and secured with metallic screws over which an isoelastic cup was attached. (C) The hip dislocated a few days later. The isoelastic socket failed and was replaced with a porous cup. (D) The graft-head incorporated with the pelvic bone

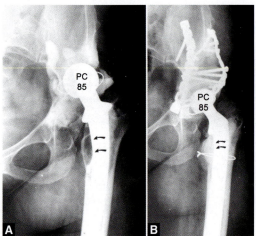

FIGS 21.10A AND B

Failed cemented total hip replacement treated with femoral autograph, reinforced with metallic plates

References*

27, 31, 35, 40, 43, 50, 57, 65, 81

---

* References provided at the end of the book after annexures.

22

Augmentation: Impaction of Morsellized Bone

The surgical technique consisting of packing of morsellized bone in a lytic femur or damaged acetabulum, usually secondary to failed arthroplasty, was first described, to the best of my recollection, by Thomas Sloof, from the Nederland, a man of impeccable integrity. Despite his solid documentation of the merits of the procedure, it has been subject to criticism by some. *The critics have argued that in the case of the femur, the newly inserted bone/cement composite often fails to maintain the position of the prosthesis and brings about its subsidence into the medullary canal or its shift into a varus attitude.*

Criticism of the procedure, when performed for deficient acetabula has received wider acceptance. My personal experience is very limited and not strong enough to make it a valid argument. I believe, however, it is a sound method of treatment when performed for the proper indications and according to the technical details described by the developers, an individual of known integrity.

Quite often I have witnessed the packing of cancellous bone throughout the entire surface of the acetabulum during revision surgery, when medial and superior migration of the prosthetic component had damaged and thinned out the acetabular walls. Packing the defect, particularly medially, makes sense. *I cannot help but wonder if "packing" throughout the entire area is always needed. I think that if there is enough bone peripherally, against which a portion of the porous cup can be placed is preferable to the pressing of the cup against cancellous bone graft throughout.* The cancellous bone is dead bone and needs to revascularize before it becomes an integral part of the pelvic bone. I suspect that the dead bone graft, incapable of osteoblastic activity until it has revascularized is simply a barrier to be overcome. If the porous cup is firmly pressed over the vascularized acetabular bone, bone ingrowth is more likely to take place at a much faster rate. *I find it difficult to believe, though some evidence to the contrary is beginning to appear, that bone ingrowth can take place when pressed against a porous surface.*

Needless to say, my question may be appropriate only regarding relatively benign situations when the protrusion is not great and there is enough normal acetabular bone against which a porous cup can be fit (Figs 21.1 and 22.2).

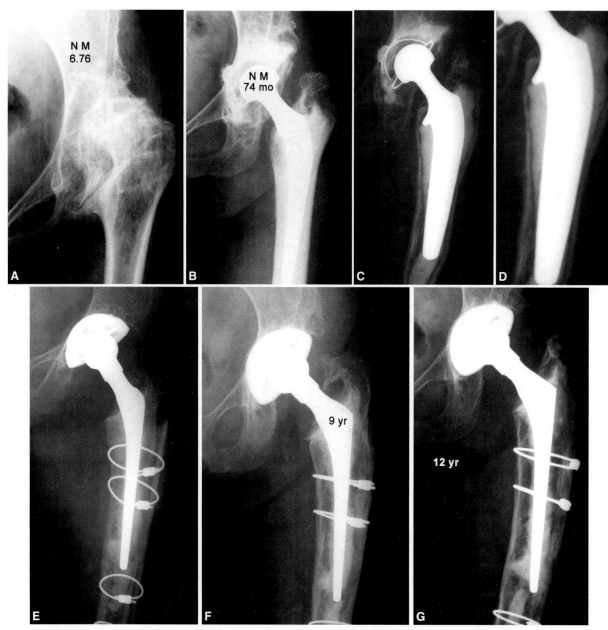

FIGS 22.1A TO G

(A) Radiograph of osteoarthritic patient. (B) Radiograph of cemented titanium total hip 6 years postoperatively. (C and D) Three years later the implant was loose and painful. The thinning of the femoral cortex was significant. (E) Radiographs obtained 3 years after morsellized bone graft impaction in the femoral canal. A cortical bone strut had been added to reinforce the femoral wall. (F) Radiograph taken 9 years after surgery showing incorporation of the grafts. (G) Radiograph obtained 12 years postoperatively. Hip has remained asymptomatic

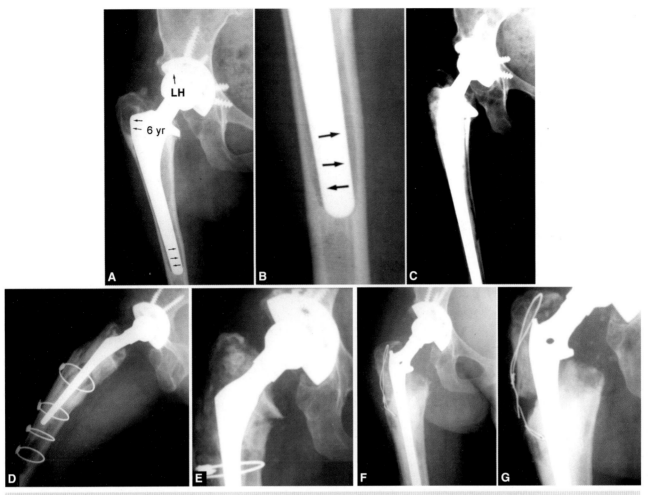

FIGS 22.2A TO G

(A to C) Radiograph of noncemented total hip prosthesis taken 6 years after surgery allegedly performed for the care of osteoarthritis. Notice the acetabular wear and he lysis in the greater trochanter and distal femur. (D) Radiograph obtained approximately 3 years after revision performed by the same surgeon using a noncemented prosthesis. Notice the severe thinning of the femoral cortex. (E and F). Radiographs taken after bone impaction procedure associated with a cortical bone strut attached to the femoral cortex. (G) A spontaneous fracture of the greater trochanter developed one year postoperatively. The trochanter was found to be extremely osteoporotic and was reattached with a wire. The wire broke and the trochanter migrated superiorly. This is the latest radiograph. The patient claims to be satisfied with the current situation, where ambulation is possible without external support and without pain. There appears to be no weakness of abduction

References*

27, 31, 35, 40, 48, 50, 57, 65, 81

---

* References provided at the end of the book after annexures.

23

Noncemented Total Hip Prostheses

There is little doubt that press-fit total hip prostheses have become the gold standard. Whether they will remain so for another 50 years cannot be predicted with certainty. We have seen many "panaceas" come and go in rapid succession. It matters not that between 2/3 and 9/10 of the blood supply of cortical bone comes from the medullary vessels. The rasping and destruction of most of the blood supplied medullary is inevitable. We have learned however, that in the absence of medullary blood supply, the peripheral vessels rapidly manage to take their place.

We have documented that in the case of a fracture of a diaphyseal bone that is rigidly immobilized there is minimal contribution to the healing of the fracture from peripheral vessels. Medullary vessels are the ones restoring viability to the bone. *On the other hand, if the fracture is not immobilized and motion at the fracture site continues, the medullary blood supply is impaired for a very long time, while the peripheral vessels immediately proliferate. The cells of the capillaries undergo metaplasia and differentiate into osteoblasts.*

It is logically, therefore to assume that the "death" of most of the cortex of the bone into which a prosthesis is driven undergoes rapid revascularization from peripheral vessels. Otherwise, resorption of bone would be seen in all instances of reamed endoprosthesis as well as in fractures treated with reamed nails.

The tight fit of a nonporous, noncemented prosthesis is not sustained indefinitely. For example, the force required to remove a nail, tightly fit in the bone immediately after its insertion, is much greater than that necessary force to remove it a few days later. The bone against which the nail rests is "dead" and remains dead for a period of time until it undergoes remodeling and revascularization. In addition it is very likely that cold flow develops after the forceful insertion of the flexible nail, resulting in a loss of the original tightness of fit. In addition, the difference in the modulus of elasticity between the bone and the implant contribute to the loosening.

I have been told that when the technique of intramedullary nailing was popularized by Kuntscher, in Germany, and his compatriots began to use it, he received several desperate calls from surgeons in the operating room who had found themselves in the predicament of not being able to either drive the nail beyond a certain point or to remove it. It is said that Kuntscher suggested that the surgeon desist in trying to solve the problem and to proceed to leaving the wound open, pack it with sterile dressings and send the patient to his hospital. Upon the patient's arrival to his institution, he did not rush him to the operating room but let him stay in bed for a few days. He then took him to the operating room where with the firm blow of a mallet he either drove the nail further or removed it. The fit of the nail was no longer as tight as it was during the original intervention.

I had similar experiences while trying to remove Austin-Moore prostheses from patients who had expired a few days after surgery. I had driven the implants very tightly into the femur and had found it very difficult to remove them at that time. Over the ensuing days the tight fit was no longer there. Food for thought. My arguments, obviously do not apply with the same degree to porous implants.

It is interesting to consider why cortical diaphyseal bone that contains an intramedullary implant for many years does not experience the changes that one sees in the nonprosthesis filled bone. Normally, as the skeleton ages, the medullary canal becomes wider as bone is lost from its endosteal surface. The thickness of the cortex obviously becomes thinner. That being the case, one could assume that "all" implants would eventually become loose. However, this is not the case. How can this phenomenon be explained? *Perhaps, because the loss of bending and compression stresses that take place under normal circumstances are replaced which hoop stresses to which the normal bone is not subjected.*

The addition of porous surfaces to the implants has proven beneficial despite the fact that the earlier experiences were less than satisfactory. Numerous investigators acknowledged that seven years after the insertion of the initial noncemented prostheses, approximately 20 percent of them demonstrated lytic changes; a much greater incidence of this complication when compared with the cemented Charnley arthroplasty. This reality proved Charnley correct, since he had long claimed that the cement was not the culprit responsible for the development of lysis, but the bearing surfaces in the acetabular side of the joint. Today, we see on with some frequency lytic complications in noncemented porous prostheses, likely to be produced from debris arising from modular components, the screw-hole interface or the porous surface of the acetabular cup or the articulating surfaces.

Bone ingrowth over a small proximal portion of the femur should theoretically produce atrophy above it due to stress shielding in that area. Parallel to it, would be an increase in the stresses below the immobilized areas of bone. *It has been well-documented, that very stiff prosthesis produce bony hypertrophy distally and some resorption of bone proximally* (See *Titanium Implants*).

In light of the originally increased incidence of lysis with porous prostheses noncemented prostheses, emphasis was directed toward the importance of the size of the pores. It was eventually agreed that the pores should not be either too big or too small. Most manufacturing adopted the resulting guidelines.

The theoretical disadvantages of press-fit implants need not be of great importance at this time. They are working very well and there is nothing to suggest that their fate will be changed dramatically in the foreseeable future.

From the technical point of view, there are issues that need not be taken lightly. At this time, there is some controversy as to the best type of prosthetic fitting is best: the line-to-line or the press-fit. With the former, the rasp and reamer used to prepare the medullary canal and acetabular cavity suggests to the surgeon the precise size of the final implant to be used. With the former, the press-fit one, the permanent implant is slightly larger than the size of the final rasp used in the preparation of the canal and acetabulum. This means that the permanent implant must be forced into the bony acetabulum and femoral canal. Once the impaction is completed the stability of the two components is very good, so much that many surgeons, under this circumstance, often choose not to insert additional stabilizing screws to the acetabular cup.

Theoretically, the press-fit method is superior since the initial stability is greater. This conclusion presupposes that maximum stability is better, something we suspect it is true, but lacks scientific evidence to support the belief. However, there are, in my opinion, some disadvantages. Forcing a metallic acetabular cup into the bony socket that is larger than the prepared cavity is possible in most instances, simply because the bone expands and accommodates the implant. *However, if the bone is very sclerotic, as it is in many younger people, the forceful hitting of the metal against the hard bone may result in a fracture of the acetabular rim, or in the case of revision surgery, when the walls of the bony acetabulum are thin and brittle. In this instance the impaction of a metal cup that is larger than the cavity easily produces a fracture that often requires additional metallic fixation.*

The possibility of fracturing the surrounding bony structures when a press-fit system is used is more common when dealing with the femoral canal. In the elderly patient with brittle bones, strong blows with a hammer against the top of the implant may cause a fracture of the femur. The same can occur when dealing with the strong cortical bone of the younger patient. I suspect that every hip surgeon has experienced this complication. A complication that requires in many instances the use of circular wires over the proximal femur to prevent further displacement of the fragments once weight bearing is introduced. Failure to recognize the fracture can result in such displacement of the fragments (Figs 23.1A and B).

We conducted extensive investigations (Figs 23.2 and 23.3) regarding the stability of noncemented femoral implants, which were published in peer-review journals.

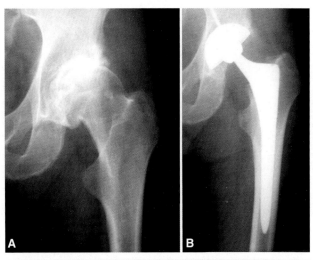

FIGS 23.1A AND B

(A) Radiograph of an osteoarthritic hip treated with a noncemented implant. (B) Radiograph obtained six years postoperatively. Notice the neutral attitude of the stem and its close contact with the femoral cortex

Among many other conclusions, we documented that considerable tightening occurs with a tightly fit stem during a 5,000 walking cycles, such that the motion of the uncemented implant was as small as that seen in the cemented stems, in the order of tens of microns.

Though several designs of noncemented prostheses had a porous surface attached to their stems covering only a small area. The vast majority of them exhibited areas where bone ingrowth took place. The most popular ones had a wire mesh that proved to be effective. Others had beads of various sizes. In the case of the acetabulum, postmortem examinations, as well as during surgical revisions, often demonstrated that bone ingrowth did not take place throughout the entire porous surface. Several times, painless and well-fixed acetabular components did not show more than 10 or 15 percent of bone ingrowth. The greatest degree of bone ingrowth was observed in the area immediately adjacent to the screws used to further stabilize the cup.

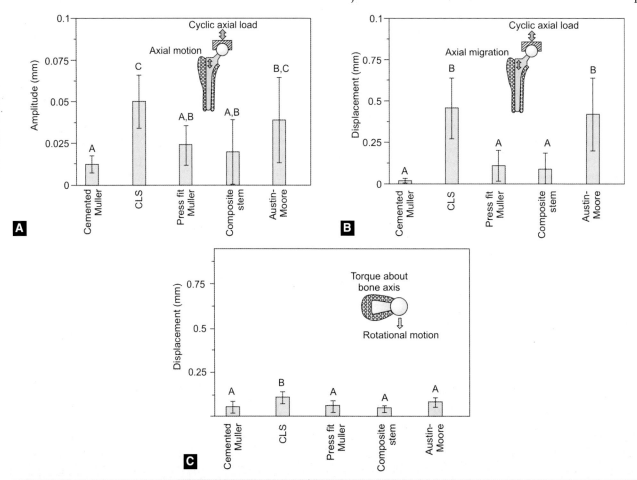

FIGS 23.2A TO C

Barographs documenting various laboratory studied regarding the stability of noncemented femoral stems (A) Axial motion (pistoning) during sinusoidal loading of 2,000 N maximum. Two stem types that do not have a letter in common (A, B, or C) had statistically different motion ($p < 0.05$). (B) Permanent axial migration due to 5,000 cycles of 2,000 N sinusoidal load. The letters A and B indicate stem types with significantly different motions ($p < 0.05$). (C) Posterior displacement of the head of the prosthesis due to 10 Newton-meters torque about the femoral shaft tending to rotate the femur externally. The letters A and B indicate stem types with significantly different motions ($p < 0.05$)

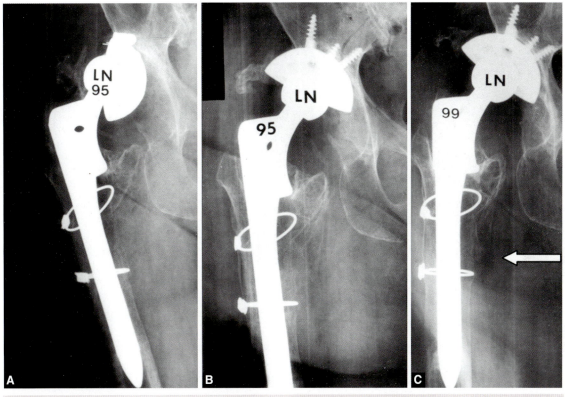

FIGS 23.3A TO C

(A) Radiograph of a totally porous prosthetic stem obtained 6 years postoperatively demonstrating severe demineralization of the proximal femur and a dislodged acetabular component. The surgery had been allegedly performed for the care of a failed intertrochanteric fracture. (B) The acetabular component was revised and anchored in a rather precarious manner. (C) Though the patient continued to be ambulatory and without pain, the demineralization progressed to a most severe degree. All laboratory studies and a biopsy failed to demonstrate infection or malignancy

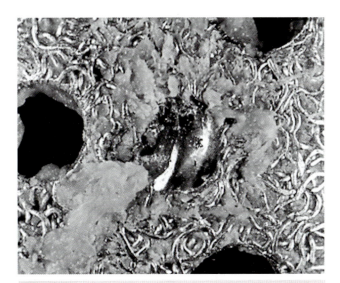

FIG. 23.4

Photograph of removed porous shell showing bone ingrowth in only small areas

Porous femoral stems also showed that bone ingrowth does not occur throughout the entire porous surface, and 'Welding spots" were readily identified, usually at the end of the porous surface (Figs 23.4 to 23.6). *This observation demonstrates that porous surfaces placed just about one inch below the collar of the prosthesis do not touch the cortex of the femur, they simply lie in a cavity created by the rasping of the canal.* These are the implants that most readily show the welding points at the end of the porous surface; that is at the point where true contact between porous metal and cortical bone meet.

This realization prompted us to design a modular femoral component that allowed the surgeon to ensure that wedges of different sizes would provide immediate contact between cortex and porous material immediately after surgery. The wedges had porous surfaces. We spend nearly two years deigning and studying prototypes of the new implant. By the time we felt comfortable with the product, the sponsoring manufacturing company decided to abandon the study because of fear that the modular wedges might become loose and generate metal debris. Despite the disappointment that the decision provoked in us, we rapidly agreed that more knowledge was needed before embarking on actual human usage.

Section 1

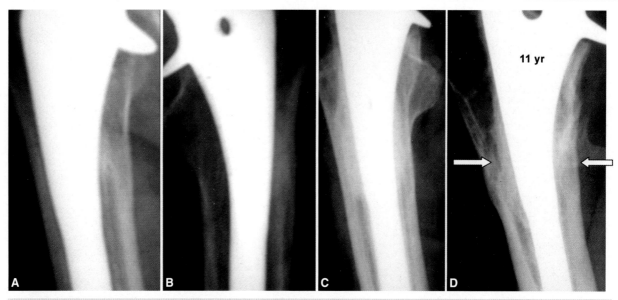

FIGS 23.5A TO D

(A) Representative radiographs of "welding points" frequently seeing opposite the tip end of the porous patch. Sometimes they appear on the medial side. (B) Other times on the lateral side. (C and D) Other times on both sides

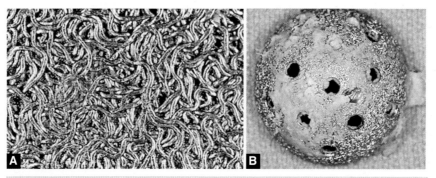

FIGS 23.6A AND B

(A) Photo of the mesh used in several noncemented implants. (B) Removed implant demonstrating small areas where bone ingrowth was taking place

It is interesting that the engineer that represented the manufacturing company and who worked with our engineers in our laboratories, left the company and moved to a different one bringing with him the prototypes we had designed. His new company proceeded to make an almost identical implant that was used by a few surgeons for a brief period of time. One of them was a former associate of mine whom I had invited to participate in the study and who later left the University to go into private practice. He traveled around the country selling the implant, but apparently was not successful in his venture. During the course of our initial studies, the SICOT meeting was held in Munich. During a visit to the commercial exhibit area I noticed that an Italian manufacturing company was displaying a product that had the same features of the implant we were trying to develop. C'est la vie! (*See Modular components*)

Though beads are still seen in certain implants, numerous reports have identified the loosening of many of them. This phenomenon may lead to their travelling to the joint and being caught between the articulating surfaces and subsequently the initiation of a third-body wear process (Figs 23.7 to 23.10).

It is almost universally accepted today that the stability of a porous cup is enhanced by the addition of screws driven into the pelvic bone. Some find this popular technique to be unnecessary and depends for fixation on the mechanical stability obtain at the time of surgery. I personally favor the additional screws, even though I have seen problems related to them in a few occasions. *The most commonly encountered is the*

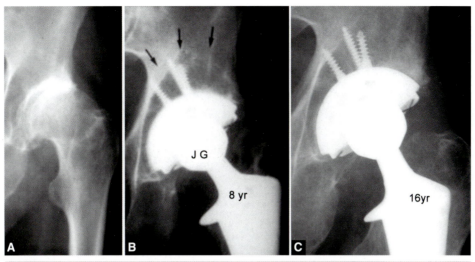

FIGS 23.7A TO C

(A) Preoperative radiograph of an arthritic hip. (B) Radiograph obtained 8 years later. Suggesting acetabular lysis. (C) Radiograph obtained 16 years after surgery indicating that lysis was not present. In retrospect it appears that what appeared to be lysis was simply osteoporosis that subsided with time

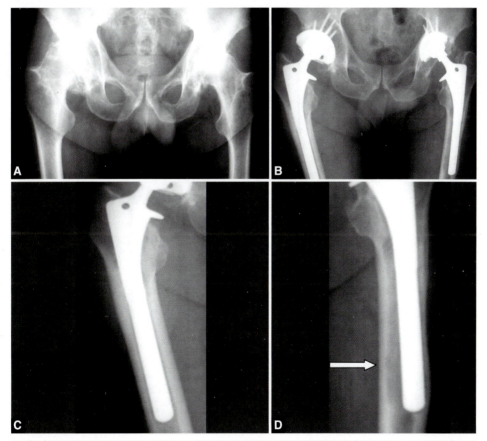

FIGS 23.8A TO D

(A) Radiograph of advanced osteoarthritis of both hips. (B) Radiograph of bilateral total hip arthroplasties using Harris-Galante noncemented implants. (C) Radiograph of right hip 7 years postoperatively. Notice the laterally located "welding spot" opposite to the distal end of the porous patch. (D) Radiograph of the left hip demonstrating lysis throughout the entire proximal femur. The implant was replaced at a later date at another institution. (See *Late Onset of Thigh Pain*)

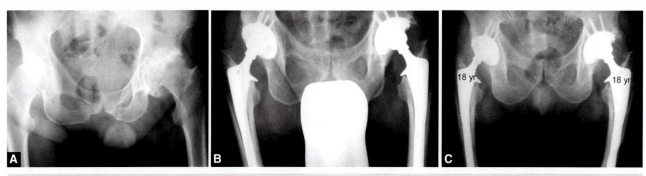

FIGS 23.9A TO C
(A) Radiographs of the osteoarthritic hips of a 48-year-old dance instructor. (B) The hips were replaced with noncemented Harris-Galante prostheses. Radiograph obtained 5 years after surgery. Notice the small areas of lysis below the collar of the prostheses. (C) Radiographs taken 18 years postoperatively. The areas of lysis do not appear top be any worse. The patient had remained extremely active and his hips were asymptomatic

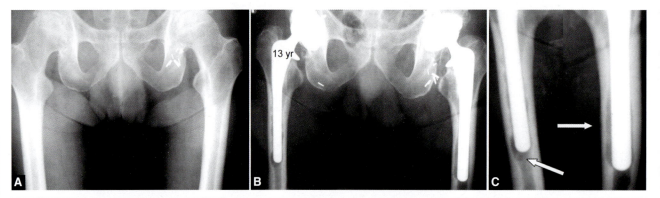

FIGS 23.10A TO C
(A) Radiograph of bilateral total hip osteoarthritis in a 52-year-old man. (B and C) Radiograph obtained 13 years later demonstrating lytic lesions in both femurs

eventual lysis resulting from the improper insertion of the screws. Suspecting that the screw had been driven to the maximum degree and not bothering to check by manual and visual examination than its head was deeply buried into the hole in the cup, the protruding head would be in contact with the plastic liner, if the forceful impaction of the liner into the metal cup was possible. It is not uncommon to find out that firmly anchoring the plastic liner into the metal cup is not possible, from failure to bury the screw head into the cup hole. Correction of this problem, them makes possible the appropriate sitting of the liner. If the sitting can be done, while the head of the screw is slightly prominent, it is very likely that plastic debris can be produced, which eventually travels to the bony acetabulum and/or the proximal femur.

Other times the imperfect placement of the screw can result of scratching of the metallic surfaces with the possibility of creating corrosion, which can eventually result in fracture of the screw. This corrosion brings about the production of metal debris responsible for lysis. This problem is more likely to occur when the porous acetabular cup is made of a Titanium alloy and he screws are made of Cobalt-Chrome or Stainless Steel. The softer Titanium, easy to scratch, begins the debris-producing phenomenon.

*References**

21, 22, 23, 24, 31, 32, 34, 35, 37, 44, 45, 48, 54, 60, 66, 72, 81, 91

* References provided at the end of the book after annexures.

24

Hybrid Total Hip Arthroplasty

A period of dissatisfaction with earlier noncemented prostheses brought about the concept of a hybrid system where the femoral component was cemented and the acetabulum component was of the porous, noncemented type (Figs 24.1A and B). At time it appeared that thigh pain was too common a feature in noncemented prostheses and that bone ingrowth, contrary to expectations had resulted in an increased incidence of femoral lysis.

I shared those concerns and began to use the hybrid system with some regularity. It did not take long, however, for us to realize that the fixation of the porous acetabulum was very good, based on the fact that we had not seen a single failure, but that the femoral components were showing a more frequent rate of loosening, as depicted by the presence of radiolucent lines around the cement.

We studied our experiences with 2 groups of patients, where 105 patients had hybrid arthroplasties and 143 totally cemented replacements. I had performed the surgeries between January 1981 and January 1992 using the same surgical approach and following an identical surgical and postsurgical protocol. The femoral component (STH-2) used in both groups was a monoblock implant made of a titanium alloy (Ti-6Al-4V) with a 28 mm diameter head, and with a 30 degree head-stem offset. The noncemented acetabular components were of the Harris-Galante design (Zimmer Warsaw).

The majority of patients had osteoarthritis, approximately 70 percent in each group. The mean age of the patients with cemented cups was 63 ± 12 years, with a median of 65 and a mode of 66 years. The mean age of the hybrid arthroplasty patients was 69 ± 9 years, with a median of 69 and 65 years. Patients under 50 years of age comprised about 16 percent of those with totally cemented arthroplasties and about three percent of the hybrid arthroplasties.

Sixty-four percent of the patients were females in the cemented group, and 76 percent in the hybrid group. The mean weight of the patients in the cemented group was 153 ± 34 lbs with a median 159

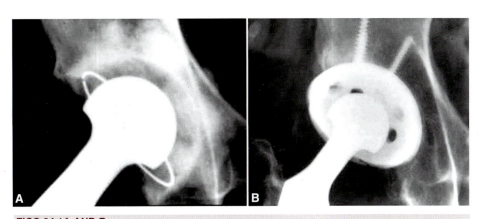

FIGS 24.1A AND B
(A) Radiograph of cemented acetabulum. (B) Radiograph of noncemented acetabulum

and a mode of 150 lbs, and that of the patients with hybrid arthroplasties was 152 ± 32 lbs, with a median of 150 and a mode of 135 lbs. The distribution of weight was normal in both groups (P = 0.9).

Figures 24.2 to 24.7 demonstrate that in all categories the incidence of abnormal; changes was higher in the hybrid group. *Particularly interesting is the much greater degree of wear in the hybrid group.* It could be argued that this was due to the fact that a titanium alloy had been used. However, this applies to both groups, to the totally cemented as well as to the hybrid. Furthermore, we had already studied the rate of wear in totally cemented titanium arthroplasties, and had found out that, though slightly higher than with other materials, it was also lower than that observed by other investigators using other materials (Figs 24.2A and B).

One needs to hypothesize on the reasons for the higher rate of complications with hybrid implants since we have no scientific explanation for such adverse effects. To simply conclude that the problems were secondary to the use of titanium is not sufficient, because other investigators, using different materials have encountered similar complications. *I admit, however, that it is possible that our higher rate of complications may be due to the use of titanium, since in totally cemented titanium total hips the rate of wear and other complications had been found to be higher than with Stainless Steel Charnley prostheses. The fact that we have on record a large number of cemented titanium total hips that have survived for a long as 30 years without any evidence of radiological changes, further confuses the issue.*

I have come to the conclusion that the information gathered from this review, may be only of historical interest. The evidence against titanium as an articulating surface cannot be dismissed.

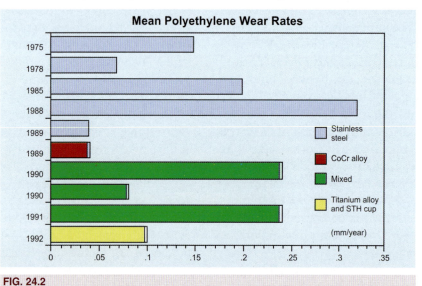

FIG. 24.2

Summarizing the reported wear rates by other investigators using 3 different materials: stainless steel, cobalt-chrome and a titanium alloy. Our data is in yellow under the name of Doctor E Ebramzadeh, who did the investigative study and compiled the data

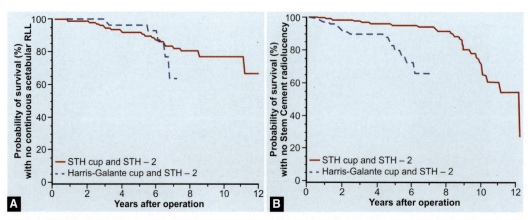

FIGS 24.3A AND B

(A) Survivorship of acetabular radiolucent lines of totally cemented prostheses and hybrid implants. (B) Survivorship comparing stem/cement radiolucent lines

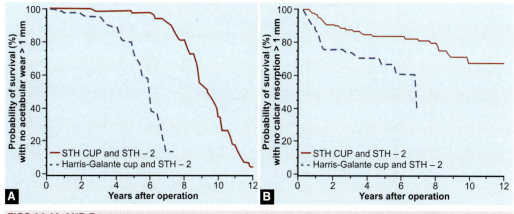

FIGS 24.4A AND B

(A) Survivorship comparing calcar resorption between the two groups. (B) Survivorship comparing wear of the polyethylene liner in the two groups. The risk of greater wear of the polyethylene liner was shown in the hybrid group, as well as that of an increased rate of calcar resorption (P < 001)

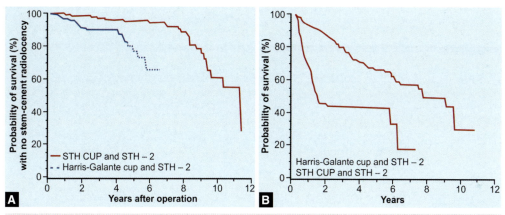

FIGS 24.5A AND B

Radiological analysis showed that the risk of developing femoral bone-cement and stem-cement radiolucent lines was greater in the arthroplasties performed with porous acetabular components (P < 0.001)

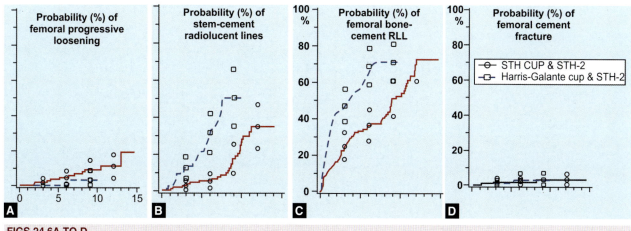

FIGS 24.6A TO D

Illustration of comparative findings between the hybrid and totally cemented total hip arthroplasties

Section 1

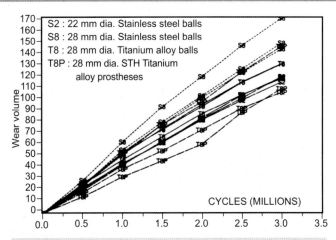

FIG. 24.7

Laboratory data indicating that under clean conditions titanium alloy prosthetic heads wear in a way comparable to other metal. This work was conducted by Harry McKellop PhD

*Reference**

112

25

An Experimental Bone-Cement Hybrid Fixation Technique

Sometime after the introduction of porous-surfaced hip prostheses into the armamentarium of the orthopedic surgeon it was realized that bone ingrowth did not always take place throughout the entire porous surface (Fig. 25.1). Postmortem examination revealed that very stable situations were created, even when no more than 20 to 30 percent of the porous material was filled with

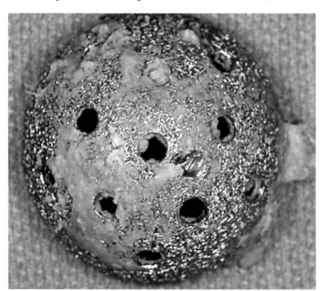

FIG. 25.1

Photograph of porous acetabular shell demonstrating the absence of bone ingrowth over a large area

new bone. In the acetabular side it was also noticed that the maximum and more consistent area of bone ingrowth was that adjacent to the screws that had been used to provide immediate fixation to the porous cup.

This finding was further supported by the identification of "welding spots" (Figs 25.2A to C) in the femoral canal that usually corresponded to the most distal end of the porous patch. In other words, it appeared that bone ingrowth was more likely to take place at points of maximum concentration of pressures. These observations prompted me to conceive the possibility of the construction of a femoral stem that had removable wedges, anteriorly and posteriorly, in order to ensure that maximum contact between the porous material and the cortical bone of the femur was obtained in all instances (See *Modular Implants*). *The traditional prosthesis that has only small areas of porous surfaces located just below the collar of the prosthesis often fails to provide contact between the pores and the cortical bone, except at its very distal end, due to the conical shape of the femur at that level. A "welding spot" develops there and it manifests itself in the form of a dense cortical bridge of bone connecting the prosthesis with the femur.*

The realization that bony ingrowth throughout the entire porous surface was not necessary to obtain adequate stability, came at the same time that concerns

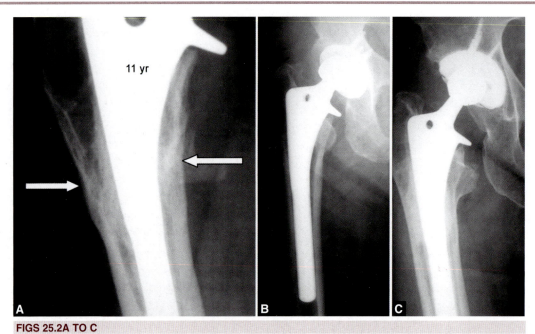

FIGS 25.2A TO C

Radiographs of noncemented Harris-Galante hip prostheses illustrating the presence of "welding spots" opposite to the porous mesh. The welding "spots" occur either medially or laterally, and in some instances on both sides

were being expressed regarding the high-incidence of lysis accompanying the original noncemented prostheses. *It then occurred to me that secure stability of prosthetic implants could be obtained by utilizing cement in combination with minimal amount of porous ingrowth using a metallic component.*

A technique was developed, consisting of the traditional cementing of the acetabulum, but preceded by the placing of one or two blocks of porous material into the pelvic bone (Figs 25.3A to C). Holes measuring one centimeter were drilled on the superior acetabulum into which the porous block was forcibly impacted untill its surface was flush with the acetabular floor. Then the acetabular cavity was cemented in the traditional manner. However, special effort was made to press the cement very firmly into the surfaced of the porous blocks.

We had already determined in the laboratory that if cement was pressed into the porous block with the pressure usually applied when pushing it into holes made in the acetabulum, only the superficial half of the block was filled with cement. The deep half of the block then remains in contact with cancellous bone.

This minihybrid system ensured that the prosthetic cup would be held in place by the cement,

but additional "welding spots" created by bony ingrowth into the metallic porous blocks would further ensure stability.

We performed the procedure in 29 instances in 27 patients with moderately satisfactory results. From this group of patients we lost 7 to follow-up after seven years of yearly radiographs. My move from California to Scotland, and then to Miami resulted in the high rate of patients lost to long follow-up. Of the remaining 20 patients the presence of radiological radiolucent lines in the acetabulum was identified in 4. Two of them were revision cases. These two patients required additional revision surgery because of acetabular and femoral failure. *If one looks only at the arthroplasties that had primary arthroplasty 25 of them did not develop radiolucent lines.* The longer follow-up was 25 years, the median was 18 years and the mode was 16 years. I abandoned the technique when it became apparent that improved porous implants were rendering good results, and the lysis that we had seen with earlier implants had been reduced significantly. The experience with the minihybrid system was an enjoyable one that shed some further light into the subject of prosthetic stability and bone ingrowth (Figs 25.4 to 25.7).

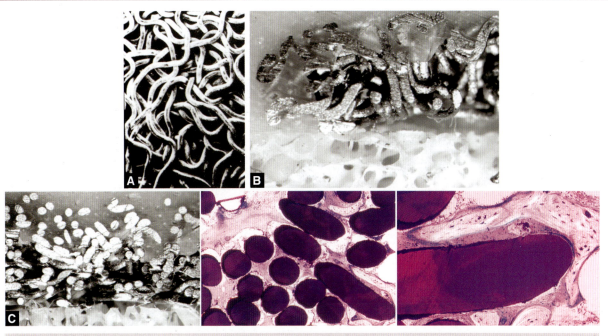

FIGS 25.3A TO C

(A) The porous surface of the metallic block. (B and C) Illustration of the degree of penetration of acrylic cement into the one centimeter porous cube. Notice that one half of the porous remain free of cement, and therefore, the other half is in contact with bone

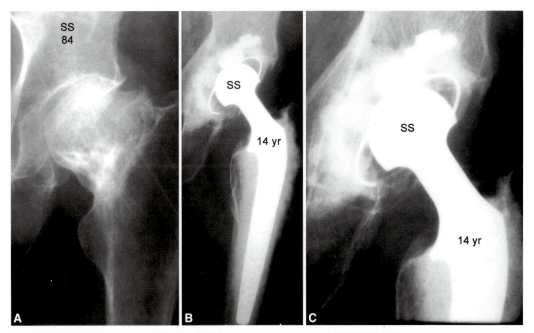

FIGS 25.4A TO C

(A) Preoperative radiograph of an arthritic hip. (B and C) Radiograph obtained 14 years after cemented total hip replacement. Two porous blocks had been inserted in the acetabulum. Good stability was maintained as depicted by the absence of bone-cement radiolucent lines

Section 1

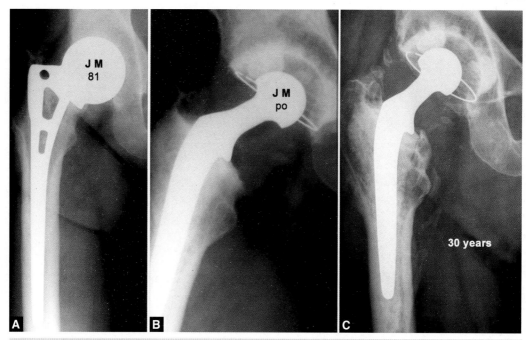

FIGS 25.5A TO C

(A) Radiograph of painful endoprosthesis that had been inserted 7 years earlier in a 26-year-old Air Force lieutenant. (B) Immediate postsurgical radiograph of the cemented titanium alloy total hip arthroplasty. A porous block was used. (C) Radiograph obtained 30 years postoperatively. Notice the absence of bone-cement radiolucent lines in the acetabulum

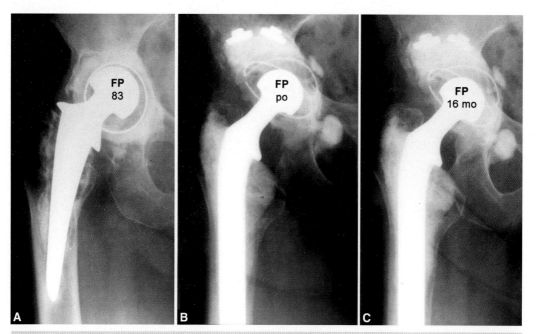

FIGS 25.6A TO C

(A) Radiograph of failed Müller prosthesis. (B) Radiograph obtained immediately after revision surgery. The deficient acetabulum had been filled with cement and 2 porous blocks had been coined in the acetabulum. (C) Radiograph obtained 16 months after surgery. The patient expired one year later

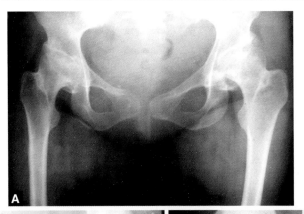

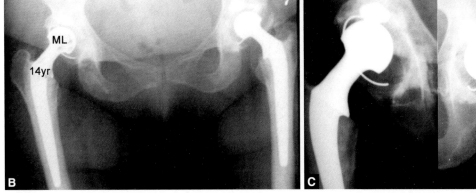

FIGS 25.7A TO C

(A) Radiographs of bilateral hip arthritis secondary to familiar osteochondrodystrophy in a woman 34 years of age. (B) Radiograph of bilateral total hip arthroplasties using porous blocks in the acetabulum obtained 20 years postoperatively. Notice the wear in both acetabula. (C) Radiographs taken 25 years after surgery. The wear in the right hip has resulted in penetration of the head through the polyethylene. Revision surgery was successfully performed at an other institution

*Reference**

50

___
* Reference provided at the end of the book after annexures.

26

Early Failure of a Series of Hybrid Total Hip Arthroplasties

Several reports have appeared in the literature in the past two decades concerning early failure of certain total hip implants (Figs 26.1 to 26.6). There is no clear explanation in many instances as to why premature failure took place. It has been speculated that in some instances manufacturing defects such as instability at the femoral head/prosthesis neck articulation leads to corrosion that produces meal debris that ultimately travels to the joint and initiates a third-body wear process. Other times, *the heads of the screws used to further stabilize the porous acetabular cup come in contact with the polyethylene liner creating plastic debris in a rapid manner.* Loosening of the liner in the metal shell has also been documented in some instances. The method of sterilization of the plastic liner has been suspected. Release of metal from the porous surface has been documented in some instances. Other investigators have identified loose grains of hydroxyapatite as the culprit. We documented the release of acrylic cement and metal particles from metal-backed acetabula in cemented arthroplasties. (See *Metal-backed Acetabula*). Efforts to eliminate early failure of total hip implants have resulted in a significant reduction in the incidence of complications.

The report, I am presenting in this chapter has eluded an explanation as to why a large percentage of

hybrid prostheses manufactured by an identified company (DEPUY), required revision within a very short period of time. The technique I used in this group of patients was the same I had used with other implants; therefore technique cannot be blamed for the bad results. The material of the femoral and acetabular components was also the same—Cobalt-chrome and high density polyethylene).

Sixty hybrid total hip arthroplasties were performed in 60 patients between June 1896 and November 1998. The surgeries were performed at Doctors' Hospital in Coral Gables, Florida. The polyethylene liners had been sterilized according to the manufactures and the modular prosthetic heads measured 28 mm. A posterior approach without trochanteric osteotomy was used in all instances.

Sixteen (32%) patients were males and 34 (68%) were females. The procedures were performed for the treatment of osteoarthritis in 55 (91.6%) instances in 45 patients; for rheumatoid arthritis in 5 (8.3%) in 3 patients; and for avascular necrosis in 2 (3.3%) instances in 2 patients.

The rehabilitation protocol consisted in the use of gradient elastic stockings during the day and their removal during the night; the frequent performance of

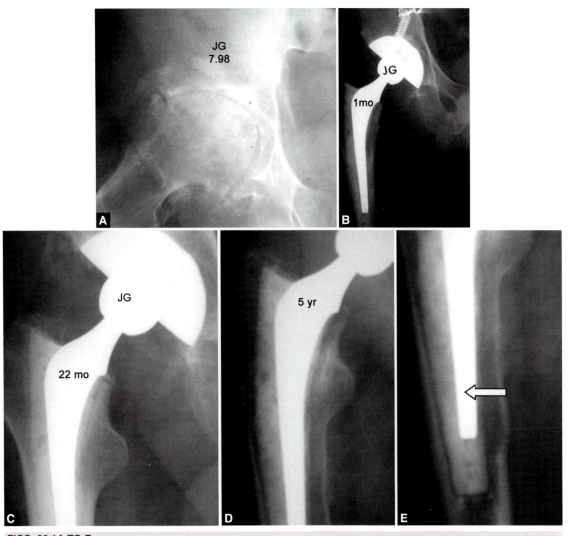

FIGS 26.1A TO E

(A) Radiograph of osteoarthritic hip in a 54-year-old man. (B) Radiograph of hybrid prosthesis obtained one month post-operatively. (C) Radiograph 22 months postoperatively. (D) Radiograph taken 5 years postoperatively. Notice the wide bone-cement radiolucent line on zone 7 of the femur. (E) Radiograph taken 5 years postoperatively demonstrating loosening of the femoral implant and lysis in the distal femur. The hip was revised at another city a few weeks later

active isometric quadriceps and gluteus maximus exercises; frequent active ankle motion, deep breathing and trapeze exercises.

Ambulation was began on the first postoperative day with the aid of a walker and gradually progressed to 2 crutches and then to one crutch whenever considered appropriate. From the 60 arthroplasties 19 (31.6%) graduated to one crutch prior to discharge from the hospital; the remaining 41 (68%) patients were discharged from the hospital ambulatory with the aid of either 2 crutches or a walker.

Following discharge from the hospital, instructions were given concerning the continuation of exercises and precautions against dislocation. An appointment to return for follow-up was made for two weeks later.

Obviously, those patients who did not live in the community were asked to graduate to nonassisted ambulation as soon as they considered their balance and muscle power sufficiently restored and to submit a new X-ray 2 months after surgery. Local patients were asked to return for a second visit 2 months later; then six months later and then on a yearly basis.

Evaluation of the first postoperative radiographs indicated that the acetabular component was 100 percent covered with bone in 58 (96.6%) instances. In 2 (3.3%) instances the coverage was less than 100 percent. The inclination of the socket was between 45 to 50 degrees in 53 (88.3%); between 35 and 40 degrees in 4 (6.6%) instances; and more than 50 degrees in 3 (5%) instances. The femoral components were in

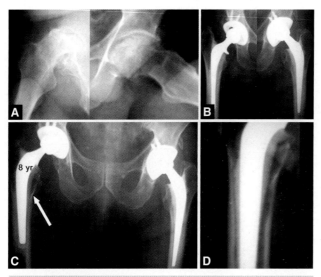

FIGS 26.2A TO D

(A) Radiographs of severe AVN of both hips. (B) Radiograph obtained shortly after bilateral total hip hybrid arthroplasty. The right hip received a stem manufactured by one company and the left by a different one. Both stems were polished. (C) Radiographs of right hip obtained eight years postoperatively. Notice the lytic lesion on the medial aspect of the proximal femur. (D) Radiograph obtained 9 years after surgery demonstrating advanced lysis throughout the entire proximal femur

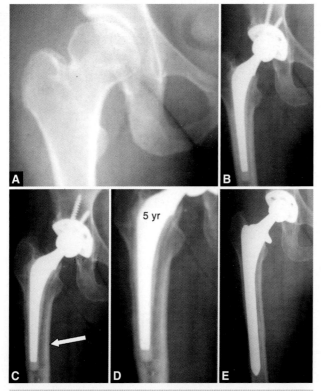

FIGS 26.3A TO E

(A) Radiograph of osteoarthritic hip in a 61-year-old woman. (B) Postoperative radiograph. (C and D) Radiographs obtained 5 years postoperatively illustrating the progressive loosening of the stem. (E) Radiograph obtained 2 years after revision surgery

neutral in 53 (88.3%) instances in slight varus in 4 (6.6%) instances; and in slight valgus in 3 (5%) instances.

The thickness of the column of cement at the level of the calcar ranged between 0 mm and 8 mm. The column measured 0 mm in 5 (8.3%) instances; between 1 and 3 mm in 10 (16.6%) instances; between 3 and 5 mm in 21 (35%) instances; and between 5 and 8 mm in 24 (40%) instances. The ratio between the diameters of the medullary canal and the prosthetic stem at 7 cm below the calcar revealed that in 34 (56.6%) instances the ratio was 50-50; in 12 (20%) instances the ratio was greater than 50 percent; and in 14 (23.3%) instances the ratio was less than 50 percent.

The column of cement ended above the tip end of the prosthesis in 3 (5%) instances; and in the remaining 57 (95%) instances extended below the tip end of the prosthesis.

The number of screws used to further secure the porous acetabular cup varied. In 2 (3.3%) instances no screws were used; in 26 (43.3%) instances 1 screw was used; in 24 (40%) instances 2 screws were used; and in 8 (13.3%) instances 3 screws were used.

In the group of 60 arthroplasties performed in 50 patients, there were no deaths during hospitalization. Three (6%) patients expired during the 1st and 2nd postoperative years. An additional 4 (8%) patients were lost to follow-up after 2 years postoperatively for reasons we were unable to identify. The remaining 53 (88.3%) arthroplasties had follow-up between 6 and 10 years.

There were no early or late infections and no thromboembolic disease.

Ten (16.6%) arthroplasties required revision surgery before the fifth postoperative day. Five (50%) arthroplasties were revised by the senior author (AS) and the remaining 5 (50%) were performed by different surgeons at other institutions. An additional 3 (5%) arthroplasties are considered possible failures-based on radiologically evidence of progressive widening bone-cement radiolucent lines. Among the revision surgeries. One (10%) revision was performed 10 months after surgery; 2 (20%) revision surgeries were performed 3 years after surgery; 3 (30%) revisions were performed 3 years after surgery; 2 (20%) arthroplasties were revised 5 years postoperatively; and 1 (10%) arthroplasty was revised 6 years after surgery. Four of the revisions were performed in 2 patients who had bilateral arthroplasties. One of them was a 58-year-old female with rheumatoid arthritis, and the other a 42-year-old male suffering from osteoarthritis secondary congenital epiphyseal dysplasia.

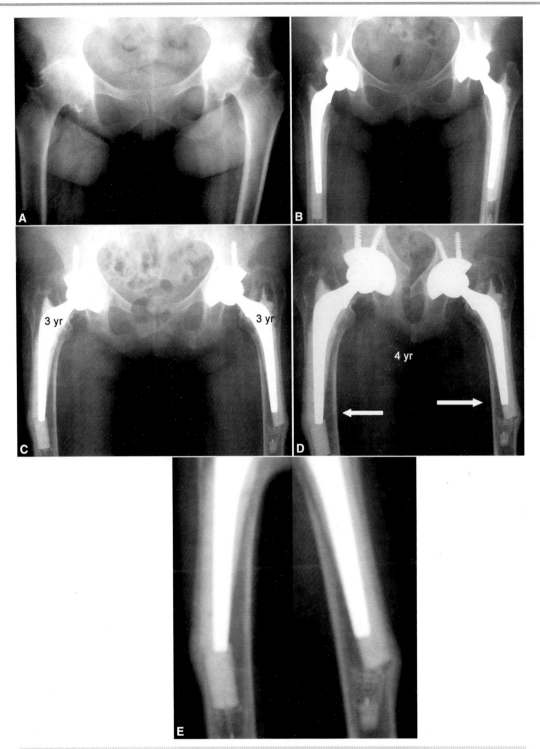

FIGS 26.4A TO E

(A) Radiograph of both hips in a 47-year-old woman suffering from rheumatoid arthritis. (B) Radiograph obtained shortly after bilateral hybrid total hip arthroplasty. (C) Radiograph taken 3 years after surgery. Notice the early signs of loosening of the femoral components. (D) Radiographs obtained 4 years after surgery. Notice the loosening of the femoral components. (E) Radiographs illustrating in greater detail the loosening of the femoral components. The patient had severe osteoporosis

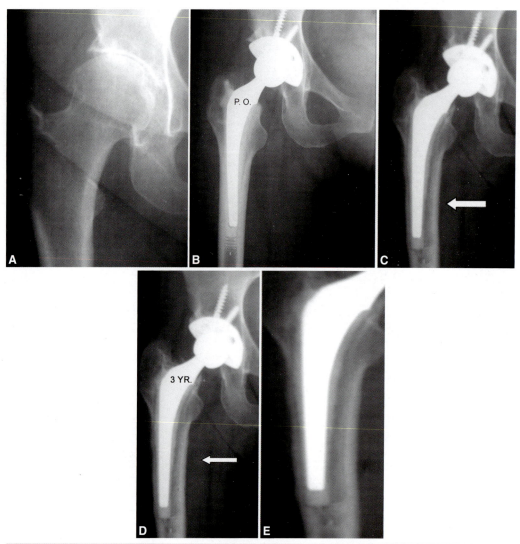

FIGS 26.5A TO E

(A) Radiograph of an osteoarthritic hip in a 59-year-old woman. (B) Radiograph obtained shortly after surgery. A hybrid implant had been used. (C and D) Radiographs obtained three years after surgery. The femoral component was loose. (D) Radiographs obtained 4 and 5 years postoperatively showing progressive loosening of the femoral stem. The hip had become symptomatic. (E) Closer views of the loose implants

All revisions were performed for loosening of the stems. The acetabular polyethylene liners were replaced in the 5 revisions, however, the porous acetabular cups were not revised as they were well-fixed and not associated with other pathology. We do not have information regarding the manner in which the remaining 5 revisions were performed. The revisions were performed 6 osteoarthritics; in 1 patient with avascular necrosis of the femoral head; and in 3 patients with rheumatoid arthritis.

Microscopic examination of tissues around the failed implants demonstrated from mild to extensive polyethylene debris. No metal debris was identified. In one instance the polyethylene component showed an indentation on its convexity created by a screw that had been left protruding.

Acetabular lysis was identified radiologically in 3 (5%) instances, measuring between 1 and 2 cm. The number of screws had been used in the revised arthroplasties was: 1 screw in 1 (10%) instance; 2 screws in 5 (50%) instances; and 3 screws in 4 (40%) instances. Acetabular wear was measured between 0 to 3 mm. In the 10 (18.8%) arthroplasties that were revised. The amount of measurable wear ranged form 0 to 3 mm. The short time of prosthetic implantation probably explains the low wear. In the 3 (5.6%) arthroplasties suspected of failing but not yet revised no measurable wear has been identified as yet.

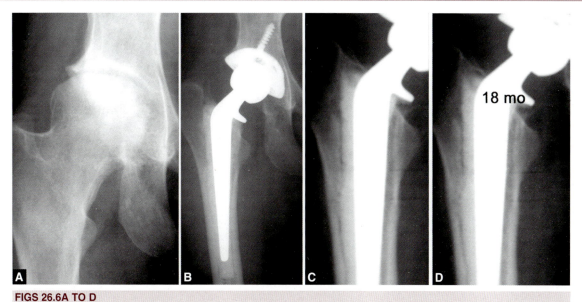

FIGS 26.6A TO D

(A) Radiograph of avascular necrosis of the femoral head in 27-year-old woman suffering from sickle cell anemia. (B) Radiograph taken a few weeks later following hybrid total hip replacement. She experienced considerable bleeding at the time of surgery. (C) Radiograph taken one year after surgery. Notice the radiolucent lines around the stem. (D) Radiographs obtained 18 months postoperatively demonstrating obvious prosthetic loosening

In the 10 revised arthroplasties the coverage of the acetabulum was complete; the inclination of the acetabulum was 40 to 45 degrees in 8 (80%) instances; between 33 to 40 degrees in 1 (10%) instance; and more than 50 degrees in 1 (10%) instance.

The femoral component was in neutral in 7 (49%) instances; in slight varus in 2 (20%) instances; and in slight valgus in 1 (10%) instance. The ratio between the diameters of the stem and medullary canal was 50 percent in 6 (60%) instances; in 2 (20%) instances more than 50 percent; and in 2 (20%) instances less than 50 percent.

Attempts to identify the reasons for the high failure rate in this group of patients have thus far eluded me.

Though, I cannot document it, I suspect a defective polyethylene liner that underwent rapid wear. However, if that were the case the rate of failure would have been grater, as it was in the case of the Teflon series performed by Charnley in the 1950's, when all of his implanted Teflon liners produced massive were and subsequent lysis. It is unlikely that the design of the stem was the responsible factor, since it was virtually identical to other prostheses manufactured by the same company.

Reference*

112

Section 1

27

Femoral Lysis

When we hear the word lysis, we assume it is in reference to total joint replacement. It is the "disease" that replaced the "cement disease", which attracted much attention in the 1970's and 80's.

John Charnley recognized and dealt with lysis during his unhappy experience with Teflon, the material he used to replace the acetabulum of his newly developed total hip prosthesis. Until the end of his career he insisted that polyethylene wear was the greatest challenge facing hip replacement surgery. It is unfortunate that for too long we ignored his warnings and chose to devote our efforts toward the design of new prostheses of different shapes and lengths, based on the presumed belief that all failures could be explained on mechanical grounds.

Now, lysis is with us even though attempts have been made to eliminate the acrylic cement, which had been mistakenly identified as the culprit. I say mistakenly, because the cement is rarely responsible for lysis. *As a matter of fact the use of non-cemented prostheses, temporarily increased the incidence of lysis.* Lysis is, in most instances, was produced by wear debris shed by the polyethylene acetabular component. This seems to be universally agreed and most research nowadays is devoted to finding materials with better wear characteristics, be it new polyethylene, ceramics or metal on metal articulations (Fig. 27.1).

The pathophysiology of lysis has been extensively covered in the literature and new knowledge continues to modify our appreciation of the phenomenon. It should suffice to say that its prevention probably rests primarily on elimination of debris from the articulating surfaces or control of chemical reactions. Interleukins and acid phosphates are at this time being feverishly studied. The debris currently identified is either polyethylene or metal. *Offensive debris may come from metal corrosion at the Morse taper of the modular prosthetic neck, other modular components in either the socket or the femoral stem, the interface between the metal cup and the plastic acetabulum, the screws used to reinforce the fixation of the acetabular shell, the porous surface of the stem and acetabulum or the stem itself.*

It is interesting to recall that in the early 1980's a passionate debate raged throughout the orthopedic community regarding the source of lysis following total hip arthroplasty. The debate took place before

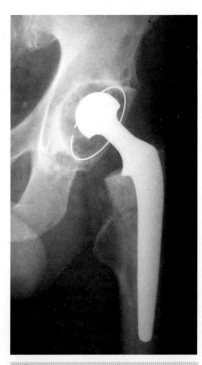

FIG. 27.1

Severe wear of polyethylene associated with relatively mild bone lysis noncemented prostheses became popular. As a matter of fact it was the debate that gave impetus to the accelerated work in the development of noncemented implants. Some strongly believed that acrylic cement was evil, as it was responsible for the increasing incidence of lysis; others argued against that premise. *In retrospect, we were forced to conclude that the cement per se was not the culprit, but an innocent bystander in the process.* When the argument gained a high pitch of controversy, a number of technical innovations were sweeping the globe: modularity, metal backed cemented acetabula, among many others. The cement found itself exonerated, others were the guilty ones.

Even today one finds orthopedic surgeons who believe that the cement *per se* produces lysis. This is not the case. *A large piece of cement implanted in soft tissues anywhere in the body does not produce an inflammatory reaction. However, a very small particle of cement can initiate a chemical/inflammatory reaction and produce lysis.* This lesson should be remembered when discussing the possible harm that metal-on-metal may do. There is abundant evidence that metals, used in orthopedic surgery, do not bring about a chemical reaction when implanted in the body. Testifying to this are the millions of plates, screws, endoprostheses that have been implants world wide over the past 100 years.

The observations I have referred to, concerning the harmless nature of large surfaces of metal or acrylic cement, but the dangers inherent in debris, prompted me to suspect that a similar mechanism may be in place when it comes to internal fracture fixation. This suspicion is supported by the fact that when screws holding a plate in place begin to loosen, one sees an area of radiolucency around them. This we have long-considered to be a mechanical phenomenon, and indeed it probably is in most cases. However, several times I have reasoned that the manner in which, and the order in which the screws loosen cannot always be explained on mechanical forces.

Therefore, I submit the hypothesis that in some instances, the bone resorption observed around the screws is lysis produced by metal debris. How this debris is produced can be explained on the grounds that even micromotion motion between the plate and the screws can generate corrosion at that level. Furthermore, it is well known that in the process of inserting screws into the bone, the drill, and/or the screws can be scratched. Systems that allow for later impaction of the bony fragments, as a result of a built-in mechanism, may perpetuate the corrosion process.

The use of interlocking screws with intramedullary mails very frequently result in scratching of the nail and screws because the targeting devices not always guarantees the smooth introduction of the screws through the nail. *Some instances of bone lysis around the screw-nail junction with intramedullary nails can be explained in that manner.*

Since there is general consensus that polyethylene debris from the concavity of the polyethylene cup is a likely etiology of lysis of the femur, it should be logical to assume that preventing the entry of debris through the top of the femur would significantly reduce the complication. Some have designed non-cemented prostheses that attempt to provide a "lid" at the level of the calcar. *Though the concept is sound, I have long-questioned the effectiveness of the system on the grounds that the very small size of the debris particles, floating in synovial fluid, find their way into the medullary canal through the space that inevitable remains between the porous implant and the cortical bone.*

This assumption prompted me to conceive a method that could more effectively seal the "mouth" of the femur, preventing therefore the entrance of debris into the bone-cement interface. I accomplished this by packing bone graft over the exposed and still viscous acrylic cement around the prosthetic stem. *Once the cement becomes hard, the bone chips are solidly fixed against it, but also in contact with the cortex of the femoral neck* (See *A Method for the Prevention of Femoral Lysis*).

I have seen a few instances of metallosis associated with noncemented Moore endoprosthesis. This phenomenon is so rare, that we have dismissed it cavalierly. I discovered the metallosis during revision surgery. Lytic lesions had formed, which I mistakenly suspected as being expressions of infection. However, infection was not found, only lysis. Up to that time I had not known that endoprostheses could produce metallosis (See *Endoprostheses*).

Polyethylenes are being frantically investigated and have been released to the public. If the alleged improved wear properties of the materials prove to be superior, a major break-through in hip and knee surgery will occur. Perhaps the most common source of complications will then be eliminated.

I remain cautious about the project, since products and concepts that had been heralded as panaceas have often disappointed us. I am particularly interested in seeing good results from this effort not only because of its clinical importance, but because the polyethylene developed by Harry McKellop and associates was conceived and tested by them in our laboratories at the Orthopedic Hospital during my tenure at the University of Southern California.

Progress will be made in the future and it is very likely that lysis will be eliminated from the scene. *However, better polyethylenes may not be the total answer. I suspect that more serious attention will have to be paid to the metal used for the implant since it is metal release that often at times damages the polyethylene, which in turn creates the harmful debris.*

Frequently, questions have been raised regarding when to intervene surgically in the presence of lytic lesions in the acetabulum or femur. There are those who say that early intervention is best; first, because lysis is often progressive, and secondly, because the condition of the bone is better. *If these two premises were always true, I would agree. However, I have seen many instances where the size of the lytic defects remained unchanged for many years* (Figs 27.2A and B). It is true that the condition of the bone is better when surgery is done early, but do we have any evidence that the surgical results are better when the size of lytic lesions differ only in minimal degrees. Is one lesion that measures two centimeters in length and three millimeters in width a more difficult one to approach surgically than one that measures a couple millimeters more in both planes?

Lysis remains the number one cause of failure of total hip implants. It has been the case since ever since the procedure was highly improved and popularized. I suspect he was the first one to recognize its importance and to experience at first hand the degree to which lysis can be a catastrophic event. After having tried Teflon as the material to articulate with the metallic femoral head, he witnessed the destruction the plastic debris was capable of producing not only in the femoral side of the joint but also in the pelvis and surrounding soft tissues (See *Charnley Prostheses*).

Charnley's subsequent experiences with polyethylene as an articulating surface proved rewarding. However, over a period of time he began to observe lytic changes (Figs 27.3A and B), though of a much less severe nature. Despite the fact that others, in other part of the world, blamed the cement for the lytic changes being observed, he maintained that the plastic liner was the culprit. He pleaded for further studies on the subject, which for the most part went unheeded. A few years later he was no longer with us.

The war around the "cement disease" raged violently for a few years. The ones who defended the cement won the final battle. While the "war" was raging, efforts were being made to develop implants with porous surfaces that would eliminate the need for cement fixation. To the best of my knowledge it was Emmett Lunceford, from South Carolina, a former student and associate of Austin T Moore, who first conducted experimental work along these lines. His premature death brought to an end his exciting work. Others stepped into the picture and carried forward his idea.

At first the new concept, the noncemented prosthesis, won the day. Initial results from its use were very gratifying. However, over a relatively short period of time, the orthopedic community began to see the presence of persistent thigh pain that required a long time for its subsidence. In addition, lysis returned. This feature vindicated John Charnley and those who had maintained that the cement was not the source of the dreadful complication. The polyethylene definitely proved to be its source.

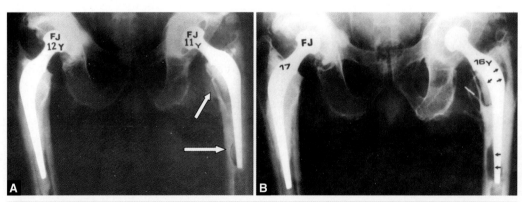

FIGS 27.2A AND B
Bilateral cemented total hip arthroplasty. Though a lytic process developed on the right hip, its progression was gradual. A chronic medical condition precluded revision surgery. The hips, however, remained asymptomatic for 20 years

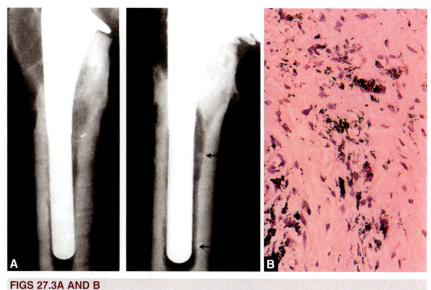

FIGS 27.3A AND B

(A) Composite illustration of noncemented total hip arthroplasty demonstrating lytic changes in the femoral cortex with eventual complete loosening of the femoral comment. Infection was ruled out. (B) Microscopic slide showing metal debris. The implant was made of a chrome/cobalt alloy

A few years after the introduction of the non-cemented prosthesis the incidence of lysis reached critical levels. Some surgeons reported an incidence as high as 25% after seven years of surgery. It was admitted by them that the pathological process was progressive in nature. In other words, a replica of the Teflon fiasco was in the making.

I have seen several porous sockets retrieved during autopsy demonstrated bony ingrowth only over a very small portion of the porous surface. Others have reported that implants found to be rigidly fixed against the underlying cancellous bone had, often, no more than 20 to 30 percent of the porous surface filled with bone. *The conclusion derived from those findings was that bone ingrowth throughout was not necessary and that its development was more likely to be seen in areas around the screws that had been used for additional stabilization. On the femoral side, bone ingrowth was not seen throughout the entire porous surface of the implant, but appeared to concentrate at the end of the porous surface.* The increased bony density at that level, the "welding points", as they were then called, was sufficient to provide the necessary stability. Concerns were voiced, however, as the possibility of unhealthy distribution of stresses throughout the femur and the likely development of stress shielding above the points of fixation.

The market has been inundated with a huge number of different noncemented prostheses. *Many of these implants have failed and were discredited within a short period of time. Some of them had been the product of thoughtful reasoning, others were simple an effort to enter into the lucrative market that total hip surgery has spawned.*

Among the most attractive concepts concerning noncemented prostheses was the Isoelastic implant, conceived by Erwin Morscher in Switzerland in the late 1970s. He felt that a prosthesis made of a material with a modulus of elasticity closer to that of bone would transfer stresses to the surrounding structures in a more physiological manner. The clinical results, however, did not match the surgeons' expectation. After a period of time loosening and lysis became apparent. The product was withdrawn from the market (See *Isoelastic Prostheses*).

I made the mistake of thinking that the occasional stress shielding we were observing with the stiff Charley prosthesis, and fracture of the stem could be reduced with the use of a Titanium alloy in preference of Cobalt-Chrome. The Titanium alloy has a lower modulus of elasticity, and is therefore capable of distributing stresses throughout the surrounding bony structures in a more physiological way. *Although the clinical results were very satisfactory for the first six years, complications began to appear. Soon we realized that the Titanium ally was subject to scratching and producing third-body particles that would eventually generate the offensive debris that produced lysis. Eventually the use of the prosthesis was discontinued* (See *Titanium Prostheses*).

There is no doubt that polyethylene debris is the most common cause of bone lysis in total hip replacement. However, *metallic debris is also produced in various degrees. Its frequency is not as great as with polyethylene, however, its significance is more likely to be greater from the clinical point of view.* There is already incontrovertibly evidence that metal debris can be harmful. Several investigators have shown changes in the soft tissues around bony lytic lesions demonstrating chromosomal abnormalities. The work of Patrick Case, in Bristol, England, is the most concerning of them all. *The chromosomal abnormalities at the same witnessed with cancerous conditions, in some instances, and other instances with congenital abnormalities.* Various metals are associated with prevalence of certain types of lysis. The recent explosion of interest in metal on metal prostheses suggests that any rapid moves made in an attempt to eliminate polyethylene should be made cautiously (See *Metal on Metal Prostheses*).

I have witnessed in numerous occasions the development of severe lysis around stems without comparable changes being observed in the opposite hip, which had been replaced at the same time with identical implants. *How can this be explained other that by suspecting that a third-body producing lysis did not appear in the non-affected side?* In one instance a very large and heavy patient showed painless femoral lysis on his left hip as early as 5 years postoperatively. The right hip demonstrated minor signs of acetabular loosening but no femoral lysis. Twenty years after surgery the lytic process in the left hip had progressed minimally and the patient was asymptomatic. Four

years later, 24 years postoperatively, he was still asymptomatic but beginning to suffer from other medical conditions that will probably take his life within a short time (Figs 27.4 and 27.5).

As I stated previously, lysis is usually produced by polyethylene, however, on occasion only metal can be identity in the tissues obtained in surgery, polyethylene being absent. The next figure is a good example of this phenomenon (Figs 27.6A to C).

I suspect I might be correct in stating that the most common site of lysis in cemented total hip arthroplasty is just above the distal end of the prosthesis. It suggests the polyethylene debris migrates distally through the bone/cement interface until its further distal motion is arrested. A plug, either plastic or bony, becomes the barrier to additional migration. Accumulation of greater amounts of debris generates the bone destructive process (Figs 27.7A to F).

The discussion of femoral lysis in total hip replacement may be summarized by saying that research and longer experiences have resulted in a significant reduction of this complication. Recent reports have indicated that with follow-ups of fifteen to twenty years, its absence has been documented in as many as 96% arthroplasties. Since some of the investigators reporting such good data are reputable and honest surgeons, one must wonder why do we continue to experiment with so many new designs. Why not use those implants and see what happens when an additional ten to twenty years have passed (Figs 27.8A to J).

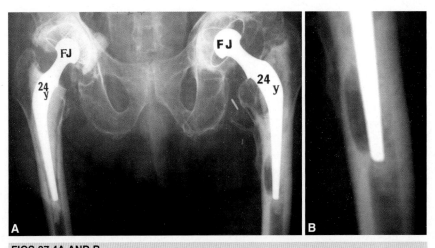

FIGS 27.4A AND B
Bilateral titanium alloy prostheses demonstrating severe, asymptomatic lysis in the left femur and early signs of loosening of the acetabulum in the right acetabulum

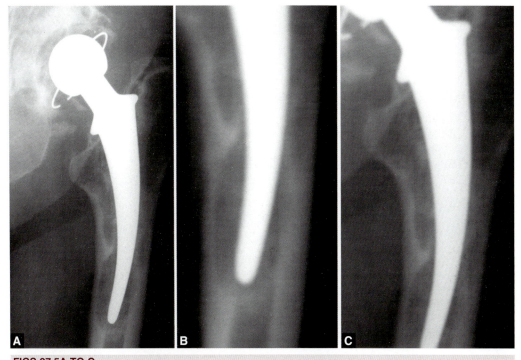

FIGS 27.5A TO C

Representative example of lytic lesions in the femoral shaft in a cemented cobalt-chrome total hip arthroplasty

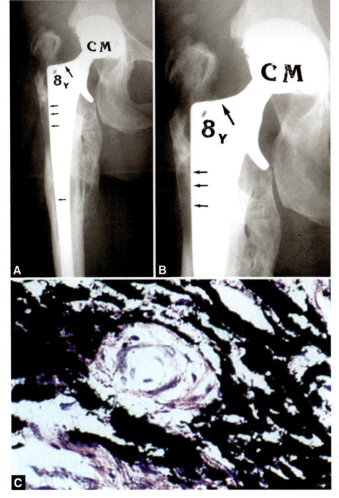

FIGS 27.6A TO C

(A) Lysis involving the greater trochanter and the proximal-lateral aspect of the femur. (B) Closer view of (A); (C) *Microscopic evidence of metal debris and absence of polyethylene debris*

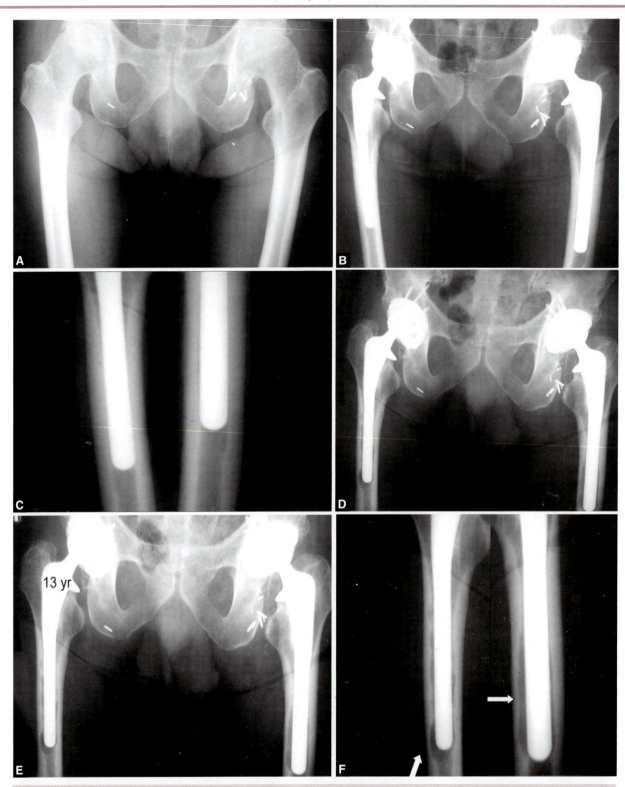

FIGS 27.7A TO F

(A) Radiograph of bilateral hip osteoarthritis in a very active 55-year-old man. (B) Both hips were replaced with noncemented Harris-Galante prostheses. (C) Radiographs obtained 5 years postoperatively showing minimal bone reaction at the distal end of the stems. (D) Radiographs taken 10 years postoperatively demonstrating early distal femoral lysis. (E) Radiographs obtained 13 years postoperatively showing further advanced femoral lysis. The patient had become symptomatic. (F) Closer view of the distal femoral lysis

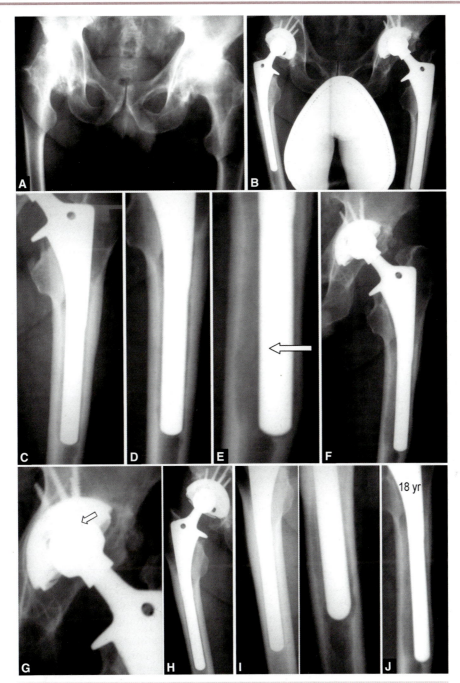

FIGS 27.8A TO J

(A) Bilateral osteoarthritis in a 48-year-old man. (B) The hips were replaced with noncemented Harris-Galante prostheses. (C to G) Radiographs of the left hip taken 5, 9 and 18 years post-operatively demonstrating progressive lysis of the femur, varus inclination of the stem and wear of the polyethylene. (H to J) Radiographs of the left hip illustrating the progressive lysis over a period of 18 years

References*

20, 22, 23, 30, 36, 39, 54, 56, 72, 81, 91, 111, 112

28

A Technique for the Prevention of Femoral Lysis in Cemented Total Hips

It is currently agreed that following total hip arthroplasty, polyethylene or metal debris depositing against the cortical femoral cortex or against the cancellous surface in the acetabulum is responsible for the production of lysis. The debris initiates a chemical reaction that in most instances is progressive in nature, and can be severe enough to loosen the prosthetic components and/or create significant bone damage. Attempting to overcome this insidious problem, new cross-linked polyethylenes have been manufactured. Though there is no long-term evidence of a superior *in vivo* performance of the new materials, their laboratory performance suggests a likely reduction in the rate of lysis. Others have developed noncemented femoral prostheses that by virtue of their design attempt to prevent the migration of debris into the medullary canal. These prostheses have porous surfaces into which bone is expected to grow, reinforcing in that manner the possibility of creating a more effective barrier. We are not aware of any attempts having been made by others in regards to cemented arthroplasties.

The technique we have used in this study, which consists of placing a bone graft over the still polymerizing cement in order to create a barrier, appears to prevent the distal seeping of debris into the bone-cement interface as depicted by the fact that lysis or radiolucent bone-cement lines have not been observed during a follow-up ranging between 3 and 14 years.

Materials and Method

Following preparation of the medullary canal, injection of acrylic cement and insertion of the prosthetic component, small fragments of bone removed from the femoral head, or obtained from the bone bank, are firmly pressed into the exposed, still doughy cement around the base of the neck of the metallic implant. *The graft particles cover the entirely exposed cement surface, and are in close contact with the cortical wall of the femur. When the cement is fully polymerized the bone graft is permanently held in place.*

We anticipate that with time the graft regains its viability from blood supply arising from the normal femoral bone. The procedure was performed in 51 osteoarthritic hips. In all instances the acetabular components were porous ingrowth implants that were fixed without cement. The first 15 (29.4%) procedures were performed at the Orthopedic Hospital of Los Angeles between July 1992 and September 1993; and the remaining 36 (71.1%) procedures were performed at Doctors' Hospital in Coral Gables, Florida between January 1999 and February 2001. The 15 (29.4%) prostheses inserted in California were made of a Titanium alloy (STH Zimmer, Warsaw); the 36 (71.1%) prostheses implanted in Florida were made of a Cobalt-Chrome alloy (Smith- Nephew, Memphis). Thirty- seven (72.5%) patients were female and 14 (27.4%) were males. The oldest patient was 88-year-old, and the youngest 49. The median age was 74 years and the modes 70 and 74 years. Twenty-one (41%) patients were 70 years of age or younger. Forty-four (86.3%) femoral stems were inserted in a neutral attitude; 4 (7.4%) stems in mild varus; and 3 (5.8%) stems in mild valgus. The femoral canal/stem ratio, measured at 7 cm below the base of the neck was 50% in 20 (39.2%) arthroplasties;

More than 50% in 26 (50.9%) arthroplasties; and <50% in 5 (9.8%) arthroplasties. The thickness of the column of cement at the level of the transected femoral neck measured < 3 mm in 10 (19.6%); between 3–5 mm in 37 (72.5%); and >5 mm in 4 (7.8%). The orientation of the acetabular component was at 45 degrees in 30 (76.4%) arthroplasties; > 45 degrees in 6 (11.7%); and < 45 degrees in 6 (11.7%) arthroplasties.

The small number of patients in this series may be explained primarily on the fact that when the study was getting underway, we had begun to perform with increasing frequency non-cemented total hip arthroplasties. The hiatus between 1992 and 1995 was due to the senior author relocating in another locality, during which time the procedure was not performed.

Results

Most patients had radiographs of their hips at one-year intervals. The longest follow-up was 12 years, with a median of 5 years and modes of 4 and 5 years. Forty-four (86.2%) patients had a minimum follow-up of 3 years. Only the results observed in this group of 44 patients with a minimum follow-up of three years are reported. Thirty-nine (88.6%) of these patients had a minimum follow-up of 4 years. The sub-group of 7 (13.7%) patients with follow-up < 3 years was made of 3 patients who expired during that period of time, and 4 patients who were lost to follow-up. Among the 44 patients with follow-up >3 years 3 (6.8%) patients have expired. One (1.9%) arthroplasty was revised six years after surgery at another institution, allegedly after rather rapid deterioration of the hip joint. The mode of failure was not known to us. There were no infections or dislocations. One (1.9%) patient had a nonfatal pulmonary embolism. In the group of 44 (86.2%) arthroplasties who had a minimum follow-up of three years, neither radiolucent lines at the bone/cement interface, nor cement/metal radiolucent lines were observed in any patient. There were no radiologically recognized fractures of the cement, migration of the stem or cancellization. Femoral lysis was not identified, unless one wishes to consider a lytic process a 3 mm resorption of the calcar seen in 1 (2.4%) arthroplasty. In this patient a titanium alloy prosthesis had been used; the stems was in neutral attitude, the stem occupied >50% of the canal at 7 cm below the base of the prosthesis and the thickness of the column of cement at the level of the transected femoral neck was <3 mm. Migration of the acetabulum has not been identified. In the group of 44 arthroplasties with follow-up > 3 years, wear of two millimeters was measured in one (2.2%) hip, 10 years after surgery. This patient did not show femoral lysis or any of the other changes discussed in the text.

At the present time lysis of the femur and/or acetabulum is one of the most common complications in total hip arthroplasty, both in cemented as well as non-cemented types. The concept of creating a physiologically constructed mechanical barrier against femoral migration of debris from the polyethylene and metal acetabular components came from the recognition of the well-accepted belief that debris was responsible for the production of lytic changes that may accompany total hip implants. We were aware of efforts to overcome the problem through the use of noncemented implants that attempt to seal the "mouth" of the proximal femur. However, we extrapolated that no matter how tightly a non-cemented prosthesis fits the medullary canal it cannot prevent the migration of microscopic particles of metal or polyethylene debris, particularly in light of the fact that bone ingrowth does not take place throughout the entire porous surface. This extrapolation is supported by the fact that noncemented prostheses have not eliminated bone lysis. In the case of cemented implants, perfect contact of cement with the endosteal surface of the femur is probably never obtained. It is likely that the temporary devascuralization of the endosteum from the mechanical and thermic injury created at the time of surgery might leave a "gap" thought which debris can seep distally. The incidence of femoral lysis in total hip replacement has been reported to range between 5% and 15%. On several previous occasions the senior author (AS) had replaced temporarily created "windows" made in the femur in order to remove cement and implants that had failed. Rather than fastening the bony fragment with wires or cables upon completion of the surgical procedure, he chose to press the removed fragment over the still polymerizing cement. The stability obtained was thought to be good. The fragment healed against the host femur in all instances (Figs 28.1A to D).

The possibility of obtaining a similar response when bone graft was pressed over polymerizing cement around a prosthetic implant attracted my attention. Since we were not in position to reproduce the technique in the hip of experimental animals we performed windows in the shaft of anaesthetized sheep, where their medullary canals had been filled with a metal rod and acrylic cement, over which bone chips were pressed prior to complete polymerization (Figs 28.2 and 28.3). Specimens obtained demonstrated incorporation of the

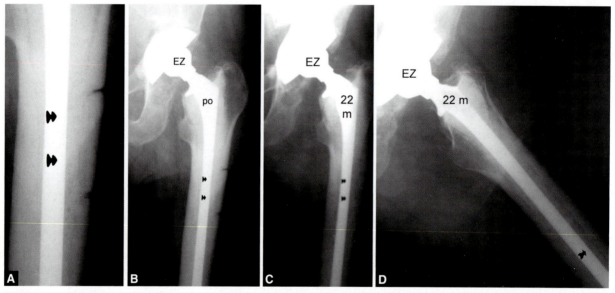

FIGS 28.1A TO D

(A) Radiograph illustrating the replacement of a window made for removal of cement during a revision arthroplasty. The bony window was pressed against the soft polymerizing cement. When complete polymerization took place the window was solidly fixed against the cement and in contact with the femoral cortex. (B) Radiograph showing the entire prosthesis and the replaced window immediately after surgery. (C and D) Radiograph obtained 22 weeks after surgery. It appears that the bony window has incorporated with the femoral cortex

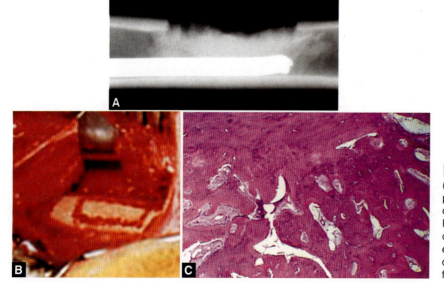

FIGS 28.2A TO C

(A) Radiograph illustrating the technique of placing bone graft over the polymerizing cement in an experimental sheep. (B) Photograph after the application of the graft over the polymerizing cement in the experimental sheep. (C) Histological demonstration of the junction between the femoral cortex and the graft

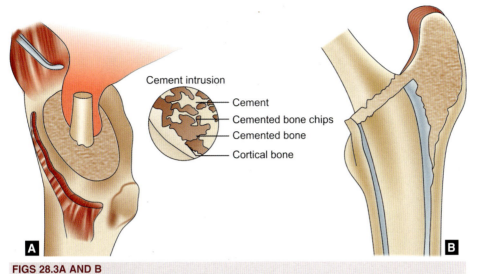

FIGS 28.3A AND B

Drawing depicting the pressing of bone graft on the still soft polymerizing cement at the mouth of the prosthesis. The fully polymerized cement holds the graft in place. The graft must be in close contact with the cortical bone of the femur. It is important to ascertain that all the bone chips are in contact with acrylic cement, for otherwise the non-cemented chips can easily fall into the joint

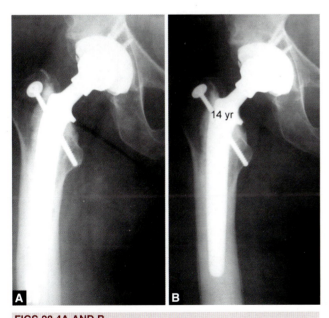

FIGS 28.4A AND B

(A) Radiograph taken immediately after surgery, during which bone graft was placed over the polymerizing cement at the mouth of the femoral canal. (B) Radiograph obtained 14 years after surgery. A titanium alloy implant was used

bone fragment with the surrounding femoral bone, in the same manner we had observed in clinical practice. The use of newly developed polyethylenes is expected to further improve the wear properties of the materials in vivo. However, sufficient time has not yet elapsed to conclude their superiority. If results from the new polyethylenes prove to be superior, the incidence of lysis will further decrease even some debris will continue to be produced. If the system we have developed provides the anticipated biological/mechanical seal, femoral lysis produced by debris should be further reduced. Questions remain concerning the fate of the bony acetabulum, since the procedure does not offer any protection to this component. However, none of our patients had shown thus far evidence of acetabular lysis. The virtual absence of lysis or bone/cement radiolucent lines in this small series composed of Titanium and Cobalt-Chrome alloys suggests the possibility that the bone graft incorporates with the viable femoral cortex, creating therefore a mechanical/physiological barrier to debris, which necessarily is generated from the acetabular polyethylene liners and metallic components. It is recognized that not enough time has elapsed to justify claims of success with the proposed technique, or that the possibility exists that the same results could have been obtained if the grafts had not been used (Figs 28.4 to 28.14).

Although CT scans have not clearly confirmed the survival of the graft because of the close proximity of the graft to the metallic stem, plain radiographs have on occasion shown the bony lid.

Hip Surgery

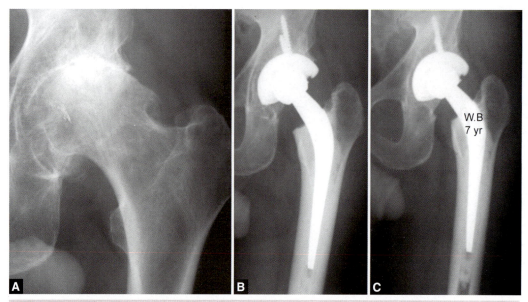

FIGS 28.5A TO C

(A) Radiographs of osteoarthritic hip in a 70-year-old man. (B and C)) Radiographs taken postoperatively and 7 years later respectively. Notice the rounding of the calcar

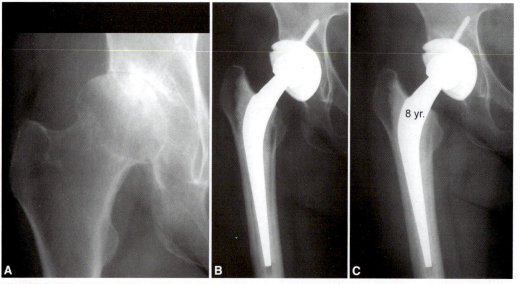

FIGS 28.6A TO C

(A) Osteoarthritic hip of a 70-year-old woman. (B and C) Radiographs taken immediately after surgery and at 8 years later respectively. A cobalt/chrome implant was used

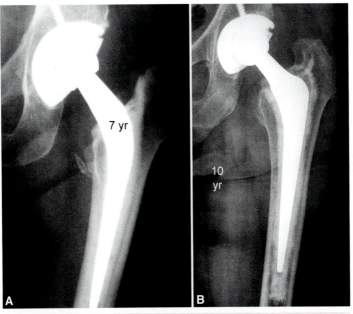

FIGS 28.7A AND B

(A) Radiographs obtained 7 years after surgery. Notice the bone graft placed over the proximal cement. (B) Radiograph taken 10 years postoperatively. The bone graft has not changed in its density

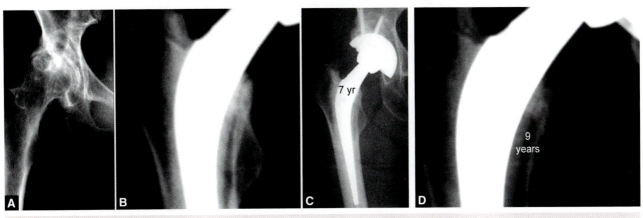

FIGS 28.8A TO D

(A and B) Radiographs taken immediately after surgery. Notice the prominent graft and a loose bony fragment medially. (C) Radiograph obtained 7 years later. (D) Radiograph taken 9 years postoperatively. A titanium alloy was used

Section 1

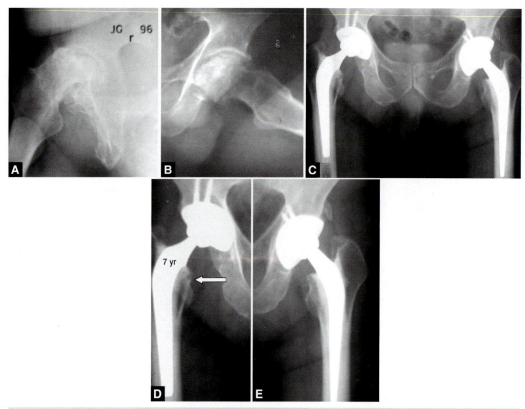

FIGS 28.9A TO E

(A to C) Radiographs of bilateral hip arthritis. (D to E) The 2 hips were replaced with two different cobalt/chrome stems. The cement/graft procedure was performed in the left hip only. Radiographs obtained 7 years posoperatively. Notice the wide radiolucent line on zone VII in the right hip

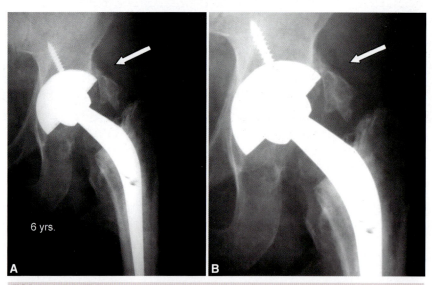

FIGS 28.10A AND B

Radiographs of arthroplasty in the left hip performed 6 years earlier. It appears that the observed ossified intracapsular fragments are an expression of bone chips that fell off after being pressed against the acrylic cement. It supports the view that only one layer of bone should pressed against cement and cortical bone

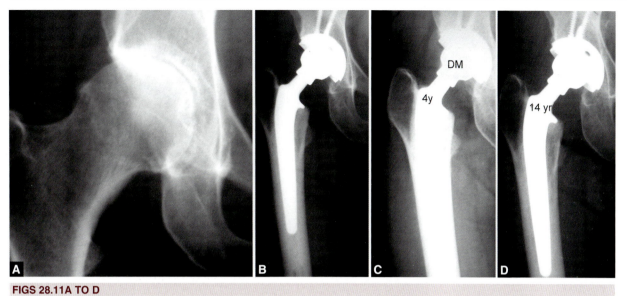

FIGS 28.11A TO D

(A) Preoperative radiograph of osteoarthritic hip in a 57-year-old woman. (B) Radiograph taken shortly after surgery of a total hip made of titanium alloy stem with a cobalt/chrome head. (C) Radiograph taken 4 years postoperatively. (D) Radiograph obtained 14 years later

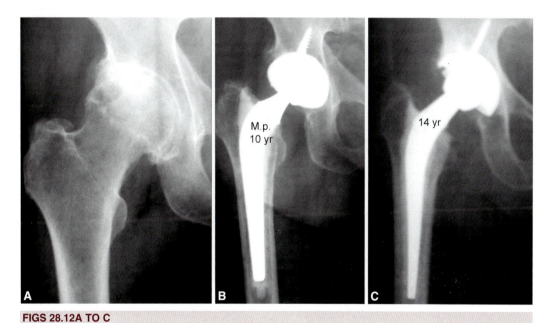

FIGS 28.12A TO C

(A) Radiograph of osteoarthritic hip of a 61-year-old woman. (B and C) Radiographs obtained immediately 10 and 14 years postoperatively. A titanium monoblock prosthesis was used

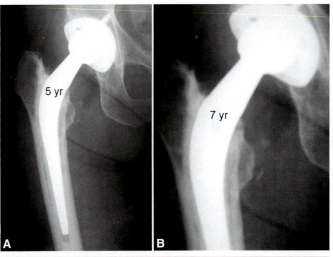

FIGS 28.13A AND B

Radiographs taken 5 and 7 years after surgery respectively. Notice the bony fragments medially

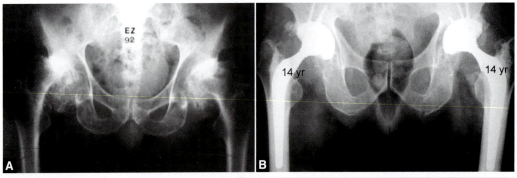

FIGS 28.14A AND B

(A) Radiograph of bilateral osteoarthritis in a 70-year-old man. (B) Radiographs of replaced hips using titanium alloy stems with cobalt/chrome heads taken 14 years postoperatively showing mild resorption of the calcar of the right hip

*Reference**

111

---

* Reference provided at the end of the book after annexures.

29

Acetabular Lysis

My personal experience with surgery in cases of acetabular lysis is limited. I have seen it in a number of instances (Fig. 29.1), but have approached the situation by surgical means in only a few patients (Figs 29.2 to 29.5) believing that the problem was not severe enough in most of them. I suspect that pain from acetabular lysis with modern prostheses is not a frequent finding and that the progression of the pathological process advances more slowly than femoral lysis.

Needless to say, large defects or rapidly increasing defects need to be handled surgically before the problem becomes a major one due to the loss of acetabular floor that would make the eventual surgical reconstruction a very difficult undertaking.

In recent days experiences with Tantalum, as the concavity of the acetabular cup, have suggested significant improvement in the density of the acetabulum surrounding the implant when compared with the more traditional Titanium alloy cup. The use of Tantalum, as a preferred metal is based to a great extent on its different modulus of elasticity. Though, enthusiastic about this work, I remain cautious, because it was the same concept that led me to introduce Titanium in hip surgery in the mid-seventies. I had surmised that some of the abnormal changes we were seeing with stiffer implants in the medullary canal could be eliminated with implants made of a material with a lower modulus of elasticity. Time proved me wrong, and have deeply regretted the Titanium experience. Is it possible that similar disappointment may be encountered after the Tantalum implants are used for a longer period of time?

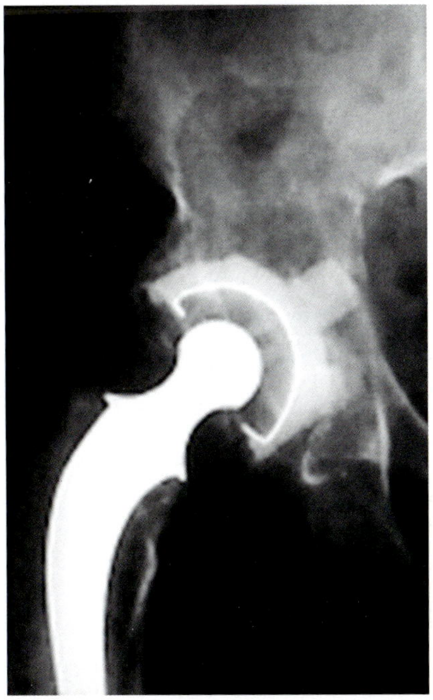

FIG. 29.1

Radiograph demonstrating lysis of the acetabulum from an early Charnley prosthesis. I suspect this is an example of a Teflon liner since I took this photograph from his file in 1970

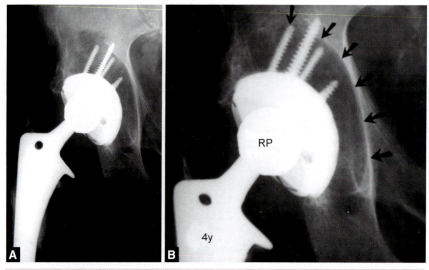

FIGS 29.2A AND B

Radiograph suggesting acetabular lysis from a noncemented Harris-Galante prosthesis. I did not intervene surgically because the patient was asymptomatic. He expired a couple of years later still without symptoms

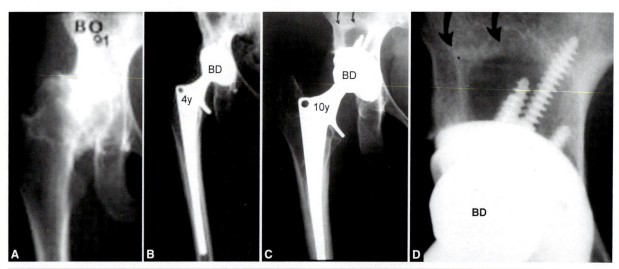

FIGS 29.3A TO D

(A) Radiograph of osteoarthritic hip in a 39-year-old woman. (B) Postoperative radiograph illustrating what appeared to be an appropriately performed arthroplasty. (C and D) Radiographs obtained 10 years postoperatively demonstrating acetabular lysis. She had become minimally symptomatic. I recommended surgery, which had been performed at another institution closer to her home. It is my understanding she did well

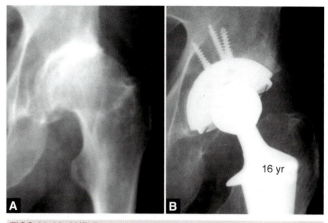

FIGS 29.4A AND B

(A) Preoperative radiograph of osteoarthritic hip in a 43-year-old man. (B) Radiograph obtained 16 years postoperatively showing no evidence of lysis. It is likely the apparent lysis suspected on the 8th postoperative year was osteoporosis that subsided with time. The patient is asymptomatic and has remained very active

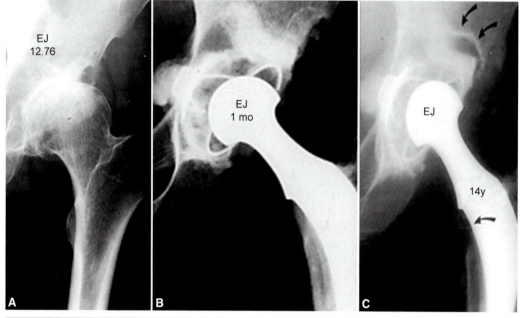

FIGS 29.5A TO C

(A) Preoperative radiograph of the arthritic hip in a 65-year-old woman. (B) Radiograph obtained shortly after surgery. (C) Radiograph taken 14 years postoperatively. Notice the lytic lesion in the acetabulum and the minimal wear of the polyethylene

*References**

36, 50, 54, 57, 70, 72, 81, 104

_____

* References provided at the end of the book after annexures.

Section 1

30

Late Onset of Thigh Pain

The incidence of pain following non-cemented total hip prostheses has decreased as newer implants have been developed. There was a time when thigh pain was identified in a large percentage of patients. The pain subsided in many instances, but several months of discomfort was a common finding. The cause of the pain that appears shortly after surgery is still unknown in some instances, particularly when all radiological and other clinical findings are negative. Early thigh pain was seldom, as far as I am concerned, a feature following cemented arthroplasties. This should be kept in mind as we ponder on the etiology of the painful condition.

It has been suggested that the pain is due to irritation of nerve endings opposite to the tip end of the prosthetic implant. Interesting histological pictures have shown strong evidence to support the thesis. The mechanism to explain the onset and some times spontaneous disappearance of the symptoms has not been offered.

There is another type of thigh pain whose etiology interests me more. That is the pain that appears years after the insertion of a prosthesis. The pain, opposite to the end of the implant, can be explained on the basis of loosening, which can be documented with X-rays. Other times, from lytic lesions at that level, produced by reaction to plastic or metallic debris.

These explanations seem to satisfy the vast majority of situations, however, I have seen on several occasions, patients where loosening of the implant was suspected, however, to find out at the time of an attempted revision procedure, that the porous prosthesis was solidly anchored in place. In those instances I had been able to reproduce the pain by pressing manually over the area identified by the patient as being the painful one.

In those instances, careful observation of radiographs obtained prior to the onset of pain had demonstrated a gradual decrease in the space between the distal end of the prosthesis and the lateral femoral cortex. This varus attitude was accompanied with sclerotic lines parallel to the distal stem, suggesting that the implant was loose in the medullary canal. However, I noticed that the sclerotic lines did not always extend above the middle-third of the prosthesis, as it should have been the case if the prosthesis was loose. The tell-tale of a pendulum motion would have shown the lines extending throughout the entire length of the stem, since not only the distal end of the stem moves; the proximal end also moves. It is logical to assume that if the stem is moving like a wind-shield wiper, the sclerotic lines would extend in declining degrees from distally to proximally, but nonetheless present throughout.

In several of those instances, I saw radiological signs indicating that the implant was solidly fixed in the femoral canal, as depicted by the identification of "welding spots" at the end of the porous surface of the implant. Furthermore, the implants, proximally, seemed to be tightly held by the surrounding femoral cortex (Figs 30.1A to G).

Several times attempts to revise the implants were unsuccessfully, since the femoral components were found to be solidly fixed. I elected at that time to apply a thick cortical tibial graft spanning the distal end of the prosthesis. The grafts were held in place with circular cables or wires. Pain subsided in all instances.

I have concluded that the displacement of the distal stem toward the lateral cortex may not always be due to stem loosening but to gradual bending of the femur secondary to the significant difference in the modulus of elasticity between the bone and the metallic implant. The bending probably produces microfractures that create the pain. The gradual bending is a form of cold flow. The addition of a very stiff cortical graft increases the stiffness of the

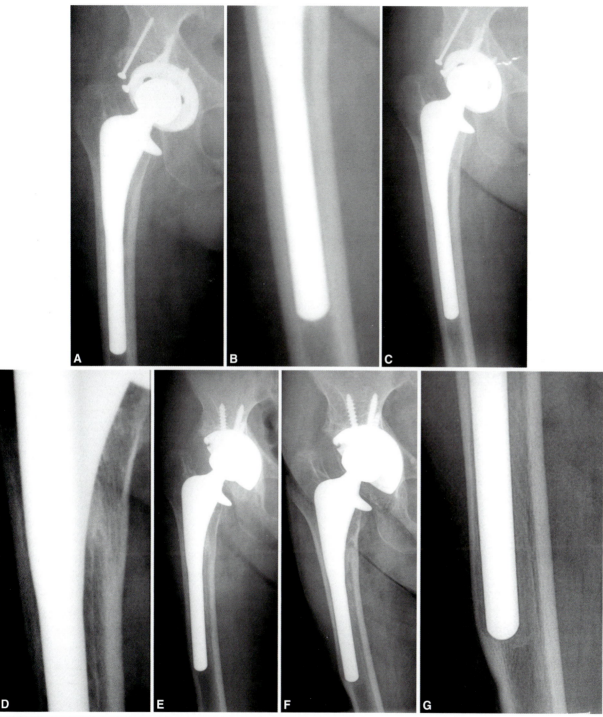

FIGS 30.1A TO G

(A) Early radiograph showing the tight fit of the stem distally. (B) Closer view showing the tight fit distally. (C) Early signs of early varus shift of the prosthesis. (D) Closer view shows the increased varus attitude of the prosthesis. Radiograph illustrating the welding spot medially at the level of the distal end of the porous patch. This indicates that bone ingrowth has taken place. (E) Attempts to remove the implant were unsuccessful. The acetabular component was replaced. Two years later the narrowing of the lateral cortex distally is obvious. (F and G) Five years later the gap between the medial wall of the femur and the prosthesis has increased, and the lateral cortex has become thinner. Pain at the level of the distal end of the prosthesis is oftentimes severe. For reasons related to a family situation she has elected not to have surgery yet

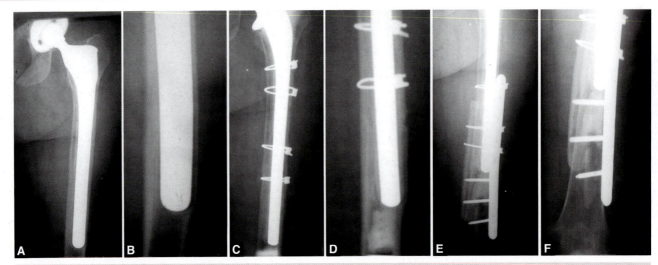

FIGS 30.2A TO F

(A) Radiographs of noncemented arthroplasty which was allegedly performed to relieve pain from a previous cemented arthroplasty that failed "because the stem was too short". The thigh pain she experienced persisted. (B) Radiograph showing what appeared to be a distal drift of the stem laterally. (C) Radiographs taken after revision with cement. At the time of surgery the cementless stem was solidly fixed to the femur. Bone ingrowth into the porous surface had taken place. The removal of the prosthesis required a Wagner, extensive trochanteric osteotomy. (D) Two years later the pain, opposite the end of the prosthesis, returned. A similar lateral displacement of the stem toward the femoral cortex was taking place. The pain had become incapacitating. (E and F) Surgery was performed revealing a fracture of the lateral cortex and protrusion of the tip end of the prosthesis at that level. In order to stabilize the facture and to stiffen the femur at that level a plate and a cortical bone graft were attached to the femur. The symptoms improved considerably but never completely disappeared. She was an elderly osteoporotic lady with multiple musculoskeletal problems, including a total knee replacement on the same side

femur at that level stopping the micro-fractures from occurring again.

The next patient was a woman in her mid-seventies who had had a revision of a painful replacement , allegedly because the "stem was too short". When I assumed her care I noticed the lateral drift of the stem toward the lateral wall of the femur. The implant was loose. I revised the prosthesis with a cemented implant. The pain persisted. I then proceeded to place a plate laterally and a cortical bone graft medially. The drifting was stopped and the pain was significantly improved (Figs 30.2A to F).

In the below-pictured instance, the pain was present in a patient 10 years after the original surgical intervention. The radiographs showed a lytic lesion opposite to the end of the implant (Figs 30.3A to F). Anticipating the pain was due to loosening, associated with polyethylene debris, revision arthroplasty was planned. At the time of surgery, I discovered that the prosthesis was solidly fixed to the bone. Having failed to remove the implant after multiple forceful blows to the implant, and concerned that perhaps inadequate exposure was responsible for my failure, I osteotomized the greater trochanter. The step did not resolve the problem. Porous ingrowth had taken place. Therefore, an alternative solution I considered, was the performance of an extended Wagner trochanteric

osteotomy. Having had previous successful experiences with the application of a bony strut over a varus-displacing prosthesis, I chose to carry-out a similar procedure. The pain disappeared, and the graft readily incorporated into the body of the femur. Twelve years later radiographs continued to show no evidence of recurrence of the lytic lesion or thigh pain. Needless to say, this instance is not similar to the one described above because in this case lysis was readily seen around the distal stem. The fact that pain disappeared following the stiffening of the distal femur speaks in favor of the possibility that difference in the modulus of elasticity between the femur and implant, made worse by the lytic defect, causing the local mechanical changes may be responsible for the onset of late pain.

The next example (Figs 30.4A to E) is similar to the one described above. It is the case of a forty-seven years old woman who developed thigh pain seven years post-operatively. Suspecting loosening of the implant, a surgeon in another city unsuccessfully attempted to revise the implant. He found the stem solidly fixed to the femoral walls. I personally made a similar attempt with an equal degree of failure. I proceeded to reinforce the femur with a thick cortical graft. Seven years later the pain had remained absent and the graft seemed to be fully incorporated.

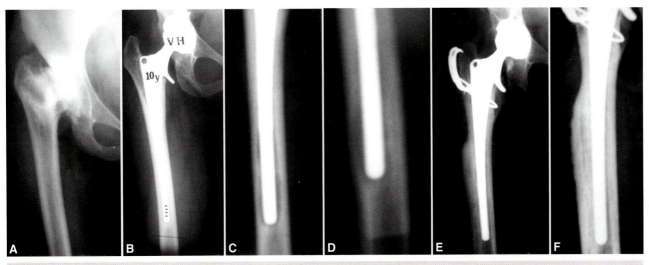

FIGS 30.3A TO F

(A) Osteoarthritis secondary to congenital hip dysplasia. (B) Radiograph obtained ten years after surgery showing tight fit of the distal stem against the femoral cortex. (C) Radiograph taken 12 years postoperatively depicting lysis around the distal stem. Notice that a tight fit has been maintained proximally. (D) Closer view of the distal stem and lytic changes at that level. (E) Radiograph obtained seven years after surgery demonstrating complete incorporation of the graft with the body of the femur. (F) Radiograph obtained 14 years postoperatively. The patient has remained asymptomatic

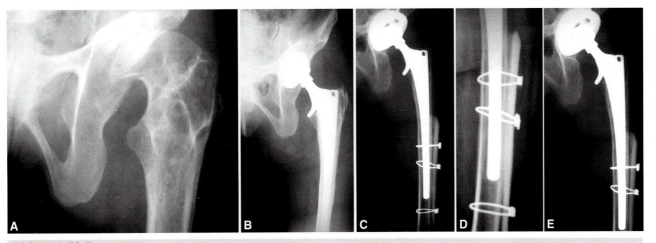

FIGS 30.4A TO E

(A and B) Radiograph of a total hip noncemented arthroplasty in a 43-year-old woman who developed thigh pain seven years post-operatively. The stem showed signs of loosening as depicted by the sclerotic lines around the stem distally. An attempt was made by another surgeon to remove the femoral component, but who found impossible to remove what appeared to be a solidly anchored implant. The thigh pain continued. Notice the tight fit of the prosthesis in the canal proximally. (C) I then performed a cortical bone grafting of the femur opposite to the distal end of the prosthesis where the pain was. (D and E) Radiographs obtained six months and five years postoperatively. The thigh pain disappeared

These observations and clinical experiences have let me to conclude that: *(1) The varus attitude of the femoral component in a total hip replacement is not always due to its loosening but maybe to a gradual bending of the bone in a varus direction.* The difference in the stiffness between the bone and the implant—the implant being stiffer- makes the gradual deformity of the bone possible. (2) A symptomatic lytic lesion at the opposite end of the implant, probably the result of a chemical reaction to debris, may be explained in some instances on similar mechanical grounds. However, this latter

explanation in itself, does not preclude the possibility that a varus force at the distal stem was precipitated by a rather sudden reduction in the stiffness of the bone at that level. It is my impression that lytic defects in the femur, away from the distal end of the implant are rarely painful. We see patients who are lost to regular follow-up visits following surgery, who many years later appear in the office complaining of pain. The radiographs demonstrate severe, wide-spread lysis, indicating that the lytic lesions had been present, but asymptomatic for a long period of time. On the other

Section 1

hand, if the lytic defects develop distally, at the level of the distal end of the stem, pain usually develops at an earlier date. As stated earlier, it is likely that the lytic defect weakened the bone at that level, permitting the creation of progressive microfractures, with subsequent bending of the bone in a varus direction.

It is probably not an unreasonable leap of faith to extrapolate that in some instances the varus loosening of cemented stems may be the result of a similar mechanical change at the level of the distal stem, bringing about softening of the bone and the resulting varus bending of the femur. I have suspected that the described mode of failure is more likely to occur in osteoporotic bones, particularly in elderly individuals, whose bones have lost the elasticity that goes along with aging.

Section 2

Specific Pathological Conditions

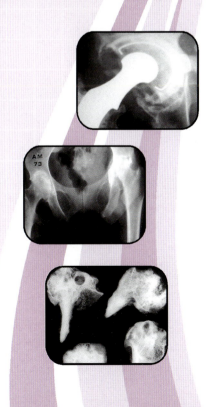

31

The Osteoarthritic Hip

John Charnley was my visiting professor at the University of Miami in 1974. While at the podium answering questions from the audience, I asked him to give us his views on whether or not some day arthritis will be preventable, or if a nonsurgical cure will be developed. Without the slightest hesitation he responded, "Never, never will there be an effective preventive measure for osteoarthritis. Osteoarthritis has been in our genes for many a millennia and it will be with us forever". He added that the same was not true for rheumatoid arthritis and that a cure for it was around the corner.

Five years later he, once again, served as my visiting professor at the University of Southern California, where I had an opportunity to ask him the same question I had asked him in Miami. His response was the same. It would have been wonderful if we had had the opportunity to ask him those questions today, when rumors of the identification of the gene that causes osteoarthritis are rampant and new medications claiming "cures" are inundating the market. Charley was right in the incredible number of issues he addressed. Perhaps this is one where he was mistaken by underestimating the forces of molecular biology and genetic engineering.

At this time our understanding of the etiology of osteoarthritis is limited. However, there are certain obvious factors that in themselves carry a great deal of weight. In the case of the hip, a shallow acetabulum is believed to predispose to the disease. This is difficult to refute. Nonetheless, how do we explain the fact that very often one hip develops arthritic changes when the shallowness of the acetabulum is equal in both hips? A mechanical explanation in this instance does not suffice.

I will now share with the readers an observation perhaps worthy of consideration. In many instances I have noticed that in the process of removing the femoral head in order to insert an endoprosthesis or a total hip implant performed following an *acute fracture of the femoral neck*, difficulties are encountered as a result of a strong ligamentum teres, requiring its section with a sharp instrument. Observation of the severed ligament oftentimes shows mild bleeding. This observation runs contrary to the popular belief that after completion of growth the blood supply coming through the ligament ceases to exist. In addition, On the other hand, I have noticed that when *the prosthetic replacement is done for the treatment of osteoarthritis*, particular if it is advanced, in the overwhelming majority of instances the ligamentum teres is no longer a barrier to the removal or the femoral head. As a matter of fact, quite often is no longer present.

These observations beg the question as to whether there is relationship between the underlying arthritic process and the condition of the ligamentum teres. What comes first, the chicken or the egg? Is there a connection between the two entities? Does the damage of the ligament contribute to the arthritic process or the arthritic process brings about damage to the ligament? Although of no practical importance, a scientific answer would be welcome.

Reinhold Ganz, from Switzerland, has recently popularized the idea that a common cause of arthritis is "chronic" impingement of the neck of the femur against the labrum during flexion/rotation of the hip. Questions remain about the long-term validity of his observations (See *Acetabular Labrum*).

Now that total joint replacement has been proven to be an effective means to restore relief to the osteoarthritic hip and knee, many have benefited from the surgical interventions. Questions linger, however, as to when to replace an osteoarthritic hip. I have struggled hundreds of times making recommendations to patients regarding the most appropriate course of action. The struggle comes from the fact that we cannot predict with certainty the course of the nonsurgically treated disease. This is particularly true for the adult patient with congenital hip dysplasia. In this instance, I am convinced that in the absence of a radiologically "perfect" relationship between the femoral head and acetabulum following closed or open reduction, with or without additional reconstructive surgery, arthritic changes are very likely to develop at a later date.

The exaggerated division of orthopaedic care into subspecialty areas has precluded a serious study of the sequella of congenital hip disease, as well as other diseases suffered early in life. The pediatric orthopedist stops seeing his patients when they reach the arbitrary age of 16 or 21 years of age. In general, they are not personally aware of late complications, and find themselves often reporting unrealistically good results. Children frequently manage to function normally and be asymptomatic during childhood and adolescence, despite the presence of deformities of the hip and other joints. It is not until they reach late adulthood that symptoms develop. I am of the opinion that if the pediatric orthopedists were better aware of the late sequella, a different approach to many musculoskeletal conditions in children could be structured.

I suspect that a better system must be developed. The Shrines Hospital system is coming closer to finding a possible solution, by virtue of the fact that, to the best of my knowledge, there are no rigid age limitations. Orthopedic investigators at the University of Iowa, where a good percentage of the patient population is local and rather stable, has been able to conduct long term studies of congenital and developmental diseases. It would be great if other institutions were to follow suit. Doctor Valentin Malagon, a most distinguished professor of orthopedics in Colombia, internationally recognized as an authority in congenital hip disease, has published a book where he deals with the disease "from the cradle to old age". His book represents a major contribution to the field.

John Charnley used to say that when a patient presents complaining of mild pain in the groin and the X-rays show early narrowing of the joint, within five years the condition would deteriorate to the point of requiring arthroplasty. Ever since I came back to America after my brief stay at his institution in England, I have tried to determine if the same pattern exists in America. I have found out that the Americans, in general, end up in surgery a lot earlier. They are not as willing to wait as long as their British counterparts.

I vividly recall Sir John Charnley telling patients who came into his clinic with obvious arthritis of the hip, limping and admitting the taking of some medication to control pain, "Go home; get yourself a cane and carry one; come back in a year". When I heard him say that to a few patients I could not understand his reasoning and thought that such an approach in the United States would be considered unkind and illogical. Further consideration made me conclude that what he was doing was to remain faithful to his firm belief that replacement arthroplasty should be offered only to those who really need it and that it should not always be the first option. If taking pain pills and using a cane provide relief, those measures should be taken first. He was keenly aware of the still experimental nature of the procedure and was not altogether sure that the artificial hip would last more than thirty years in the very active individual. *Furthermore, he knew that osteoarthritic patients frequently experience periods of exacerbation and remission. Many times, the disease process "burns out" and disabling symptoms virtually disappear.*

I have tempered the temptation to operate on many occasions by remembering that there are exceptions to the rule and that not everyone with mild osteoarthritis of the hip requires surgery three to five years later. I have seen patients who have gone a lot longer without aggravation of symptoms. *Patients with bilateral osteoarthritis, who had one hip replaced and obtained good clinical results, often find themselves complaining very little about pain on the opposite arthritic hip. I wonder if there is some chemical factor that explains this phenomenon.* I have made the same observation while dealing with rheumatoid patients.

Another reason for not performing the prosthetic replacement early is that we cannot guarantee a good clinical result, despite the relative predictability of the operation. Complications following surgery can and do occur in a percentage of instances. If one adds to the very low incidence of infection, nerve palsy, dislocation, heterotopic bone, thromboembolic disease in its various manifestations, early loosening, subsequent revisions and other problems, one must conclude that replacement arthroplasty should not be taken lightly.

I must admit, however, that my attitude about the issue of when to operate on a painful, osteoarthritic patient has changed, as I have been able to observe that the prognosis following total replacement has gotten so much better and the complication rate has been reduced rather dramatically. *That being the case, how can the orthopedic surgeon tell an individual with mild radiological osteoarthritis, but with disabling symptoms, to postpone the surgery for another year or more? Does that advice make sense? What is it to be gained from spending another year in pain when in fact the operation will be performed in another year or two?*

The etiology of osteoarthritis continues to elude us, which to some extent explains the pessimism expressed by Sir John Charnley, which I discussed at the beginning of this chapter. Trueta, from Oxford, in my opinion, conducted very elegant and persuasive work dealing with the pathology of osteoarthritis and the circulation of the femoral head. He made impressive observations. *The one which has been indelibly stereotyped in my mind, is his observation that the narrowing of the joint space of the hip in idiopathic osteoarthritis, as we see it in radiographs, is not in all instances the result of wear of the articular cartilage, rather its replacement with bone growing from the subchondral region. This bony substitution gives the radiological appearance of cartilage erosion from wear against the opposing acetabular surface.*

I suspect it would be wrong to conclude that all "osteoarthritic joints" are the result of ossification of the cartilage from vessels that grow from the subchondral bone. *Nonetheless, it is probably the most common explanation in the case of the truly idiopathic type of osteoarthritis.* I do not find it difficult to picture an intraarticular fracture leading to osteoarthritis at a later date due to bone growth into the cartilage from the subchondral bone. Likewise, the constant friction between two rough surfaces, as in the case of a fracture, could lead to osteoarthritis through a mechanical mode.

Osteoarthritis can develop from a violent impaction force over normal cartilage that produces—as it has been proven in laboratory studies—where subchondral bone replaces the damaged cartilage. The frequent picture of late radiological arthritic changes seeing following Colles fractures (impaction fractures) supports this view. Our obsession with mechanics and our desire to explain everything on mechanical bases has blinded us in more than one occasion. This is true in most areas of orthopedics, be it in fracture care, prosthetic replacement, spine surgery and many

others. Hopefully, the day will come when orthopedists will reason with greater emphasis on biological basis.

I am hesitant to discuss recent work done regarding cartilage transplant or the placing of chondrocytes at the level of the damaged cartilage. I question of we have made any further progress since Pap, from Hungary, did his work back in the 1960s. My knowledge in this area is minimal. Nonetheless I am skeptical, based on the reading of the literature on the subject.

I do not wish to leave out completely the nonsurgical measures that can be taken regarding the role that oral medications and intra-articular injections play in the management of osteoarthritis. Unfortunately I do not possess the necessary knowledge to intelligently render an educated opinion. However, I have dealt with many arthritic patients that I treated nonsurgically and had the opportunity to observe their response to the nonsurgical modalities I had prescribed. In addition, I had the opportunity to know and observe the work of several rheumatologists from whom I have the greatest respect. From them I have learned a great deal.

In recent years we have witnessed in the United States a series of scandals dealing with the usage of nonsteroidal analgesics that claimed spectacular long-lasting good results in the care of osteoarthritis. It has been documented that some of these drugs, such as Vioox, are responsible for a high number of cardiac problem, of which the manufactures of the products were aware but failed to acknowledge. The news of this development did not surprise me at all, since the overall conduct of the pharmaceutical industry has been seriously tarnished for a long time. A huge percentage of medications advertise to help, if not to totally eliminate arthritis, are nothing but nostrums, false panaceas, with no value whatsoever to the patients, only to the their manufactures. The problem has been further aggravated by the more recent practice of direct industry advertisement to patients through television. The promotion of products through such a medium has been most effective, as patients literally demand from doctors' prescription of medications of unproven or dangerous properties.

Something similar can be said about the use of intra-articular injections, which when abused can do harm and in some instances deprive patients of the benefit of surgical treatments that may be clearly indicated. I suspect that the indiscriminate use of intra-articular injections must be tempered and placed in its proper place. The problem is that the practice is a very lucrative one for the physicians, since many patients, unaware of other options, continue to return to their offices seeking the temporary relief the injections provide.

We have witnessed during the past yew years the wide use of orally ingested chondroitin sulphate and glucosamine. The oral medication has been advertised as if it were a miracle drug. *However, prospective, randomized, placebo-controlled studies have indicated that placebos are equally as effective.*

One of the most abused medical modalities carried out in the United States at this time following hip replacement is prolonged rehabilitation therapy, particularly in the form of physical therapy. This practice is so pervasive that failure to prescribe it is, in the eyes of patients, tantamount to poor practice. They expect it and demand it under virtually all circumstances. In a number of occasions I have "lost" patients to other surgeons, on whom I had planned to operate, because they had "learned" that I did not routinely prescribed prolonged supervised physical therapy following hip replacement arthroplasty. The fact is that most such patients receive the necessary physical therapy treatment while in the hospital, and go home within a few days independent and well informed regarding the necessary precautions and progressive activities. *They want the expensive daily visit to the physical therapy facility where they carry out the same exercises they, unsupervised, can perform at home. This trend has serious economic implications that need to be addressed.*

It is commonly believed that muscle strengthening exercises are helpful in slowing the progression of osteoarthritis of the hip or knee. Many patients acknowledge improvement, and rightly so. I wonder, however about the mechanism that leads to the perceived improvement, *as I ask myself how a stronger muscle improves the condition of an arthritic joint. I have concluded, rightly or wrongly, that it is not the muscle strengthening that appears to be helpful, but the prevention or correction of limitation of joint motion that is achieved in the process of strengthening muscles. Therefore, the greatest benefit is gained by preventing and fighting the ubiquitous stiffness of the joint and correcting early contractures.*

I have noticed orthopedic residents, as well as physical therapists, advising arthritic patients on the conduct of exercises emphasizing the benefits of bicycle riding. *Though I see no harm in doing such an exercise, the pedaling of the vehicle does not subject the affected hip or knee joint to reaching maximum flexion and extension, which is after all what is needed.* For whatever reasons, the individual developing osteoarthritis of these joints, first experience stiffness and then pain upon the initiation of function. Subconsciously, they avoid the motions and the degrees of motion to which the affected joist respond with pain.

In the case of the hip joint, the first motion that is lost is and later becomes a permanent feature, is internal rotation. *I do not think that the absent internal rotation is due to a special pathology affecting that motion, only that internal rotation is the motion the hip joint needs the least.* Therefore, unintentionally the early arthritic avoids that motion. Avoiding other motions is more difficult than for example, flexion of the hip. The sitting position forces the maintenance of hip flexion, explaining why flexion is the last motion to be lost. To a lesser degree is external rotation, a motion that is essential for normal walking, and a motion that is reinforced by virtue of the fact that at heel strike the extremity is forced in that direction. I have noticed that the second motion to be reduced is that of abduction, since as in the case of internal rotation, it is not needed to the same degree as flexion of the hip.

Bony spurs are frequently found in the osteoarthritic hip joint. It is commonly believed that the spurs are responsible for the limitation of rotation of the hip. I do not think this is true from the outset. The spurs are not the case of limitation in the early stages of the disease. They form at a later date and then perpetuate the limitation of motion. The spurs are the result of traction on the bone at the level of the attachment of the capsule. The stiffness produced by the inflammatory arthritic process results in a loss of elasticity of the capsule. Any voluntary or involuntary rotational motions further place tension on the inelastic capsule, pulling on the bone, and then creating the spurs.

A comparable phenomenon occurs in the knee joint, and probably in all arthritic joints. During the early stages of the arthritic process, patients experience stiffness, and then pain, when the knee is fully flexed or extended. This explains the characteristic flexed-knee gait of the arthritic. The fact that pain occurs when the knee is forced into full flexion or extension, leads to an unconscious avoidance of such motions, creating a permanent deformity. Encouraging these patients to do bicycle exercises has only minimal benefit. The exercise increases the amount of synovial fluid and provides some temporary relief, but does not do any good in preventing or correcting permanent limitation of motion. *To accomplish such prevention or cure, the joint must be flexed and extended fully.* Although reaching those desirable degrees of motion may be uncomfortable and many times impossible at first, repeated attempts in that regard usually pay high dividends.

I have attempted to correlate the radiological changes in the osteoarthritic hip, as well as in other arthriditis, with histology and photoradiography of the excised femoral head. My efforts have been futile for the most part. The gross appearance of the head as observed with the naked eye is frequently deceiving. Sections of the head show degrees of pathology that varies tremendously from one hip to the next. The following radiological, microscopic, histological and surface photos (Figs 31.1 to 31.9) illustrate the point.

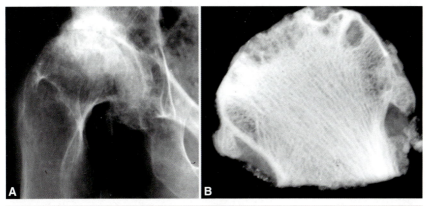

FIGS 31.1A AND B

(A) In this instance of idiopathic osteoarthritis is difficult to attribute a shallow acetabulum as the genesis of the arthritic process. (B) The cystic nature of the disease, as demonstrate in the radiomicrograph, cannot be guessed from the plain films

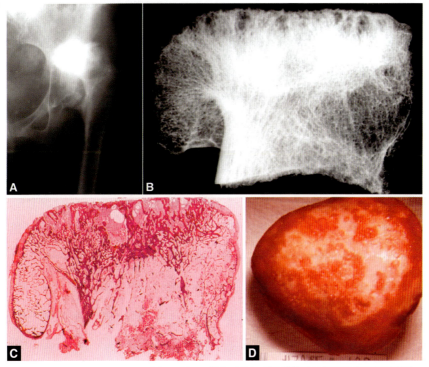

FIGS 31.2A TO D

(A) Radiograph of an osteoarthritic hip, secondary to congenial hip disease. (B) Photoradiograph of section of the femoral head illustrating multiple cysts. (C) Corresponding histological slide showing the multiple cysts. (D) The gross appearance of the removed femoral head. Notice the multiple ulcerated areas, which may be a component in the production of pain

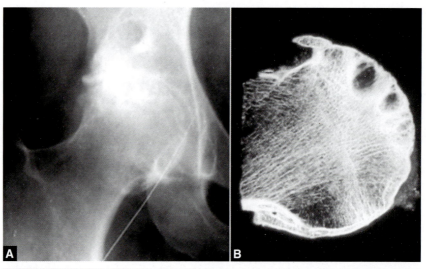

FIGS 31.3A AND B

(A) Radiological appearance of an osteoarthritic hip showing narrowing of the joint space throughout. (B) The articular cartilage seems to have been completely replaced with subchondral bone

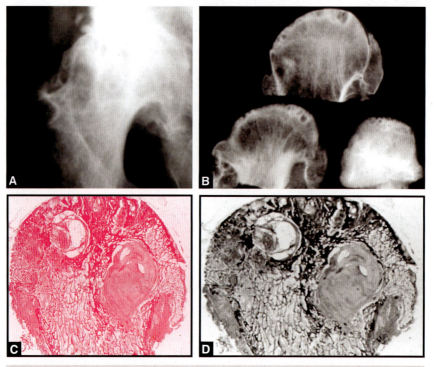

FIGS 31.4A TO D

(A) Radiograph of osteoarthritic hip in a 59-year-old man. (B) Cross-sections of the femoral head illustrating the replacement of articular cartilage with bone, the multiple cysts and the bony spurs. (C and D) Histological pictures of section of the femoral head that best illustrate the cystic changes

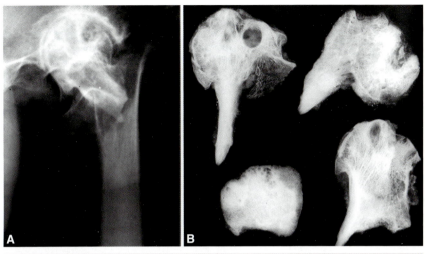

FIGS 31.5A AND B

(A) Radiograph of a base of the neck fracture that occurred to a man with existing arthritic changes. (B) Radiographs of the removed femoral head and neck illustrating the cysts and cartilage changes

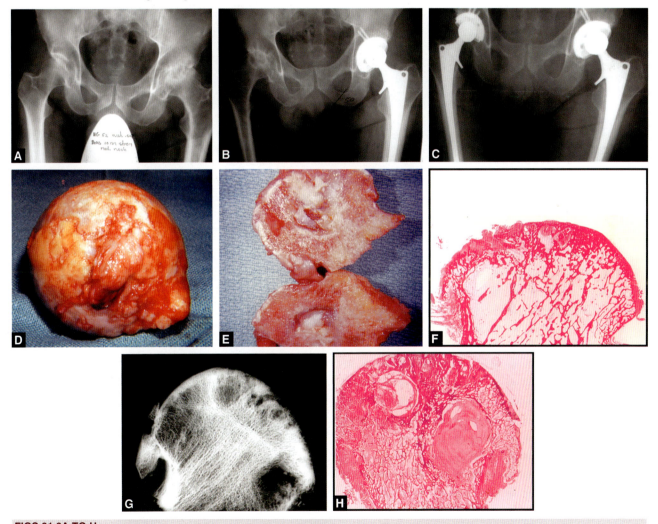

FIGS 31.6A TO H

(A) Radiograph of arthritic hips of a 49-year-old physician at the time the symptoms were becoming disabling. (B and C) Radiographs illustrating Bias noncemented prostheses. (D to G) Gross appearance of the femoral heads at the time of surgery. (H) Gross views and histological pictures of the transected femoral heads

Section 2

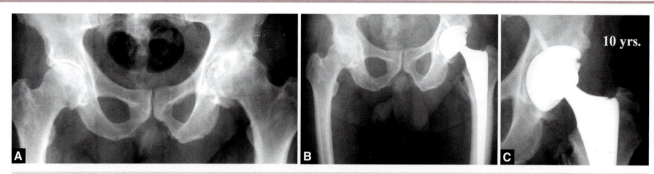

FIGS 31.7A TO C

(A) Radiograph of osteoarthritic hips with the left being symptomatic. (B) The left arthritic hip was replaced with a noncemented prosthesis. (C) Radiograph taken nine years after surgery. Notice the wear of the polyethylene liner. The right hip is minimally symptomatic

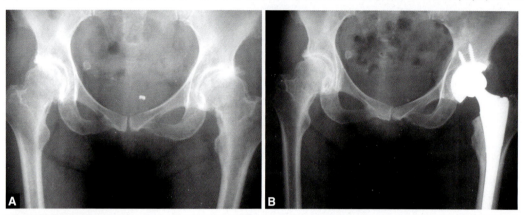

FIGS 31.8A AND B

(A) Radiograph of bilateral hip osteoarthritis in a very active 60-year-old woman with allegedly equally painful hips. (B) Radiograph obtained 5 years after surgery. The pain on the right hip improved significantly following replacement of the left hip

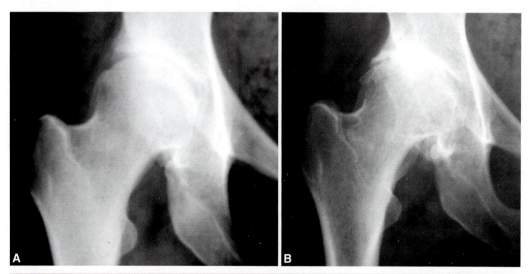

FIGS 31.9A AND B

(A) Radiograph of hip showing early osteoarthritic changes and minimal symptoms. (B) Radiograph obtained 4 years later depicting further narrowing of the joint space. The symptoms had become more incapacitating. This patient represents the most common pattern of deterioration

*References**

10, 46, 51, 52, 58, 59, 70, 76, 104, 114

---

* References provided at the end of the book after annexures.

32

The Acetabular Labrum

Very little attention was given in the past to the acetabular labrum in regards to its integrity and possible role in the development of degenerative osteoarthritis. Only a few papers had appeared in the literature dealing with the subject.

Having followed the recent interest in the subject during the past ten years I have become increasingly convinced that *in many instances osteoarthritis is preceded by acute or chronic damage to the labrum either in the form of a tear or a dislocation.* Many patients who experience pain in the groin, which is aggravated by flexion and rotation of the hip but who do not show radiological evidence of arthritis, eventually develop radiological changes.

I have referred for arthroscopy a few patients with painful flexion of the hip on whom the diagnosis of a damaged labrum was conformed. They all experienced significant relief, but several of them eventually developed the classical radiological and clinical picture of osteoarthritis. It appears that *if the arthroscopic procedure does not reveal articular cartilage damage, the prognosis following surgery is usually good.* However, if the cartilage is damaged the procedure fails to provide long-term relief of symptoms. I do not have personal experiences with the procedure; however, I feel that the prognosis following arthroscopic treatment of a damaged labrum is similar to the one I have personally observed following removal of loose osteo or osteochondral bodies in the hip. Patients experience relief of pain for a period of time, but the symptoms often recur and obvious osteoarthritis becomes evident (See *Synovial Chondromatosis*). *Perhaps, an analogy can be made with the fate of many patients with torn knee menisci, who, contrary to popular views, do well following meniscectomy if the pathology is entirely limited to the meniscus. If there are already arthritic changes in the knee at the time of excision, or the cruciate ligament is also injured, the prognosis becomes guarded.*

As it is true with so many new techniques, arthroscopy of the hip is being abused by some. I know of an orthopedists who claims that within a period of a couple of years he had arthroscopically treated hundreds of patients "suffering from diseased acetabular labrum." I am concerned not only because he practices as an itinerant surgeon, but also because I have seen a couple of his patients where, in my opinion, the arthroscopic procedure was not indicated. They had moderately advanced osteoarthritis readily visible in plain radiographs at the time of the arthroscopic intervention. Within the subsequent six months both patients had their arthroscoped joints replaced. The possibility exists that the itinerant surgeon is correct in his aggressive approach and that he may be blazing beneficial trails. However, I doubt it.

Reinhold Ganz, a most distinguished orthopedist from Switzerland, has presented some very interesting and convincing evidence regarding the etiology of labrum pathology. *He believes that there is no primary lesion of the labrum except for strictly traumatic cases of hip dislocation or similar conditions.* He says that in dysplastic hips there can also be labral lesions secondary to rim overload caused by the instability generated by the lack of a well covered head. In impingement, either cam or pincer type, the labral lesion is secondary to the lump or decreased anterior femoral-neck offset in the former, and to an increased coverage of the head which, induces impingement to the neck in full range of motion in the latter. In cases of cam impingement, where a lump on the femoral head exists, this bump is covered by normal articular cartilage suggesting this deformity is primary and not secondary to either an old slipped capital femoral epiphysis or different type of deformity. In cases of pincer impingement, the problem is also a primarily deep acetabulum with a prominent posterior acetabular wall mainly. In cam impingement, the acetabular lesion starts in the labral-chondral junction from inside out, and in pincer impingement the trauma to the labrum is direct and injures it to the point of making it atrophic.

I am not totally comfortable with his theories, despite the fact that Ganz is one of the most resourceful and brightest hip surgeons I have ever met. Some of his ideas regarding the acetabula labrum do not seem to square off with the fact that valgus femoral necks, by virtue of their increased length, permit the hip a greater degree of motion and therefore diminishes any possible early contact of the neck against the acetabular labrum. These are the patients who, in my opinion, most frequently demonstrate labrum pathology. On the contrary, patients with varus hips are the ones who should experience early abutment of the neck of the femur against the pelvic bone. These people do not seem to be the ones commonly suffering from labrum-like symptoms.

Section 2

33

Acetabular Impingement

Among recent contributions to the understanding and etiology of hip pain has been the recognition that under certain circumstances the lateral aspect of the femoral head may abruptly impact against the border of the acetabulum, initiating articular damage leading to eventual arthritic changes. Radiologically, a lump on the femoral neck at the level of impaction suggests the pathology.

The condition may be diagnosed from various radiological views in patients who experience painful limitation of rotation and/or flexion of the hip. However, I have noticed from presentations made by others that most of the representative examples were hips with moderately excessive valgus rather than varus, which in my view should be the ones to "impinge" first. I cannot help but wonder what comes first, the chicken or the egg? Is the lump on the femoral neck present for many years but asymptomatic until for some reason its impingement against the acetabulum becomes symptomatic, or is the impingement the source of the "lump"?

To reinforce my uncertainty is the fact that osteoarthritis of the hip is less frequent among Orientals. These people frequently "sit" on their calves with their hips flexed to a maximum. Obviously this position is more likely to create impingement between the femoral neck and the pelvis. The more valgus the neck the more room is available before it impinges against the acetabulum. Why is it then that most

patients with the impingement syndrome have valgus rather than varus necks? It should be the other way around, since the varus hip impinges on the acetabulum sooner. The varus necks should have a higher incidence of arthritis, which indeed is not the case.

A number of reports have appeared in the literature illustrating the pathological changes and various techniques to correct the situation. The removal of the prominent new bone restores a congruent environment, which theoretically should result in permanent elimination of the painful symptoms.

The follow-up of adequate duration in a large number of patients is not as yet available. However, mid-term follow-ups have been encouraging. Recurrence of symptoms and the reappearance of the femoral head lump have been low. Complications from surgery, such as avascular necrosis, have not been reported, but caution must be exercised to prevent damage to the retinacular vessels.

This operation holds good promises, which along with increasing knowledge of the role of the labrum plays in the etiology of osteoarthritis is likely to have a major impact in the future of hip surgery. The increasing evidence that despite progress in the field of total hip replacement, but eventual failure of many of them after prolonged usage, gives further credence to surgical procedures that do not require the sacrifice of essential joint structures.

34

Destructive Osteoarthritis

I had the opportunity to see and treat a few patients suffering with the "destructive" type of osteoarthritis of the hip. Most of them were older females. The symptoms were severe and the deterioration of the bone took place in a very short period of time.

In "destructive" osteoarthritis the hip joint initially resembles very aggressive rheumatoid or septic arthritis. Gouty arthritis can also give the same radiological picture. The joint space disappears rapidly and the femoral heads seems to melt before your eyes

(Figs 34.1A and B). On two occasions, at the time of surgery, *I encountered a large collection of purulent-looking fluid upon entering the joint. In one instance there were large loose cartilaginous fragments that resembled tuberculous arthritis.* All cultures were negative for infection and laboratory and clinical tests ruled out rheumatoid arthritis (Figs 34.2A to F).

I wonder what causes this bizarre type of arthritis, and suspect that its classification as "osteoarthritis" is probably inappropriate.

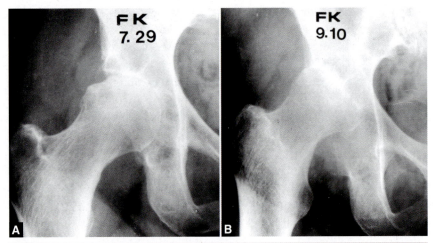

FIGS 34.1A AND B

Radiographs of the right hip of a 63-year-old woman taken less than 2 months apart. The diagnosis of destructive osteoarthritis was made. Upon entering the joint a large collection of purulent/looking material was encountered, Cultures were negative

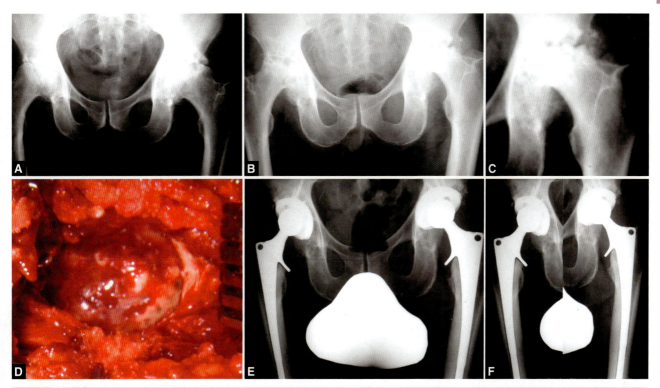

FIGS 34.2A TO F

(A and B) Radiographs of arthritic hips in a 60-year-old man. Notice the relatively mild arthritic changes. (C) Radiographs obtained seven months later. The change was dramatic. (D) Photograph of the floor of the acetabulum demonstrating aggressive inflammatory changes. (E and F) Radiographs taken 1 and 15 years respectively after the surgical replacement. The left hip demonstrates early lytic changes in the proximal femur. The hips are still asymptomatic

35

Ankylosing Spondylitis

Ankylosing spondylitis is a terribly incapacitating disease, particularly when involves not only the spine but other joints as well. I have seen a few patients whose spines were fused from the skull to the sacrum, and their shoulders, knees and hips were also ankylosed. I first had that experience when I was a young resident under Austin Moore. He replaced both hips in a severely disabled 40-year-old man using his prosthesis, but the operated joints promptly ankylosed again. That experience, supported by other surgeons' experiences, led me to believe that replacement arthroplasty in patients suffering from this disease always had a poor prognosis.

On three occasions I have seen spontaneous fusion of the hip following total hip arthroplasty, however, none of these patients were diagnosed as having Ankylosing spondylitis. *In these instances, the only thing that impressed me was the fact that they had an unusual degree of pain postoperatively that was out of proportion. They began to form bone very early after surgery until the joint finally fused completely* (Figs 35.1A and B) (See *Heterotopic Bone*).

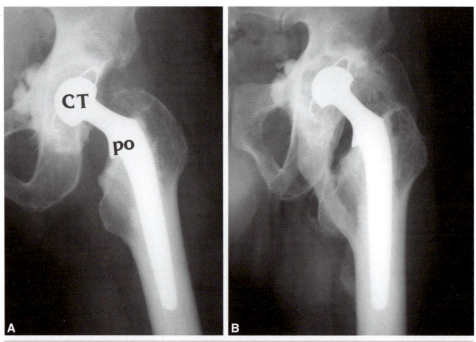

FIGS 35.1A AND B

(A) Immediate postsurgical radiograph of the hip of a patient with osteoarthritis. (B) Radiograph obtained three months postsurgery. Notice the massive heterotopic bone that spontaneously fused the joint

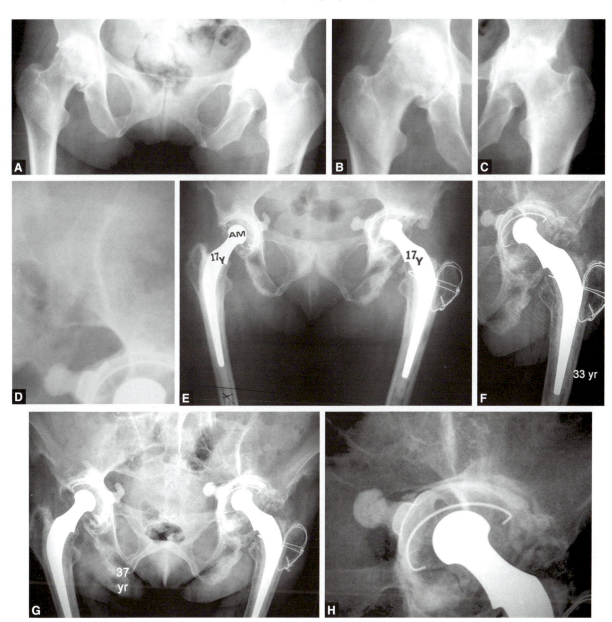

FIGS 35.2A TO H

(A) Radiograph of hips of a 24 years of woman suffering from severe ankylosing spondylitis. Her twin sister (shown in the next page) suffered the condition to a similar severe degree. (B and C) Closer view of both hips. Notice the protrusion of the acetabulum of the left hip. (D) Radiograph of fused sacroiliac joints. (E) Radiograph of bilateral Charnley arthroplasties obtained 17 years after surgery. (F) Radiograph taken 33 years postsurgery. (G and H) Radiograph obtained 37 years postoperative. The protrusion on the left side has gotten worse and the hip has become symptomatic. Patient has refused surgery

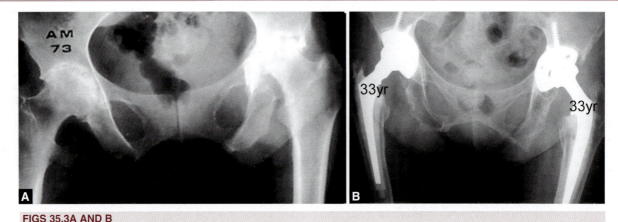

FIGS 35.3A AND B

(A) Radiograph of arthritic hips of 24-year-old woman, suffering from ankylosing spondylitis. The similar problem her twin sister had was described above. (B) Radiograph obtained 33 years postoperatively

It is usually believed that results from total hip surgery in patients with ankylosing spondylitis is different from other patients suffering from osteoarthritis. I am not sure this is the case. My experiences have not supported that theory. I do not know if my happy experiences were due to the fact I have not replaced a sufficiently large number of hips with this disease, or simply because I have been lucky. These patients received Indocin as prophylaxis, and only one patient received prophylactic radiation therapy.

Two of the patients I am presenting in this chapter were twin sisters who developed the symptoms in their early 20s. Both had their spines fused from the skull to the sacrum. One of them had limitation of motion of the shoulders but had normal knees. The other sister had trouble with her knees but to a moderate degree. The first sister had bilateral Charnley arthroplasties that have remained asymptomatic for 35 years, despite the fact that her left hip has demonstrated protrusion of the acetabular component (Figs 35.2A to H). The second sister who was operated three years later had titanium monopolar total hips, using noncemented acetabulum on one side and an isoelastic acetabulum on the other side. This isoelastic component was revised because of loosening 3 years later with a noncemented socket (Figs 35.3A and B).

36

The Rheumatoid Hip

Since the rheumatoid arthritic patients are usually the most disabled among all arthritic patients, it is logical to assume they would be the ones to benefit the most from replacement arthroplasty. To a great extent this is true; however, until now it appears that the prognosis from total hip arthroplasty is not a good as it is when the procedure is performed in osteoarthritic patients. This was definitely the case with endo-prostheses where it is well-known that boring of the prosthetic head into the pelvic bone takes place at a faster pace. This phenomenon was explained on the assumed, but not proven premise, that the rheumatoid patient undergoes osteoporosis as the disease progresses, while the osteoarthritic has a tendency to develop sclerotic changes. Though these mechanical/metabolic intrinsic changes are a reality, the reasons behind the phenomenon are likely to be more complicated. Other factors not fully understood at this time are probably involved.

The above comments regarding the behavior of implants in rheumatoid patients apply to a greater degree to cemented arthroplasties, which are the ones

with which I am able to provide long-term results. I believe at this time that the use of noncemented prostheses has dramatically improved the prognosis of hip arthroplasty in the care of the rheumatoid patient, who in addition to being the most disabled, is also, as a rule, the youngest. I do not have a clear explanation for this salutary experience. Acrylic cement can stabilize a femoral or acetabular implant equally as well. Osteoporotic changes that develop following implantation should affect the two environments in a comparable manner. One might even suspect that bone ingrowth usually present in noncemented prostheses may be compromised, preventing the benefits it normally provides. The many drugs that rheumatoid patients usually receive, many of them known to inhibit bone ingrowth, may theoretically, preclude permanent stable fixation. This apparently is not happening.

As it is true with just about every observation we make regarding the prognosis from arthroplasty, I have been able to follow a number of rheumatoid patients (Figs 36.1 to 36.12) for as long as 34 years.

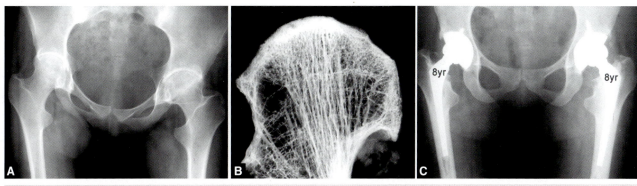

FIGS 36.1A TO C

(A) Radiographs of rheumatoid arthritis affecting both hips in a 24-year-old woman. (B) Photoradiograph of sectioned femoral head following bilateral simultaneous hybrid total hip replacements. (C) Radiograph obtained eight years postoperatively

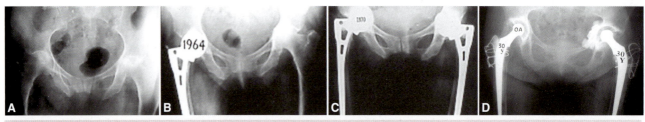

FIGS 36.2A TO D

(A) Radiograph of both hips affected with rheumatoid arthritic in a woman 30 years of age. (B and C) I replaced her right hip with an endoprosthesis in 1964 and her left hip in 1964. (D) Radiograph of both hips following revision of painful endoprostheses at 10 and 20 years postoperatively respectively

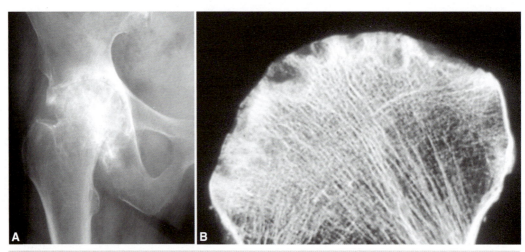

FIGS 36.3A AND B

(A) Radiograph of rheumatoid arthritic hip. (B) Cross-section of the arthritic femoral head

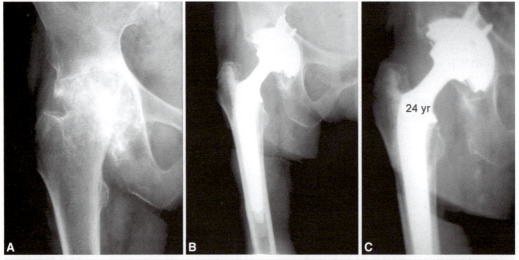

FIGS 36.4A TO C

(A) Radiograph of rheumatoid arthritic hip in a 72-year-old woman. (B) Radiograph obtained 10 years postsurgery.
(C) Radiograph taken 24 years postsurgery. The patient was not X-rayed again and died at the age of 100

Section 2

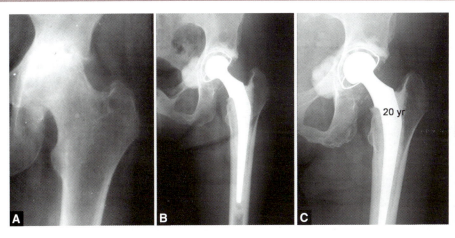

FIGS 36.5A TO C

(A) Immediate preoperative radiograph of a rheumatoid hip in a 45-year-old woman. (B) Radiograph obtained five years post-operatively. (C) Radiograph taken 20 years postoperatively. Notice the minimal wear and the presence of a thin bone/cement radiolucent line in the acetabulum

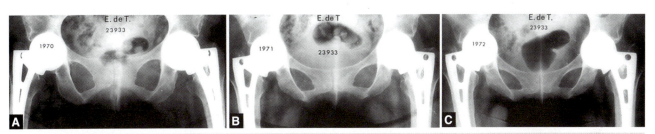

FIGS 36.6A TO C

Radiographs of bilateral Austin-Moore endoprostheses obtained in 1970, 1971 and 1972 respectively in a 39-year-old woman with rheumatoid arthritis. The initial surgery was performed in 1968. Notice the progressive boring of the prostheses into the acetabulum. She became severely incapacitated and was confined to a wheel-chair because of multiple joint involvement. She expired eight years later

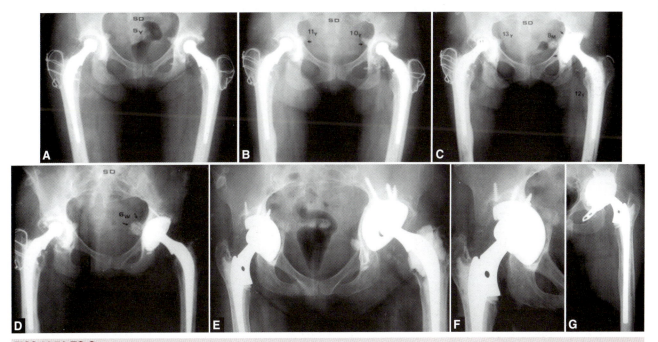

FIGS 36.7A TO G

(A) Radiograph of bilateral Charnley arthroplasties performed in a 30-year-old woman with rheumatoid arthritis, who had multiple joint involvement. This radiograph was taken 8 years postoperatively. (B) Radiograph obtained 10 and 11 years after surgery respectively. (C) Radiograph obtained 13 years after surgery, and shortly after revision of her left hip with a noncemented acetabulum. (D) Radiograph demonstrating loosening of the right acetabulum. (E) Radiograph taken 30 years after the initial surgery and revision of both femoral and acetabular components. (F) Radiograph showing further protrusio of the right socket into the acetabulum. (G) Radiograph obtained 32 years postoperatively after further revision surgery using once again acetabular graft and a plate

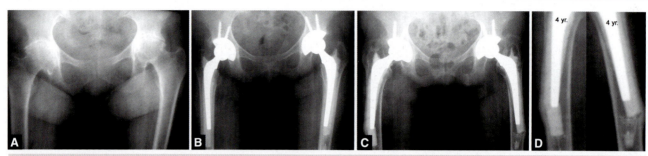

FIGS 36.8A TO D

(A) Radiograph of rheumatoid hips in a 53-year-old woman. (B) Radiograph obtained shortly after bilateral hybrid arthroplasties. (C) Radiographs taken four years after surgery showing loosening of both femoral components. (D) Radiographs documenting the progressive nature of the loosening of the femoral components

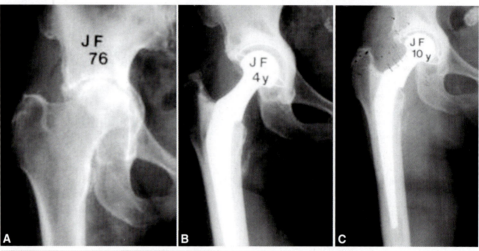

FIGS 36.9A TO C

(A) Radiograph of rheumatoid arthritic hip in a 50-year-old woman. (B) Radiograph obtained 4 years post-total hip cemented titanium monoblock arthroplasty. (C) Radiograph obtained 10 years postoperatively

Section 2

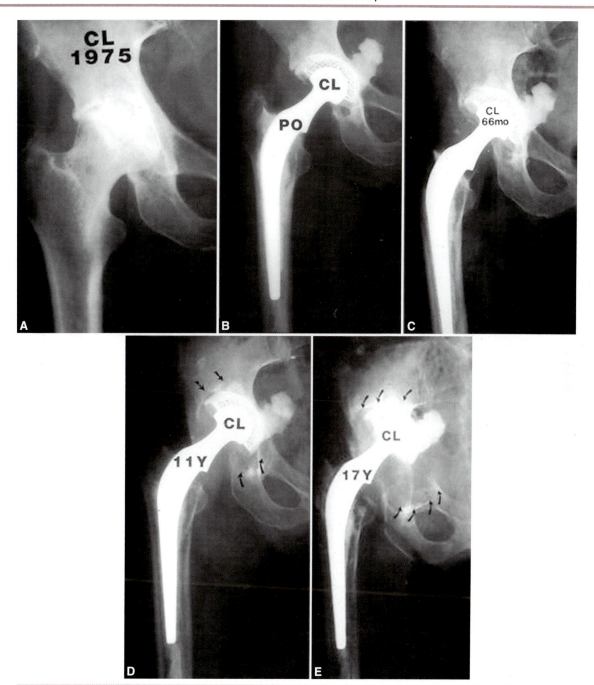

FIGS 36.10A TO E

(A) Radiograph of rheumatoid arthritic hip in a 19-year-old woman. (B and C) Radiographs obtained postoperatively and five and one half years postoperatively respectively. (D) Radiograph taken 11 years after surgery showing failure of the acetabular components. (E) Radiograph taken 17 years postoperatively showing massive acetabular lysis and femoral loosening. At this time I lost the patient to follow-up and she was subsequently operated upon by another orthopedists. I am not aware of the final outcome

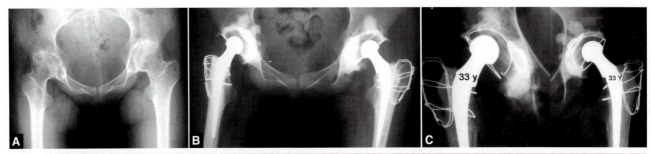

FIGS 36.11A TO C

(A) Radiograph of rheumatoid hips in a 21-year-old woman. (B) Radiograph of both hips following simultaneous bilateral Charnley arthroplasties. (C) Radiographs of both hips taken 33 years postoperatively. Notice the wear of the polyethylene acetabula

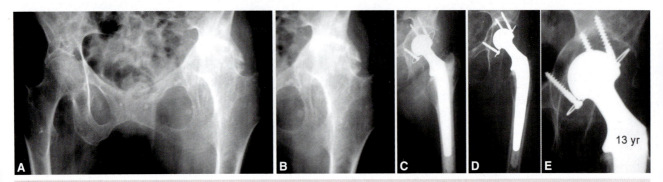

FIGS 36.12A TO E

(A and B) Radiographs of rheumatoid arthritic hip in a 45-year-old woman. (C) Radiograph obtained six months after surgery. An isoelastic acetabulum had been used. (D) Radiograph obtained three years after surgery. Notice the early loss of demarcation around the acetabular cup. (E) Radiograph showing a fracture of the ischial ramous as a result of a fall. Radiograph obtained 13 years after surgery. Further loss of demarcation can be noticed. Patient expired shortly afterwards

Many of them still show pristine radiographs with complete absence of signs of loosening.

I am not aware of any special surgical details that are unique to the surgical replacement of the rheumatoid hip. There are however, certain considerations that must be kept in mind. Often, rheumatoid patients present themselves with bilateral hip involvement, associated with flexion contractures of varying degrees. *Replacement of one hip and the resulting elimination of the contracture do not permit the patient to benefit from the mobility gained in the operating room, because the other hip, still with a contraction deformity, precludes the maintenance of the gained motion.*

The joint with the greatest limitation of motion dictates how much the operated hip can flex. This is vividly demonstrated during sitting: the limited degree of motion present in the no-operated hip determines the degree of motion the improved hip can reach. Therefore, it is desirable to either perform simultaneous bilateral arthroplasty or to replace both hips within a relatively short period of time (See *Bilateral Total Hip Arthroplasty*).

References*

10, 51, 52, 58, 76, 77, 104

---

* References provided at the end of the book after annexures.

37

The Dysplastic Hip

Segments of the following narrative were taken from my contribution to Professor Valentin Malagon's book on *The Dysplastic Hip. From the Cradle to Old Age.* Doctor Malagon was a most distinguished orthopedist from Bogota, Colombia and past-president of the Latin American Orthopedic Association (SLAOT). His long-standing interest and contributions to the understanding and treatment of the dysplastic hip has made him one of the most prominent leaders in this field. He has granted me permission to reproduce segments of my contribution to his book.

Orthopedics, as a distinct branch of medicine, came into being less than two hundred years ago. Its name clearly indicates that the initial intent of its founders was the care of the musculoskeletally disabled child. Over time it began to include within its territory adults with other musculoskeletal disabilities. Nonetheless, for all practical purposes the practice of orthopedics has been divided between children and adult disorders.

This division has served well the disabled child. People and institutions dedicated to the study and care of problems within a given category usually lead to progress. *However, the trend toward subspecialization in orthopedics has been, in my opinion, overly exaggerated to the point that the profession has been fragmented, weakened and trivialized.*

The training of the orthopedic resident has long called for separate periods of time devoted to the musculoskeletally disabled child, usually at the beginning and end of their supervised education.

Since, orthopedics has become a discipline heavily driven by technology, it has experienced a growing neglect of the biological foundations of the profession. This trend has affected especially adult orthopedics. Pediatric orthopedics, for a long time remained relatively impervious to the trend, traveled the high road, and preserved the biological approach to medicine. More recently, however, the commercialization of medicine and the major influence that the manufacturing industry of orthopedic implants has had in the education of the orthopedist has affected pediatric orthopedics as well. The current trend to approach many simple fractures in very young children by surgical means is a good example.

It was because of the separation between adult and children orthopedics that pediatric orthopedists paid little attention to the long-term results of congenital hip disease. Regulation and tradition precluded them from continuing the care of their patients beyond the completion of skeletal growth. Their publications therefore often dealt with results that did not provide data that extended beyond the ages of 16 to 20 years. In turn, adult orthopedists seldom knew much about the etiology of the arthritic conditions of the patients they were treating. At best they speculated that some kind of problem had affected them either at birth or some time during their childhood or adolescence.

This gap of knowledge involved a variety of disorders. Patients, who early in life suffered from Perthes disease or slipped capital epiphysis, and later developed degenerative joint disease, were often not in a position to provide their physicians valuable information. Those with congenital conditions found it even more difficult sharing light into their original problems.

The Sequelae of Congenital Hip Dysplasia and Dislocation in the Adult

It is not uncommon to find in the orthopedic literature reports of excellent results obtained in a high percentage of patients with congenital hip disease, who, however, had not as yet reached maturity. Many of those excellent results are often determined on the basis of absence of pain and good joint function.

A moderately shallow acetabulum observed in infancy and adolescence, not always results in late degenerative osteoarthritis as demonstrated by the fact that many adults so afflicted live long lives without ever developing arthritic problems.

Little is known as to the precise features under which a dysplastic acetabulum leads to joint degeneration. The most common explanation given for this sequella is a resulting mechanical environment where stresses on the articular cartilage are abnormally concentrated. However, articular cartilage tolerates enormous forces without experiencing pathological changes. Obesity with its parallel increased in the forces to which lower extremity joints are subjected, have also been implicated as possible factors. However, individuals who reach their twenties weighing no more than 150 pounds, but 20 to 30 years later weigh 250 pounds do not necessarily develop arthritis. In the ones who develop the condition, many of them experience pathologic changes in only one hip. If increased stresses on the articular cartilage were the definitive cause of the disease, then the abnormal changes should have occurred bilaterally.

Athletes who subject their joints to stresses manifold greater than those experienced by their more sedentary counterparts are not known to have a higher incidence of arthritis. Those athletes, who experience arthritic changes in later years, are more likely to have been subjected to direct trauma to the affected joint.

Therefore, there is no solid data to support the theories that increased stress on the hip's articular cartilage is a proven cause of osteoarthritis. There is only anecdotal, suggestive evidence.

The infant suffering from congenital hip dislocation, who is subjected to surgical reconstruction, frequently does well-clinically and radiologically into late adulthood if a congruously stable joint is obtained at the time of surgery and it is maintained during the time required for collagen tissues to regain maturity. In the absence of such congruous stability a residual instability persists, leading to late arthritic changes.

With the occasional exception of the totally dislocated hip, where there is no contact between the femoral head and the acetabulum, patients with subluxated hips experience limitation of abduction of the hip. This lack of abduction places valgus stresses on the knee joint, which over time leads to a valgus deformity, ligamentous instability and subsequent joint degeneration. The normal side of the body may also experience secondary mechanical changes that may result in arthritic changes in the knee joint.

Low-back pain is a frequent complication, which is also explained on mechanical grounds. Secondary scoliosis and degenerative disk disease are the usual clinical and radiographic manifestations.

There is no data to indicate that the often seen shortening of the involved extremity in itself is a cause of arthritis either in the hip of knee in the ipsilateral side.

Malrotation of the femur is commonly seen in arthritic hips secondary to congenital hip disease; and this abnormality can be seen also associated with flexion contracture of the hip joint and shortened adductor musculature.

The degree of symptoms experienced by the adult patient suffering from osteoarthritis secondary to congenital hip dysplasia should be the most important factor in determining the need for surgical treatment. The surgeon cannot reach a sound conclusion-based entirely on radiological findings, for after all, it is the patient not the X-rays who suffers the pain and experiences the disability.

Totally dislocated hips are very often associated with minimal pain. It is not uncommon to see patients with high bilateral congenital dislocation of the hip ambulate with an obvious limp, but without pain. Some of these people, however, as they get older begin to suffer from sacroiliac and low-back pain as well as knee pain. If obesity is also present, the disabling symptoms increase.

Osteoarthritis of the hip is associated with progressive limitation of motion. However, not all motions suffer that fate in identical patterns. Internal rotation is the motion that first demonstrates a loss of range. It is also true that in most instances, internal rotation, when clinically tested, produces the most pain. *I suspect that since internal rotation of the hip is the motion least important in daily activities, the patient subconsciously avoids such motion.* Flexion, on the other hand, is often preserved even in the most advanced cases. The fact that sitting forces the hip to flex ensures the preservation of this motion. Abduction frequently loses range of motion, probably for reasons somewhat similar to the ones that cause limitation of internal rotation. Shortening of the adductor musculature and an associated flexion contracture of the hip are commonly seen.

It has become increasingly evident that for all practical purposes there are at this time only two surgical methods of treatment for the care of the arthritic hip resulting from congenital hip disease: osteotomy and total joint replacement. Fusion of the hip joint is seldom performed.

Osteotomies are not performed very frequently, particularly in the United States. This is an unfortunate pattern in light of the evidence that the procedure, if performed correctly and for the appropriate pathology, provides very good and long lasting results.

Osteotomies preserve biological structures that are not subjected to the mechanical changes affecting surgical implants. *In the event of failure of the osteotomy to provide long lasting relief, the preservation and/or restoration of more desirable bony anatomy ensures a better prognosis for the eventual prosthetic arthroplasty.*

Certain osteotomies, popular in the past, were associated with a high degree of unsatisfactory results. Undue emphasis was placed on femoral osteotomies, rather than on acetabular osteotomies where most problems arise. Currently, a renewed interest in acetabular osteotomies is largely due to the work of pioneers like Latournel, Wagner, Ganz and Matta (See *Pelvic Osteotomy*).

The fact that replacement arthroplasty has become a procedure associated with few early complications and provides almost immediate relief of symptoms, has made the arthroplasty approach the most popular one. Total hip arthroplasty is more popular, not only because of is high success rate, but also because it brings to the surgeon much higher financial compensation.

It has been approximately 45 years since total hip arthroplasty was introduced in the United States. Initially, the operation was performed almost exclusively in older people. In the younger individual, following Charnley's advice, total joint replacement was discouraged. Nonetheless, a number of younger people have received the implant, giving us an opportunity to study the behavior of the implant and that of the surrounding tissues over a long period of time.

Charnley stated that no total hip arthroplasty performed in young athletic individual could last 30 years. Today we have seen a number of patients who

30 years after surgery maintained excellent use of the joint while carrying out very active lives. Many of them indulge in some athletic activities, such as skiing and tennis. Though there are exceptions, *I doubt, however, that many patients following a total hip arthroplasty have succeeded in preserving the integrity of the artificial joint after being involved in sports such as competitive tennis, basketball or football.*

Since, total hip arthroplasty cannot be guaranteed to last the life span of the young adult, is theoretically best to recommend to patients to postpone the surgical procedure until the symptoms are no longer controllable with symptomatic medications and the use of external support. Some nonsteroidal anti-inflammatory medications are making it possible to assuage symptoms in a more effective manner. However, more recently several of the most popular nonsteroidal anti-inflammatory medications have been found to have undesirable side effects, such as coronary disease. Repeated intra-articular injections of cortisone carry the potential complication of introducing an infection into the joint. An infection that may not manifest itself acutely but remains dormant until a surgical intervention is carried out.

Not infrequently, the presence of constant pain and disability forces patients to avoid exercise, resulting in generalized muscle atrophy and obesity. The latter may expedite the collapse of the joint. The associated reduction in activity can also make matters worse. It is a mistaken popular belief that rest is beneficial to osteoarthritic joints. The opposite is true: osteoarthritic joints that maintain good range of motion last longer and the severity of the pain is of a lesser magnitude.

There are factors that often justify the performance of total hip arthroplasty in younger people. How can a surgeon condemn a young person to additional years of pain, disability and the use of external support, knowing that eventually the symptoms will become more severe? Can the surgeon justify the recommendation to postpone surgery simple because of a concern about the number of years that the implant will serve well? Neither is rushing younger patients into having surgery an appropriate approach. *Oftentimes, acute episodes of exacerbation of pain spontaneously subside.* In addition, many osteoarthritic hips never develop severe pain and incapacitation. Furthermore, the fact that major complications from surgery are always possible, justify the postponement of surgery for reasonably longer periods of time.

Section 2

Contrary to the case of the individual with disease in the hip joint that can only be treated by means of arthroplasty, for others with still minimal but progressively disabling pain, osteotomy is the treatment of choice. *Osteotomy, however, should be performed early; otherwise, the final result from surgery may be seriously comprised* (See *Acetabular Osteotomy*).

Several surgical approaches for the performance of total hip arthroplasty have been widely discussed in the literature. Each has its advocates and the results obtained with each one of them are probably comparable.

We will describe in some detail only the two surgical approaches with which I have the greatest experience: the transtrochanteric lateral approach described by Charnley and the posterior approach without trochanteric osteotomy. After performing nearly 700 arthroplasties using the Charnley's approach, I abandoned the technique in preference for the posterior approach without trochanteric osteotomy. The Charnley approach dislocates the hip anteriorly, the posterior approach posteriorly.

What prompted me to abandon the Charnley approach was the realization that the trochanteric osteotomy was associated with complications referable to the fixation of the trochanter, particularly wire fatigue, delayed union and nonunion. Most of these complications are rarely serious but represent an unnecessary inconvenience. The fact that protection against nonunion requires a longer period of relative gluteal muscles inactivity, is often considered by many as an undesirable feature. *The nonunited trochanter predisposes to subsequent dislocation from the loss of the tethering effect that the attached trochanter provides.*

The two approaches provide comparably satisfactory results in a very high percentage of patients. The degree of exposure to the acetabulum and femoral canal is also comparable.

An observation made by others, and later supported with my own experiences, relates to the higher incidence of thromboembolic disease when the hip is dislocated anteriorly and held during surgery in extreme positions of external rotation and flexion. It appears that such a position creates a temporary "kink" in the femoral and popliteal vessels producing damage to their walls.

Since, the various surgical techniques have been widely publicized there is no need to cover every detail of the operations. I will limit my comments to a few specific points, which I consider most important for their successful completion (See *The Posterior Approach*).

With the lateral transtrochanteric approach, in order to properly expose the acetabulum and femoral shaft it is necessary to flex the hip to 90 degrees and to rotate the leg externally to a point where the foot faces the ceiling. *This position is likely to damage major vessels and set the stage for thromboembolic complications.* In order to lessen the likelihood of such problems it is desirable to relax the extreme external rotation position whenever possible, and return to it only during the critical times when it is absolutely necessary (See *Thromboembolic Disease*).

Using the posterior approach, following dislocating the hip posteriorly the hip may be kept in almost full extension during the preparation of the acetabulum and the securing of the acetabular component. This position does not place the femoral or popliteal vessels under unfavorable conditions.

During preparation of the femoral component there is no need to acutely flex the knee. It is only during the few minutes that are required to drive the cement and/or prosthesis into the canal, that 90 degrees of flexion of the hip is necessary.

Since it is anticipated that careful templating of the acetabulum and femur was carried out prior to surgery, the surgeon should know in advance as to where he intends to place the artificial implant.

To appropriately determine the placement of the acetabular cup, the type of pathology must be considered. The Crowe classification of hip dysplasia is simple and practical. It divides the pathological condition into four categories:

1. A shallow acetabulum without subluxation.
2. A subluxated hip, but with significant contact of the head with the acetabulum.
3. Significant subluxation of the head but with residual small area of contact of the head with the acetabulum.
4. Complete dislocation and without contact of the head with the acetabulum.

Full exposure of the acetabulum is essential. Appropriate retractors must be used but care should be exercised to avoid injury to the major vessels and nerves. This is more likely to happen, not only during their introduction in front of the anterior wall of the socket but also during the conduct of the operation, when the assistant must maintain anterior retraction of the soft tissues.

When cement is used, leakage of the material into the surrounding tissues should be avoided to prevent thermal injury to the femoral and sciatic nerves (See *Peripheral Nerve Injury in Total Hip Surgery*).

When using noncemented acetabular components, which are stabilized with metallic screw, care must be exercised to avoid injury to major intrapelvic vessels and nerves. *Screws should be reserved for the superior and posterior regions of the acetabulum* (See *Vascular Complications in Total Hip Surgery*).

Considerable debate has ranged over the years concerning the value of placement of the prosthetic socket at the level of the original acetabulum. The data thus far published suggest that it is best to avoid a high axis of rotation when placing the socket higher on the pelvic bone. Such high position is almost always associated with a residual limp. The long-term stability of the implant is probably more precarious.

However, placing the acetabulum lower, at the level of the original acetabulum, is not always possible. The thickness of the pelvic wall may be too thin, precluding anchorage of the implant even after attempting bone grafting surgery.

Medialization of the acetabulum is always desirable. However, in the performance of total arthroplasty in the presence of shallow acetabula, this is not always possible for the reasons mentioned above. The surgeon finds it necessary to accept a thin pelvic wall, unless major additional bone grafting is carried out.

Reaming of the acetabulum must be done carefully to avoid perforation of the pelvic floor. Several surgeons have reported perforation of the floor with resulting massive tear of major vessels and/or nerves. A catastrophic complication (See *Vascular Complications in Total Hip Arthroplasty*).

If deepening of the acetabulum cannot make possible the placement of a socket that is fully covered with bone it is necessary to use a bone graft. In most instances a segment of the removed femoral head is used. Its contact with the pelvic bone should be as great as possible and its anchorage made secure.

It is wrong to be satisfied with a small cavity into which to place the prosthesis, in order to avoid the performance of a graft. A small socket requires a thin polyethylene liner that is likely to wear more rapidly. At least six millimeters of plastic material are necessary. Various X-ray views must be obtained to evaluate the thickness of the pelvic bone at various levels. CT scan is most informative.

In instances where deepening of the acetabulum to an ideal depth is not possible, the acetabular component is often found to have been anchored in place in more than the accepted 45 degrees of inclination. Though we have observed that cemented acetabula placed at a 90 degrees angle of inclination functioned as well as those placed at 40 degrees of inclination, we do not know if a longer follow-up will support the initial the shorter period of observation.

It is generally agreed that the acetabular component should be given between 15 and 20 degrees of anteversion. However, in the case of the congenitally dysplastic hip rigid figures must be ignored. The surgeon must accommodate the developmental changes that have occurred over the course of years. Trial reductions determine the best orientation of the acetabulum.

Congenital hip dysplasia is often associated with developmental malformation of the pelvis and femur. Therefore is of extreme importance to ascertain that at the time of anchoring of the prosthetic implant the appropriate amount of anteversion is obtained. It is desirable to temporarily fix the acetabulum in place until trial reductions of the hip is attempted. Significant secondary changes in the femoral component, such as malrotation, often call for accommodations that affect both sides of the joint.

Since many patients suffering from congenital hip disease have corrective surgery performed during infancy or childhood the anatomy of the pelvis and/or femur may be significantly altered. Different types of osteotomies of the acetabulum or pelvis distort the anatomy of the area, which require careful identification of important landmarks. Failure to do so might lead to serious complications (See *Acetabular Osteotomy*).

If the surgeon anticipates the need for additional support of the acetabular component, because of its shallowness, there is one main option: the use of bone autograph or bone allograph. Most often the patient's own femoral head is carried out, obviating in this manner the more expensive and riskier use of bone allograph. Particulate grafts have been used, but have not as yet become popular.

It is feared that bulk allographs may undergo resorption, leading to shortening of the extremity and loosening of the implant. Though the results have been, in general satisfactory, their long-term follow-ups, has indicated to some investigators the presence of complications. Lee, Cabanela et al, from a review of 102 consecutive primary and revision total hip arthroplasties performed with bone graft found "no difference in failure rate between primary and revision hip arthroplasty, type of deficiency, or amount of graft coverage". They added, "Although early results are encouraging, acetabular loosening increased significantly with longer follow-up evaluation; however, graft incorporation was successful and facilitated subsequent revision surgery".

It is clear that different and opposite opinions still cloud the issue. Additional long-term follow-ups will eventually be able to shed meaningful light into the issue.

If the autograph is chosen it is best to mark the superior articulating surface of the femoral head, immediately preceding the complete dislocation of the hip, in order to achieve the greatest eventual contact of that surface against the pelvic bone with the least difficulty.

Once the superior portion of the femoral head has the articular cartilage removed, it should be temporarily stabilized against the false acetabulum using Steinman pins. Reaming of the graft can then be carried out with greater ease.

The graft once reamed to accommodate the prosthetic component must be stabilized with screws that connect it with the underlying pelvic bone. If a noncemented component is chosen, the screws that are driven into the holes of the implant may be used to provide fixation to the graft as well.

If a cemented component is chosen, the graft must be stabilized with screws independently.

The use of cement to build a roof to a dysplastic acetabulum has been criticized is considered by some as being inferior to autographs or allographs. This criticism should be tempered in view of the fact in many instances they have served well (See *Fractures of the Acetabulum*). The use of cement eschews the problems associated with resorption of the graph, which is a known possible complication.

Not every dysplastic acetabulum requires a bone graft. Slightly uncovered components function well. Often grafts are used that serve no mechanical purpose, since they fail to provide effective mechanical support.

When using noncemented acetabular components, complete bony coverage of the implant is not essential. Bone ingrowth throughout the entire surface of the metal is not necessary for adequate stability since it is well-known that bone ingrowth in porous acetabula is rarely complete. Postmortem examinations of removed implants have revealed that small areas of bone ingrowth provide effective "welding" between the porous cup and the underlying bone.

Surgeons worry about problems that might result from attempts to gain length during the performance of total hip arthroplasty in patients with osteoarthritis from congenital, developmental or traumatic conditions, when significant leg length discrepancy is present. The possibility of stretching the major nerves, particularly the sciatic nerve hovers over the mind of the operating surgeon.

Though there are relatively new and effective methods designed to monitor the condition of the sciatic nerve during surgery, there are simple guidelines that ensure with some reliability the protection of the nerve.

A carefully conducted preoperative physical examination is most helpful. *The dislocated or subluxated hip that has very limited flexion is the one least likely to tolerate significant lengthening of the leg.* If 90 or more degrees of passive flexion can be obtained implies that the sciatic nerve has been subjected to constant stretching during the patient's daily activities. On the contrary, the hip that has poor flexion suggests that the sciatic nerve has been deprived of such physiological stretching. Sudden attempts to lengthen the extremity result in subjection of the nerve to stresses, which its fibers cannot tolerate.

In order to gain as much length as possible during the surgical procedure, it is necessary to avoid pressure of retractors against major nerves. Therefore, long incisions are preferable. Short incisions require forceful soft tissue retraction to obtain adequate exposure of the various bony and soft tissue structures.

Structures that appear to limit manual attempt to regain length should be severed. Often, the iliopsoas muscle requires its severance from its insertion as well as the adductor muscles. The latter require a separate surgical incision, made either prior to the initiation of the surgery or after its completion. Stripping of the gluteus medius insertion on the pelvic bone is frequently necessary. It must be performed with care in order to avoid damage to the inferior gluteal nerve. In extreme situations tenotomy of the hamstring muscles may be necessary.

If the length to be gained is moderate, the adductor surgery can be performed after the major surgery has been terminated. Otherwise it is best to carry out the adductor tenotomy prior to the major event. The capsule must be completely released anteriorly and posteriorly.

Of major importance is the release of the gluteus maximus muscle from its insertion on the femur. Without this step it is virtually impossible to identify the other adjacent muscular structures in need of surgical release, and to permit visual and finger contact with the nerve. The nerve that becomes too taut may be easily damaged; being able to feel it at all times helps in determining whether additional soft tissue releases are necessary.

Following completion of the surgical procedure it is best to reattach the gluteus maximum muscle with some tension to prevent the appearance of an atrophied buttock. Failure to repair the muscle, however, does not seem to affect the power of the muscle.

On occasion is necessary to shorten the femur in order to be able to place the artificial acetabulum at the level of the original one. This can be done with or without trochanteric osteotomy. It is best to carry out the procedure without the trochanteric osteotomy to avoid the problems often associate with the fixation of the trochanter on its new bed.

Since the patient and surgeon wish to achieve equalization of length, trial femoral prostheses of various lengths must be available. If the reduction is very difficult with a given neck-length implant, a shorter one must be accepted. However, *if reduction with a neck that seems to be too long can be accomplished without excessive force, the hip should be held in flexion for a few minutes without making any attempts to extend the knee joint.* It is often possible to observe that those few minutes bring about gradual stretching of the remaining soft tissues without compromising the sciatic nerve. In those instances it is better to maintain the hip and knee in flexion after the patient leaves the operating room. Gradually, the joints can be extended. Elevation of the head of the bed with the knee in extension should be forbidden under these circumstances, since elevation of the trunk places stretching forces on the sciatic nerve.

The precautions I have outlined above help to protect the sciatic nerve, but do nothing to ensure protection to the femoral nerve. Whatever maneuvers are carried out to protect the sciatic nerve are likely to adversely affect the femoral nerve. For example, flexion of the knee relaxes the sciatic nerve but stretches the femoral nerve. Contrariwise, flexion of the knee hip relaxes the femoral nerve but stretches the sciatic nerve (See Peripheral Nerve Injury During Total Hip Replacement).

It is possible that the femoral nerve tolerates tension better than the sciatic nerve, since postsurgical femoral palsy is rare. A more logical explanation is the fact that the femoral nerve, for all practical purposes does not extend below the knee joint. The bifurcated sciatic nerve reaches the distal aspect of the foot. The common peroneal nerve is relatively fixed behind the fibular neck, so when the nerve is stretched, tension at the level of the fibular neck occurs. *This explains why traumatic or sciatic nerve palsy frequently affects only the peroneal component of the sciatic nerve.*

The most common complication encountered during surgery for advanced osteoarthritis of the hip resulting from congenital hip disease, is the failure to recognize the developmental changes that affect the femur. Femoral malrotation is common, leading to the possibility of placing the prosthetic component in an abnormal attitude.

Often, the size of the medullary canal is small and its identification and enlargement may be difficult. When the prosthetic component is of the noncemented type, excessive reaming might render the cortexes of the bone, not only weak but also avascular.

Many adult patients have the prosthetic replacement after having had a variety of surgical procedures performed early in life. Certain rotational or angular osteotomies may require correction prior to the performance of the total joint replacement. Attempt to carry out the procedure before correcting those deformities may result in perforation of the cortex of fracture of the femur or ultimate undesirable deformities.

Special attention must be paid to the anteversion of the femur since excessive anteversion is common in congenital hip dislocation. Attempts should be carefully made during the trial reduction to ensure that the patella faces the same direction of the opposite patella; otherwise an excessive internal rotation deformity of the leg will be detected during ambulation. This iatrogenic complication leads to subsequent painful knee instability.

We have data to justify rendering judgment regarding the fate of the Charnley prosthesis, performed with trochanteric osteotomy, because with this prosthesis a 35-year follow-up has been reported. Though a small percentage of them failed as a result of wear or loosening, the long-term results have been satisfactory (See *Long-term Follow-up of Charnley Prostheses*). However, since in the case of the dysplastic hip the operations were performed when many of the patients were still very young, it is impossible to tell that another 10 to 20 years of prosthetic usage will not alter unfavorably the final outcome.

Section 2

It can be concluded that total hip arthroplasty is an acceptable method of treatment for osteoarthritis secondary to congenital hip subluxation and dislocation. However, the procedure is no a panacea; failure of the components and surrounding bony structures occurs with some frequency; and the long-term outcome is not yet known. Though newer implants and additional basic research are likely to improve the results, the enthusiasm with modifications must be accepted carefully.

Secondary knee osteoarthritis, also explained on mechanical grounds, is a very common sequella of congenital hip disease, and likely to develop when the hip point suffers from limitation of abduction and rotation. Patients who eventually require replacement arthroplasty of both joints seldom reach an excellent clinical result.

Several times, I have reported on my personal experience with total hip arthroplasty, However, a deliberate effort was never made to study those patients who had the operation performed for the treatment of osteoarthritis secondary to hip dysplasia. I recently completed a careful review of 135 total hip arthroplasties that had a minimum follow-up of 15 years and a maximum of 33 years. Among these patients 71 patients had suffered from osteoarthritis. Of these patients 17 had been diagnosed as having the arthritic condition as being secondary to congenital hip dysplasia. It is very likely that many conditions classified as primary osteoarthritis were in actuality secondary to congenital hip disease. It is often difficult to tell the true etiology of the pathological condition because of changes that develop over a period of many years. Primary osteoarthritic hips often subluxate and in some instances to a severe degree. In those instances one may be correct in assuming that the condition was secondary to congenital disease.

Our study attempted to identify the technical details that may have been responsible for the long-term survival. Some very interesting observations were made. For example, it was found that (93%) hips had 100 percent coverage of the acetabular component, while 9 (6.6%) hips had between 80 and 90 percent coverage. The inclination of the acetabular component was between 40 and 50 degrees in 88 percent hips. The orientation of the femoral component was neutral in 112 (82.9%) hips; in varus in 13 (9.6%) hips; and in valgus in 10 (7.4%) hips. The percentage of medullary canal occupied by the femoral stem 7 centimeters below the collar of the prosthesis was more than 50 percent in 110 (81.4%) femurs; in 13 (9.6%) femurs the prosthesis filled less than 50 percent of the canal; and in 12 (8.8%) femurs 50 percent of the canal was occupied by the femoral component.

Wires used to stabilize the osteotomized greater trochanter were identified as having broken in 13 (9.6%) patients.

The thickness of the column of cement at the level of the transected femoral neck measured between 3 and 5 millimeters in 84 percent radiographs; between 0 and 3 millimeters in 11.8 percent radiographs; and more than 5 millimeters in 3.7 percent radiographs.

No migration of the acetabular component was seen in 130 (96.2%) radiographs; migration of less than 5 millimeters was measured in 4 (2.9%) radiographs; and in 1 (0.7%) radiograph migration of more than 5 millimeter was recorded.

A continuous bone-cement radiolucent line in the acetabulum was seen in 8 (5.9%) radiographs while no continuous lines were seen in 127 (94%) radiographs.

Bone-cement radiolucent lines in the femur, measuring more than 1 millimeter, were seen in 6 (4.4%) radiographs while no bone-cement radiolucent lines were seen in 129 (95.5%) radiographs.

Metal-cement radiolucent lines in the femur were seen in 3 (2.2%) radiographs while no metal-cement lines were seen in 132 (97.7%) radiographs.

Fractures of the cement in the femoral side were seen in 5 (3.7%) radiographs while no fractures were observed in 130 (96.2%) radiographs.

Neither acetabular nor femoral lysis was observed in this group of radiographs, unless one chooses to consider radiolucent bone-cement lines as an expression of bone lysis.

The cement extended distally to just above the tip end of the prosthesis in 12 (9%) radiographs; to the level of the prosthetic tip in 10 (7%) radiographs; and below the prosthetic stem in 113 (84%) radiographs (Figs 37.1 to 37.28).

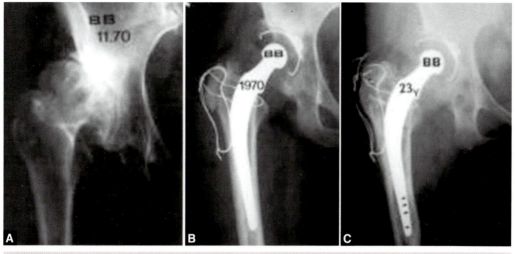

FIGS 37.1A TO C

(A) Radiograph of osteoarthritic hip, secondary to hip dysplasia in a 55-year-old woman. (B) Radiograph obtained shortly after surgery. Notice the absence obtained barium in the acrylic cement. A new acetabulum was surgically created. (C) Radiograph obtained two years postoperatively showing no gross evidence of wear or acetabular loosening. The femur shows early lytic changes distally

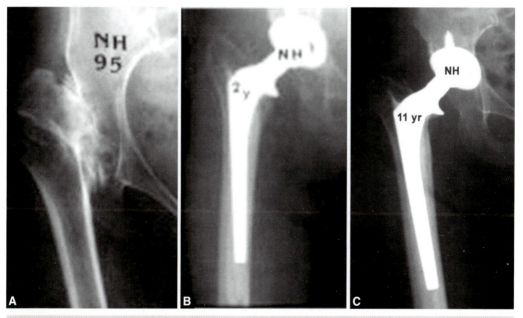

FIGS 37.2A TO C

(A) Radiograph of osteoarthritis in a 61-year-old woman secondary to congenital hip dislocation. Prior to surgery she has significant leg shortening, an adduction contracture of the hip, and significant limitation of motion. (B) Radiograph showing the postoperative radiological appearance of the hip. The old acetabulum was used to place the noncemented shell. The adductors were released as well as the iliopsoas. (C) Radiograph obtained ten years postoperatively. The length of the leg was increase by 1 inch, and the range of motion, though limited for a long time, eventually reached 80 degrees of flexion and perhaps some 10 degrees of abduction. The patient has remained very unhappy, primarily due to her inability to done her shoes in the way she used to do it before surgery. She did it the way patients with fused hips do it

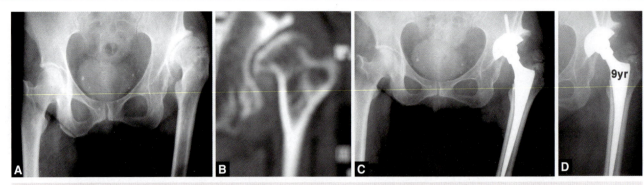

FIGS 37.3A TO D

(A) Radiograph of congenital hip dysplasia in a 67-year-old woman. (B) CT scan of the hip. (C) Postoperative radiograph showing the location of the noncemented porous shell in the old acetabulum. The adductor muscles were released. The length of the extremities became equal, and the pelvic obliquity corrected spontaneously. (D) Radiograph obtained 9 years postoperatively. The patient regained power of abduction and after a few months she was able to active contract the iliopsoas muscle

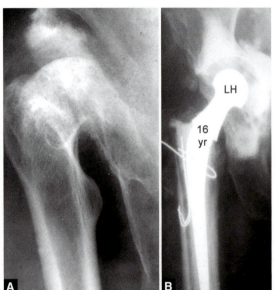

FIGS 37.4A AND B

(A) Radiograph of arthritic hip secondary to congenital hip dysplasia in a 64-year-old woman. (B) Radiograph obtained 16 years postoperatively. The patient was lost to further follow-up

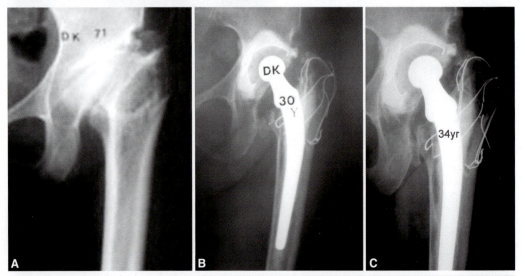

FIGS 37.5A TO C

(A) Radiograph of arthritic hip, secondary to congenital hip dysplasia in a 35-year-old woman. (B) Early postoperative radiograph of the Charnley arthroplasty taken 30 years postoperatively. (C) Radiograph obtained 34 years after surgery. The patient has remained asymptomatic, though displaying a gluteal lurch

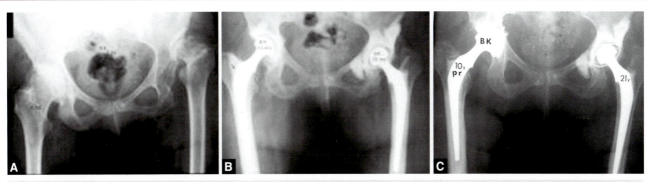

FIGS 37.6A TO C

(A) Radiograph of both hips in a 58-year-old woman illustrating the arthritic right hip with a deep acetabulum and a completely dislocated hip on the left. (B) Radiograph showing early signs of failure of the right hip. (C) Radiograph obtained 10 years after revision of the right hip using a noncemented acetabular shell. The left hip was replaced 27 years earlier

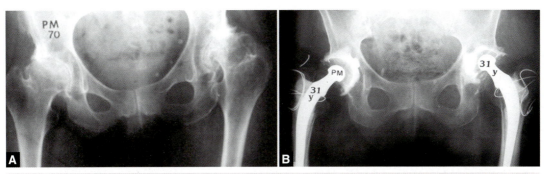

FIGS 37.7A AND B

(A) Radiograph of bilateral osteoarthritis of the hips secondary to congenital hip dysplasia in a 52-year-old woman. (B) Radiographs obtained 31 years postoperatively. Charnley arthroplasties were performed simultaneously. Notice the evidence of minimal wear and no signs of lysis or failure. The patient expired two years later

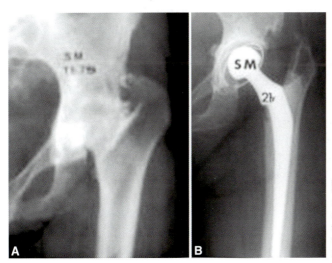

FIGS 37.8A AND B

(A) Radiograph of arthritic hip joint probably secondary to epiphyseal arrest following closed treatment of congenital hip dislocation in a woman 40-year-old. (B) Radiograph obtained 21 years postoperatively

Section 2

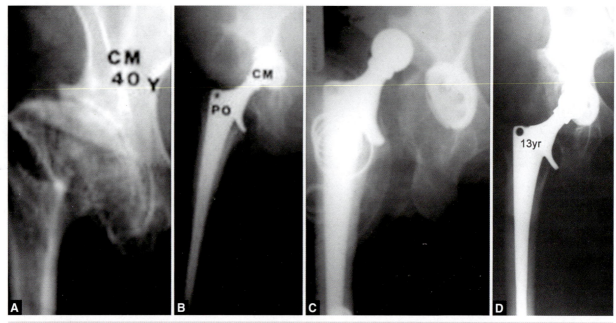

FIGS 37.9A TO D

(A) Radiograph of osteoarthritic hip secondary to congenital hip dysplasia in a 43-year-old woman. (B) The hip was replaced with a noncemented Bias prosthesis. Unfortunately a very small socket was used in preference to the placement of a bone graft to make possible a more desirable bigger acetabular shell. (C) The hip dislocated a few days postoperatively. (D) Radiographs taken 13 years postoperatively

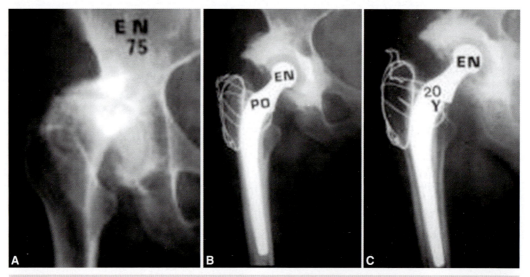

FIGS 37.10A TO C

(A) Radiograph of arthritic hip secondary to hip dysplasia in 59-year-old man. (B) Postoperative radiograph of the Charnley arthroplasty. The acetabulum was not deepened enough. The coverage of the acetabular component was completed with acrylic cement. (C) Radiograph obtained 20 years later with no gross evidence of wear or other complications

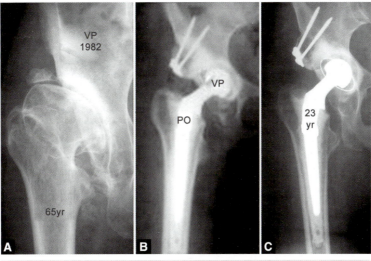

FIGS 37.11A TO C

(A) Osteoarthritic hip secondary to congenital hip dysplasia. (B) At the time of prosthetic replacement, the femoral head was use to provide better coverage of the acetabular component. (C) Radiograph taken 23 years after surgery. She recently had a knee replacement

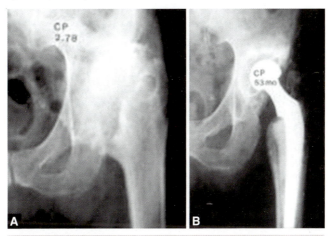

FIGS 37.12A AND B

(A) Severely advanced osteoarthritis. (B) The plastic acetabular component was placed at the level of the original cavity

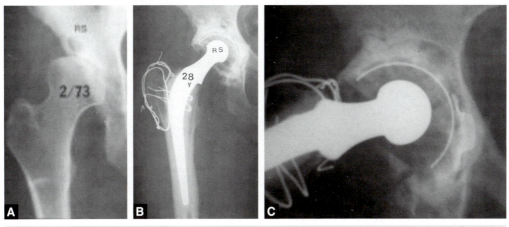

FIGS 37.13A TO C

(A) Osteoarthritic hip secondary to dysplasia. (B) Radiograph obtained 28 years after surgery. (C) Radiograph taken 35 years postsurgery. The hip shows signs of loosening and lysis. Pain has developed. Surgery is likely to be needed in the near future

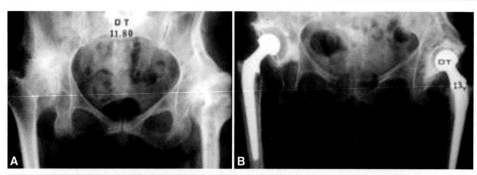

FIGS 37.14A AND B

(A) Osteoarthritis of both hips secondary to hip dysplasia. An acetabular osteotomy had been performed early in her life. (B) Thirteen years after surgery the patient has remained asymptomatic

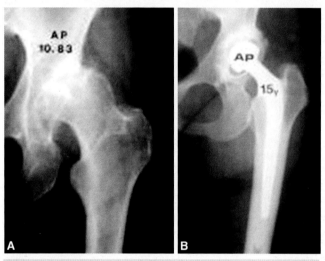

FIGS 37.15A AND B

(A) Osteoarthritis secondary to hip dysplasia. (B) Fifteen years postoperatively there is no evidence of failure and the patient has remained asymptomatic

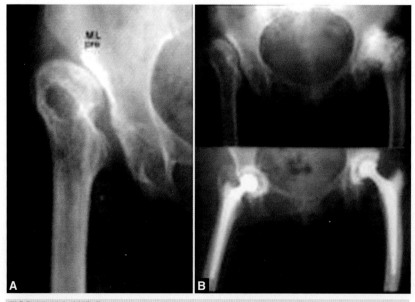

FIGS 37.16A AND B

Preoperative radiograph showing the right hip dislocated and the left demonstrating advanced osteoarthritic changes. The acetabular component was place at the level of the original acetabulum

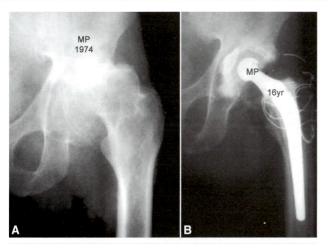

FIGS 37.17A AND B

(A) Advanced osteoarthritis with significant degree of subluxation of the hip. (B) Sixteen years post Charnley arthroplasty the radiograph shows no evidence of complications and the patient has remained asymptomatic

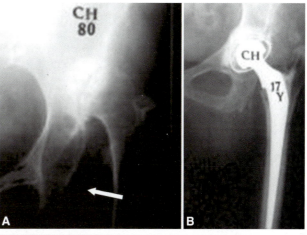

FIGS 37.18A AND B

(A) Dislocated hip allegedly sustained at approximately 10 years of age. (B) Seventeen years post-total hip replacement of the hip has remained asymptomatic. Notice what appears to be avulsion of the tip of the trochanter. This displacement did not seem to affect the power of abduction

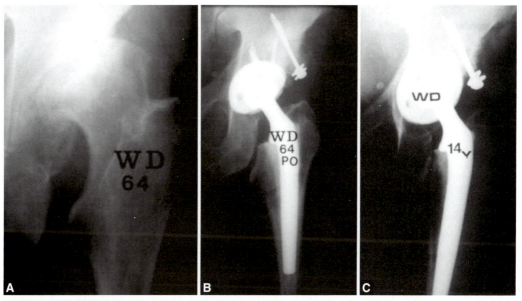

FIGS 37.19A TO C

(A) Radiograph of osteoarthritic hip secondary to congenital hip dysplasia. (B) Radiograph taken shortly after surgery. A bone graft was use to provide better acetabular coverage. (C) Radiograph obtained 14 years later

Section 2

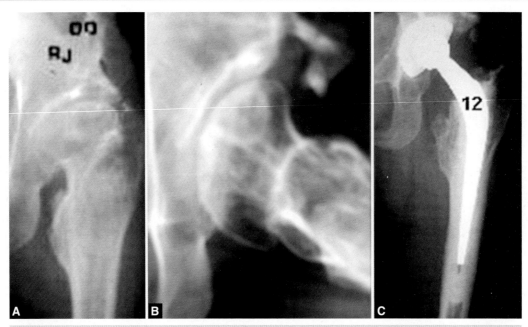

FIGS 37.20A TO C

(A) Radiographs of osteoarthritic hip in a 39-year-old woman, secondary to congenital hip dysplasia. (B) Radiograph obtained shortly after surgery. (C) Radiograph taken 12 years postoperatively. The patient has remained asymptomatic

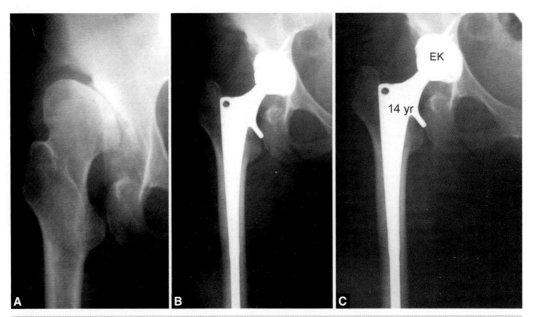

FIGS 37.21A TO C

(A) Osteoarthritis secondary to congenital hip dysplasia in a 29-year-old woman. (B) The hip was replaced with a noncemented Bias prosthesis. He experienced an episode of posterior dislocation which never recurred. (C) Radiograph taken 22 years postoperatively. The hip is allegedly symptomatic

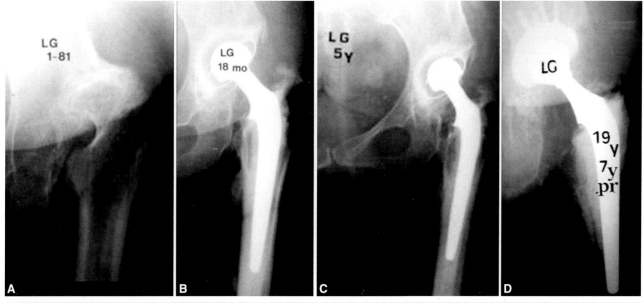

FIGS 37.22A TO D

(A) Radiograph of osteoarthritic hip secondary to congenital hip dysplasia in a 54-year-old woman. An acetabular osteotomy had been performed during her early adult life. (B) Radiograph taken a few months after arthroplasty. (C) Radiograph obtained 5 years postoperatively. (D) A revision arthroplasty was performed due to acetabular and femoral components failure. The films showing the failed implants were lost. This film (D) was taken seven years after revision

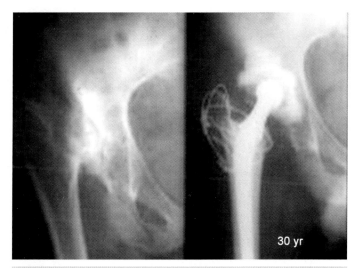

FIG. 37.23

Composite radiograph of osteoarthritic hip secondary to congenital hip disease in a 55-year-old man and a Charnley arthroplasty performed 30 years earlier

Section 2

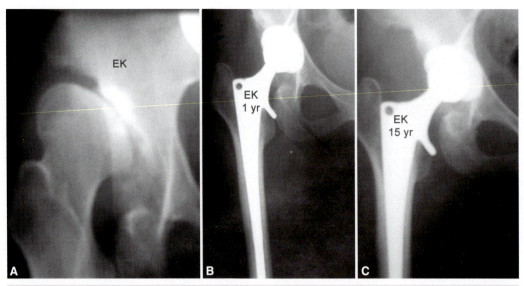

FIGS 37.24A TO C

(A) Radiograph of congenital hip dysplasia in a 50-year-old woman. (B and C) Radiographs obtained 1 and 15 years postoperatively respectively. A Bias noncemented prosthesis had been used. Notice the mild subsidence of the stem into the medullary canal. The hip has remained relatively asymptomatic

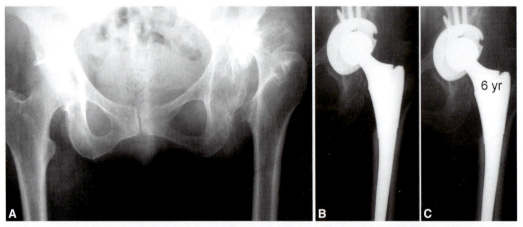

FIGS 37.25A TO C

(A) Radiograph of congenitally dislocated hip in an active 63-year-old woman. (B) Radiographs taken immediately after surgery showing the placement of the acetabular component at the level of the original socket. (C) Radiograph obtained 6 years postoperatively

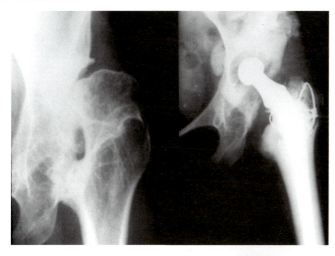

FIG. 37.26

Composite radiograph of severe osteoarthritis secondary to congenital hip dysplasia in a 69-year-old woman showing the high placement of the cemented polyethylene socket. The patient was lost to follow-up two years after surgery

FIGS 37.27A AND B

(A) Radiograph of dysplastic hip with secondary osteoarthritis in a 75-year-old woman. (B) Radiograph of Charnley arthroplasty obtained ten years postoperatively. The patient died shortly afterwards

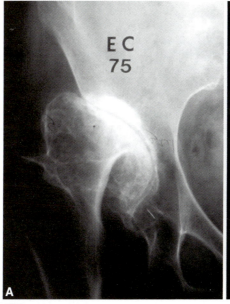
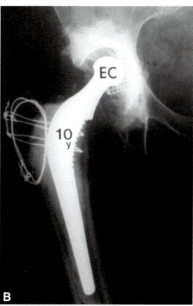

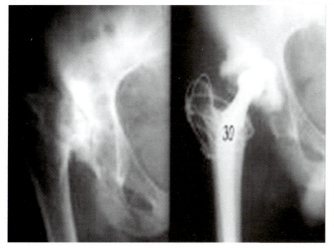

FIG. 37.28

Composite radiograph of osteoarthritic hip secondary to hip dysplasia in a 45-year-old woman. The X-ray was taken 15 years postoperatively. Patient was then lost to follow-up

*References**

10, 77, 104, 114

* References provided at the end of the book after annexures.

Section 2

38

Avascular Necrosis

One of the yet to be conquered frontiers in orthopedics is "Avascular Necrosis" of the femoral head. After many years of feverish attempts to find answers about its true etiology and management we still are puzzled by its elusive nature. Reports abound of promising solutions, be it core decompression, osteotomies or grafting of various types. The fact remains that there is not as yet a method of treatment that consistently renders good results. To complicate matters, we now know that there is a previously unrecognized condition called "transient osteoporosis" that gives similar clinical and imaging changes. *Such a revelation makes one wonder how many of the reported successful procedures performed for the care of avascular necrosis were carried out in patients with "transient osteoporosis", not with avascular necrosis.*

The more core decompression procedures I see, the greater my lack of enthusiasm with this approach. In too many instances a second and more definitive procedure becomes necessary. The decompression seems to be most effective in patients who do not need the procedure.

I participated in an effort to duplicate the results reported by Sugioka using his osteotomy. I had heard him illustrate his very good results on several occasions. Our attempts resulted in failure. We either did not know how to carry out the procedure appropriately or the osteotomy was performed for the wrong reasons and in the wrong patients.

I have personally become skeptical about the true value of many surgical approaches in vogue; this in spite the fact that I am familiar with the various reports in the literature and have personally performed some of them. I have seen very satisfactory short-term results from vascularized fibular grafts performed in patients with grades I and II disease, but have serious doubts

concerning their effectiveness in grades III and IV. Even the proponents of the graft have expressed the same reservations.

James Urbaniak, a most credible former professor and head of Orthopedics at Duke University, has reported very impressive results from vascularized fibular grafts. Subsequent ankle pain has been reported by others. I was surprised to hear about this complication, because my experiences with osteotomies of the fibula in the treatment of tibial nonunions had not shown ankle pain as a problem. The few patients, who had pain, eventually, and within a relatively short-time, rid themselves of the discomfort. Perhaps the same is true for those who had their fibulae transplanted.

We all seem to believe that a well-established AVN if left alone eventually demonstrates the classical collapse of the femoral head, particularly if a "crescent sign" has already appeared on the lateral X-ray of the femoral head. *I have seen probably half a dozen patients with "obvious" radiologically diagnosed AVN, who without treatment of any kind never demonstrated progression of the disease or collapse of the femoral head.*

I remember the case of an alcoholic man (Figs 38.1A to C) I presented at an Academy meeting in Miami Beach in the early 70's to a panel of gurus of hip surgery in those days. Upon looking at the projected X-rays, there was unanimous consensus that the pathology causing the radiological signs was characteristic of AVN. When asked about their preference for treatment some of the panelists agreed that prosthetic replacement was the treatment of choice. One panelist suggested mold arthroplasty; another one mentioned osteotomy and a third-one thought that fusion was probably a good option. He backed-down as the discussion continued and he was

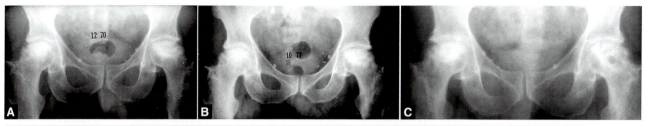

FIGS 38.1A TO C

(A) Radiograph of alcohol induced bilateral avascular necrosis of the femoral heads in a 36-year-old man. The symptoms were minimal. (B) Radiograph obtained two years later. The symptoms had remained tolerable and the patient walked without external support. (C) Radiograph taken six years after the initial films. The clinical condition had remained essentially unchanged

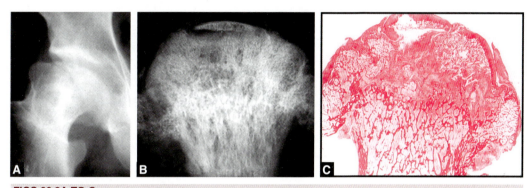

FIGS 38.2A TO C

Radiograph of avascular necrosis of the femoral head, radiograph of a section of the removed femoral head, and histology of the necrotic head respectively

reminded that the incidence of bilateral disease was as high as sixty percent. Doctor Lazansky, from New York, an early disciple of Charnley, recommended total hip replacement. Most of the panelists were not as familiar with the new procedure as Lazansky was.

After listening to the various recommendations, I informed the experts that the X-rays they had reviewed had been taken five years earlier. He had not had surgery of any kind. I summoned the patient to the stage. I suspect he had imbibed a few drinks on the way to the hotel, which helped make his performance all the more entertaining. He ran the distance and once there he proceeded to squat down a few times, spread his legs apart and ran down the steps. He denied any pain. I then proceeded to flash on the screen recent films that showed no progression of the disease process and a perfectly round head. I followed him for several years until he disappeared (Figs 38.2A to C).

I have another patient, a bartender, who in the late 1960's presented himself with pain in both hips. A diagnosis of bilateral AVN was made, which I proceeded to treat with an endoprosthetic replacement of his most painful joint. Histological sections of the femoral specimen showed large necrotic areas and the subchondral "fracture" (Figs 38.3A to C). Over the

ensuing months the nonoperated hip showed spontaneous clinical improvement, so much so that we decided to postpone surgery on that side. Three years later the Austin-Moore replacement became painful and bored into the pelvis. The painful condition was approached by replacing the endoprosthesis with a Charnley total hip arthroplasty, which within a relatively short-time showed signs of loosening, fracture of the cement and distal migration of the femoral stem. However, the symptoms ranged from minimal to nonexisting at times. Twenty-two years later he died. X-rays had been taken a few months before his death. The "failed" arthroplasty had become stable many years earlier and never showed any evidence of further mechanical loosening or lysis. The opposite hip, the nonoperated one, never collapsed and maintained the mild loss of sphericity that appeared on the original radiographs.

These and other experiences (Figs 38.4 to 38.17) have convinced me that there is much we do not know about the subject and that it will be a long-time before the final word is written.

I would not be surprised if total hip arthroplasty becomes the universal treatment for virtually all patients with avascular necrosis. For practical purposes, that is the case

Section 2

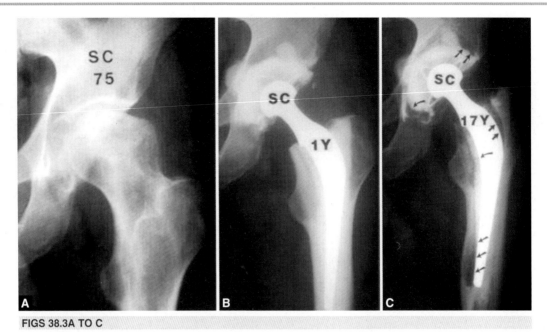

FIGS 38.3A TO C

(A) Preoperative radiograph of hip with avascular necrosis. (B) Radiograph obtained one year ATE surgery. (C) Radiograph taken 17 years postsurgery illustrating the extensive lytic lesions in the femur and loosening of the acetabulum

today. If the results from this operation continue to improve, there is no reason to doubt that the procedure will ultimately displace all others. The road to such destination is, however, rough and full of obstacles.

During a panel discussion at an Academy's annual meeting in the late 1980's, the four panelists agreed that the incidence of lysis in their respective patients with avascular necrosis, who had been treated with cementless total hip arthroplasty, was 25 percent at the end of the seventh postoperative year. When, I pursued the discussion and asked them if they felt that lysis was progressive in nature, they all agreed it was. That meant that the chances were that most of the young patients reported in their series would eventually require additional surgery.

I took advantage of the agreement between the panelists so I, as moderator, could try to get them to share their views on related issues. I remarked that they had agreed that lysis occurs in 25 percent of the patients with cementless prostheses at seven years after surgery. Therefore, what bizarre logic could justify the use of such implants when the incidence of lytic changes with cemented prostheses was so much lower? Without giving them a chance to answer the question, I added, "Why use noncemented implants in these younger patients realizing that sooner or later they will have secondary surgery which oftentimes is

likely to be very difficult to perform and requires major bone reconstruction"?

I suspect that I was not quite as candid as I should have been. I personally have no answers to the problem and find it very difficult to decide what is best for these patients. For a few years I performed hybrid arthroplasty in most instances (a cemented femoral component and a noncemented acetabular cup). During the past 20 years, I have been using noncemented implants in virtually all instances, based on frequent reports that the "new" implants have solved many of the previous problems. They have indeed improved significantly.

In regards to the behavior of avascular necrosis, there is not much solid information up to this time. Most of what the "experts" say is based, to a great extent, on hypothesis and speculations. I have remained attracted for many years to the ideas on the mechanism of progression of AVN described by Glimcher, from Boston, in the 1960's. He said, and rightly so, that a dead, avascular femoral head does not collapse as long as it is dead. It is only when vessels succeed in restoring blood supply to the dead structure that the, now softer, bone collapses under the weight of the body. This hypothesis probably explains the situation of my previously above mentioned patients who never showed bony collapse. It can be safely suspected that

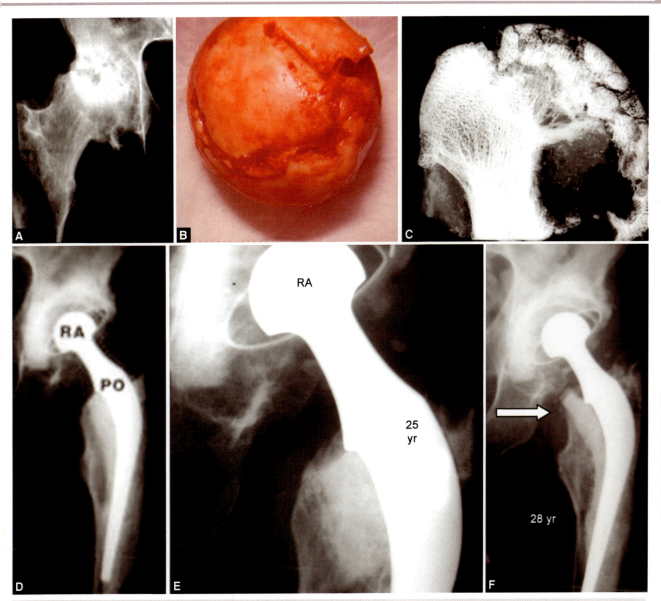

FIGS 38.4A TO F

(A) Avascular necrosis in a 38-year-old patient with acromegaly. (B) Photograph of the removed femoral head. (C) Radiograph of a sectioned femoral head. (D) Radiograph obtained postoperatively. (E) 25 years postsurgery. (F) Radiograph obtained 25 years later. Radiographs taken 28 years after surgery showing the loose femoral component and lysis over the distal-medial aspect of the femur. The acetabular component has not shown evidence of wear or loosening

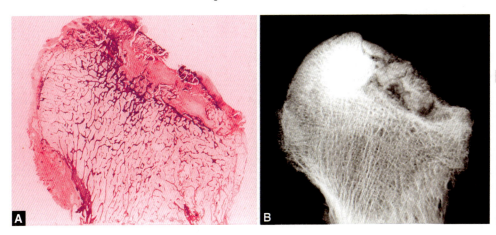

FIGS 38.5A AND B

(A) Microscopic slide of avascular necrosis in a patient with AIDS. It takes a great leap of faith to believe that this type and depth of lesion treated with currently available grating techniques can provide a clinical result comparable to total hip arthroplasty. (B) Photo radiograph demonstrating the depth of the avascular lesion

Section 2

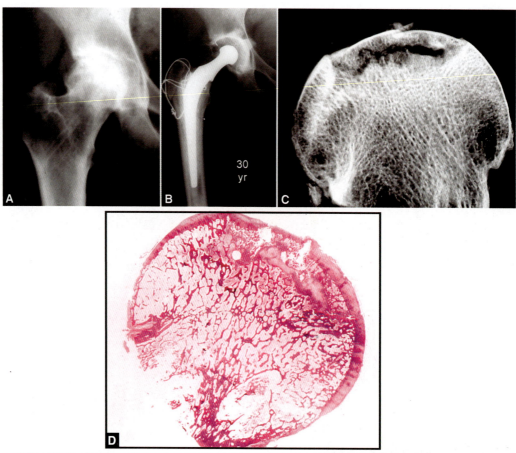

FIGS 38.6A TO D

(A) Radiograph of avascular necrosis of the femoral head. Radiological appearance is rather benign. (B) The hip was replaced with a Charnley arthroplasty 33 years earlier. (C and D) Radiograph and histological sections of the excised femoral head

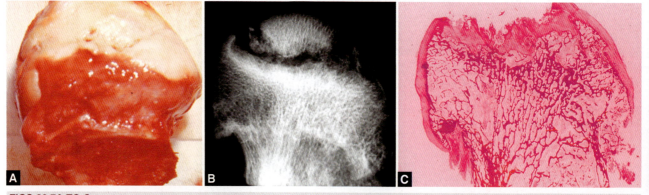

FIGS 38.7A TO C

(A) Gross appearance of avascular necrotic femoral head showing significant amount of inflammatory soft tissue reaction. (B) Photo radiograph showing the large separated segment of bone and cartilage. (C) Microscopic slide depicting the size and depth of the necrosis. The patient died one year later from AIDS

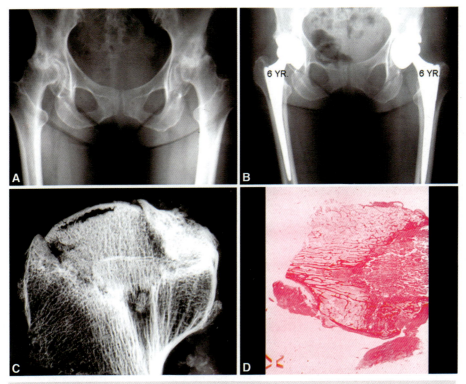

FIGS 38.8A TO D

(A) Radiograph of bilateral avascular necrosis probably secondary to chronic alcoholism. (B) Both hips were replaced with noncemented prostheses. (C and D) Closer view of the right and left femoral heads. Cross-section of the left femoral head illustrating the fracture of the bone at one level. Corresponding microscopic slide of the defect

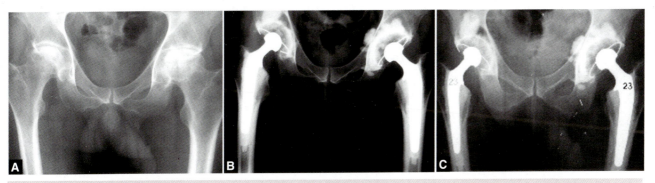

FIGS 38.9A TO C

(A) Radiograph of bilateral avascular necrosis in a surgeon 44 years of age. (B) Closer view of right and left femoral heads. (C) Radiograph obtained 23 years postoperatively

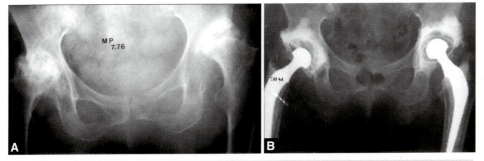

FIGS 38.10A AND B

(A) Bilateral idiopathic avascular necrosis in a 56-year-old woman. (B) Radiograph showing the bilateral cemented titanium total hip prostheses taken 20 years postoperatively

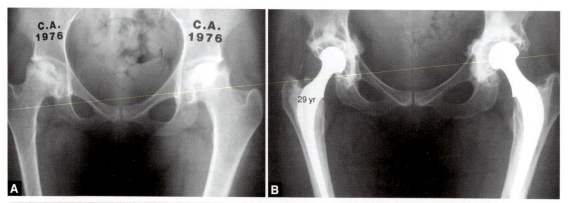

FIGS 38.11A AND B

(A) Radiograph of bilateral AVN secondary to lupus in an 18-year-old woman. (B) Radiographs obtained 29 years postoperatively

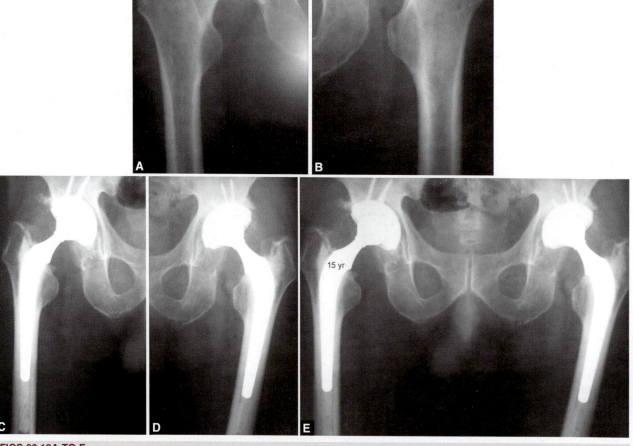

FIGS 38.12A TO E

(A and B) Radiograph of bilateral avascular necrosis in a 54-year-old man. (C and D) Radiographs of right and left hips following bilateral total hip arthroplasties using titanium stems with modular cobalt-chrome heads. (E) Radiograph obtained 15 years later

Section 2

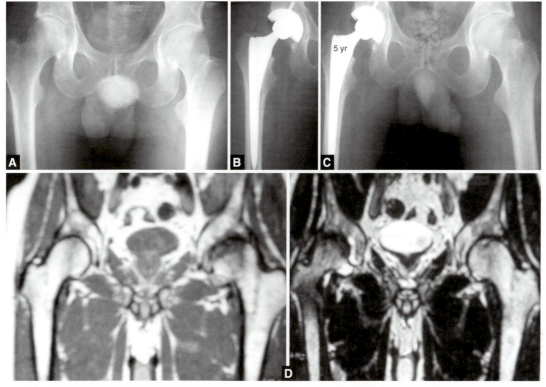

FIGS 38.13A TO D

(A) Radiograph of avascular necrosis. Hip remained symptomatic throughout. (B) Postoperative radiograph. (C) Radiograph obtained 5 years later. (D) MRI obtained prior to surgery

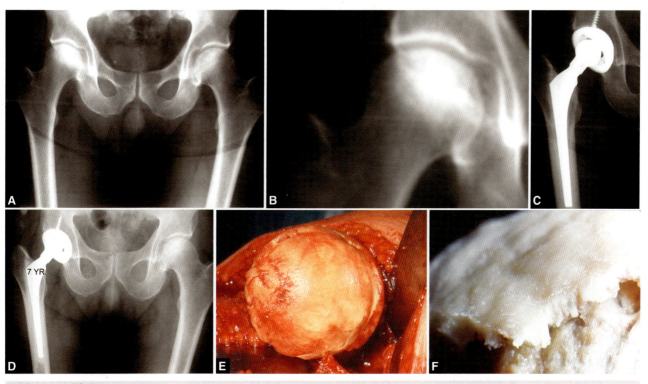

FIGS 38.14A TO F

(A) Avascular necrosis of the right hip probably secondary to cortisone injections in a 48-year-old man. (B) Close view of damaged femoral head. (C) Postoperative radiograph following hybrid arthroplasty. (D) Radiograph obtained 7 years postoperatively. (E) Photograph of thee excised femoral head. (F) Appearance of the subchondral defect frequently found in advanced avascular necrosis

Section 2

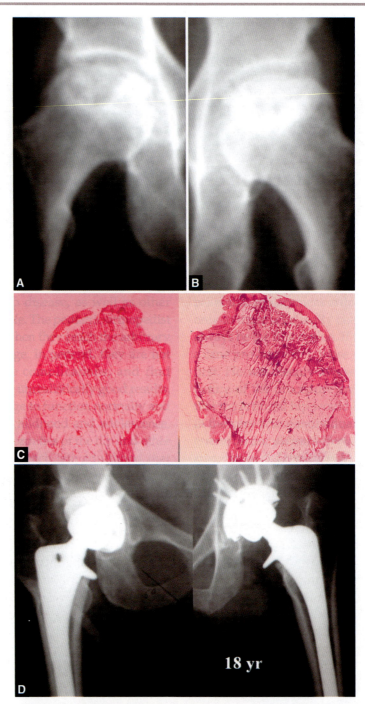

FIGS 38.15A TO D

(A and B) Bilateral avascular necrosis probably secondary to alcoholism. (C) Microscopic slides of avascular necrosis. (D) Radiographs obtained 18 years postoperatively. Notice mild wear of the polyethylene liner in the right hip

revascularization never took place and the dead head remained dead and therefore, like the dog's toy, hard and strong. He jokingly remarked that the "avascular" bone the dog plays with in the backyard of the house never collapses.

Another good example to support the fact that an avascular femoral head does not collapse as long as it remains avascular, is the fact that the femoral head of an individual who sustains a completely displaced femoral neck fracture, which is not reduced and is allowed to remain totally

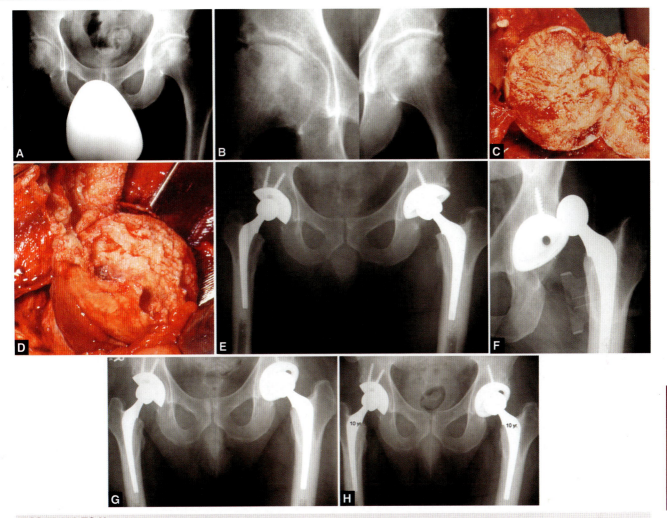

FIGS 38.16A TO H

(A and B) Radiographs of bilateral avascular necrosis of the femoral heads secondary to alcoholism in a 35-year-old man. (C and D) Gross appearance of the femoral heads with a grade IV avascular necrosis. *To expect a satisfactory result from an osteotomy or core decompression is wishful thinking.* (E) Radiographs of both hips after the performance of bilateral hybrid arthroplasties. (F) The left hip dislocated 2 months after surgery while the patient was heavily intoxicated. It was suspected the acetabulum did not have sufficient anteversion and that a revision of the acetabulum was appropriate. (G) Radiograph taken 2 years following revision surgery. (H) Radiograph obtained 10 years postoperatively

separated from the femoral neck, never collapses. If one looks at X-ray films of that hip several years later one sees the uncollapsed head in the acetabulum. Collapse does not take place because blood supply never invaded the femoral head.

Some have tried to fill the curetted femoral head with bone graft, but with disappointing results; others have packed the "empty" head with acrylic cement with similarly poor outcomes. I personally worked in the laboratory dealing with the subject of acute fractures of the femoral neck. I was hoping to develop a method that would allow us to remove all bone from the femoral head and place the remaining cartilaginous shell over a metallic prosthesis. It was an exercise in futility.

I am forced to conclude that in light of the increasingly high success from prosthetic arthroplasty,

it is becoming difficult to justify the performance of more conservative procedures that, even in the best of hands, often fail to render good long-term results.

Quite recently, I was shown the following radiographs of a 25-year-old man who developed pain in both hips. The films show large lytic cavities that may militate against the diagnosis of AVN. However, that was the diagnosis made by the radiologist and plans had been made to perform total hip arthroplasty. Unfortunately, I have no information as to the surgical findings and final diagnosis. I am concerned that the true pathology is something more serious, such as a malignant degeneration of a benign condition. In one occasion I saw a young man with somewhat similar findings being finally diagnosed with AIDS. Too far fetched (Figs 38.18A and B)?

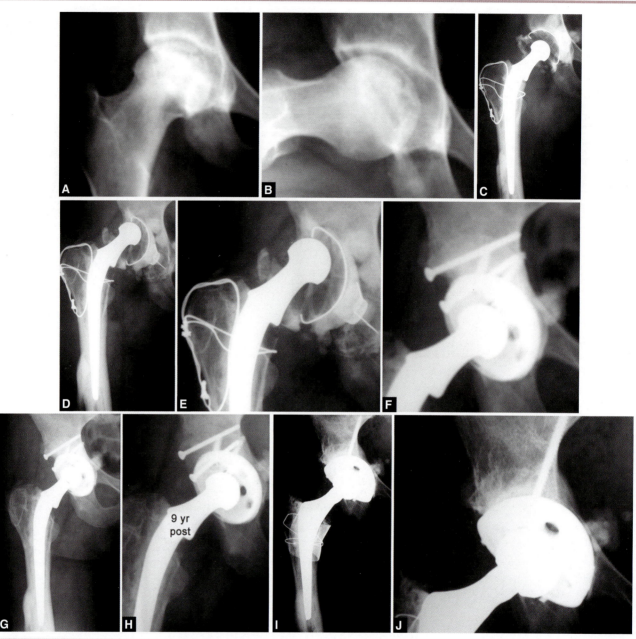

FIGS 38.17A TO J

(A and B) Radiographs of avascular necrosis of the femoral head secondary to sickle cell disease. The Charnley arthroplasty was allegedly performed when the patient was 20-year-old. (C) Radiograph obtained 10 years postoperatively. (D and E) Radiographs taken after sudden onset of pain appeared without trauma or infection six months later. The acetabular component had dislocated. I revised the hip and found out a membrane at the bottom of the socket that suggested its long-time presence. (F) Radiograph obtained postoperatively showing the graft, I used to provide appropriate coverage of the new porous acetabulum. (G and H) Radiographs obtained 9 years after revision surgery suggesting good incorporation of the graft. (I and J) Over a period of twelve months the hip failed and required additional surgery that was performed by another surgeon in a different city. He revised the acetabular and femoral components. The patient has done well according to a telephone conversation one year after surgery

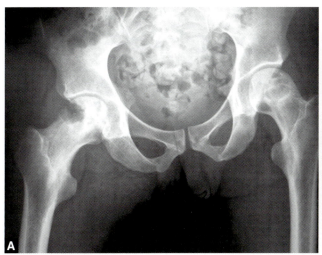 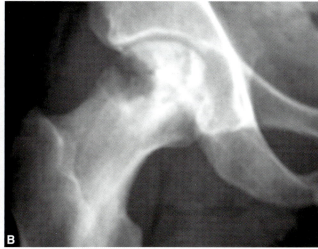

FIGS 38.18A AND B

(A) Radiograph of both hips showing changes that have led the radiologist to interpret as avascular necrosis. (B) A closer view showing the large lytic lesion in the right femoral head. Could this be something else rather than AVN or in addition to it?

References*

10, 77, 104

_____

* References provided at the end of the book after annexures.

39

Slipped Capital Epiphysis

I suspect a large percentage of people who experience slipped femoral capital epiphysis in their teen years and end up with some deformity eventually develop arthritic changes (Figs 39.1 to 39.7). I have observed that these people begin to experience symptoms sooner than those who had suffered from Perthes disease. I have no reasonable explanation as to why this is the case. *It is possible, however, that the deformity of the femoral head in Perthes disease takes place at an earlier age and in a more gradual manner, during which time the acetabulum undergoes parallel accommodating changes.* In the case of slipped epiphysis, such gradual changes do not occur gradually. If the femoral head undergoes collapse as a result of avascular necrosis, the acetabulum does not have time to experience favorable changes.

It is well-known that a relatively high percentage of patients with slipped epiphysis develop avascular necrosis and some of them also experience chondrolysis. It was suspected for a long time in North America that the prognosis from surgical treatment was worse in the black race. This turned out to be inaccurate. More careful studies failed to reveal any different between the white and dark races.

One thing I was personally able to observe, and the point had been made by others, is that *chondrolysis does not seem to occur in hips that had not been either*

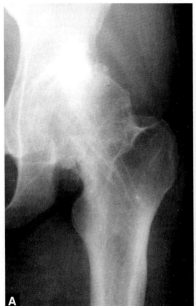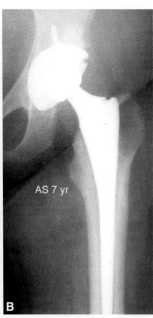

FIGS 39.1A AND B

(A) Radiograph of osteoarthritic changes in the hip of a 38-year-old woman who became disabled 20 years after surgical pinning of a surgically treated slipped capital femoral epiphysis. (B) Illustration obtained seven years after surgery

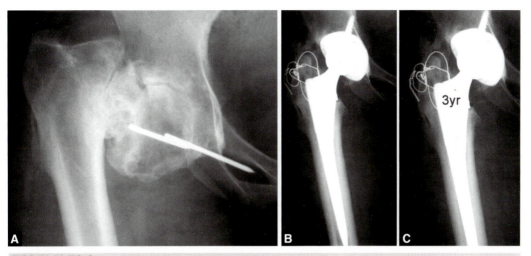

FIGS 39.2A TO C

(A) Radiograph of the hip of a 25-year-old obese woman taken 15 years after surgical treatment of slipped capital femoral epiphysis. There was a rather fixed adduction contracture, an external rotation deformity and significant shortening of the extremity. (B) Radiograph obtained a few months after surgery. *Osteotomy of the greater trochanter was performed because of the fixed external rotation and to facilitate exposure of the acetabulum and proximal femur. After stripping of soft tissue, adductor and iliopsoas tenotomy, the legs were made equal in length.* (C) Last radiograph of the hip obtained three years after surgery. Patient was lost to follow-up

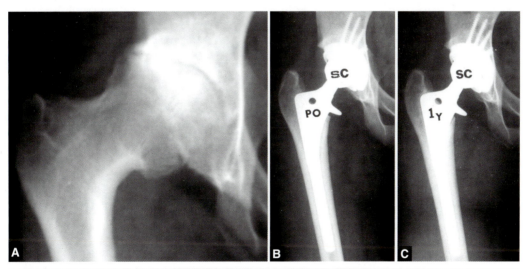

FIGS 39.3A TO C

(A) Radiograph of the arthritic hip of a 30-year-old black man taken 15 years after surgical treatment of slipped epiphysis. The condition had been allegedly treated by manipulation and cast immobilization. (B) Radiograph obtained shortly after surgery. The external rotation and significant ankylosis were overcome. (C) Radiograph obtained one year postoperatively. The patient was lost to follow-up

manipulated or operated upon. A slipped femoral capital epiphysis that is left untreated and the deformity is allowed to develop will be associated with permanent deformity and some shortening of the extremity, but free of chondrolysis.

It is believed, though not scientifically proven, that perforation of the articular cartilage at the time of pinning may lead to chondrolysis. There is some anecdotal evidence to support the concept, but not sufficient to make it impermeable.

The frequently encountered external rotational deformity accompanying long-standing bony changes requires attention when a prosthetic replacement procedure is being performed. The surgeon must ascertain that the component enters the femoral canal in a manner that accommodates the femoral retroversion, and the likely changes in the femoral shaft. Since the acetabulum may also show major structural changes, the position of the acetabular component has to be critically established. Trial reduction of the hip often shows limitation of

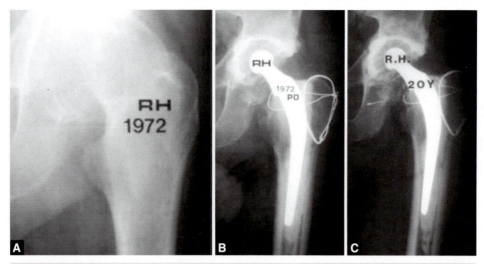

FIGS 39.4A TO C

(A) Radiograph of the osteoarthritic hip in a 54-year-old man secondary to slipped capital femoral epiphysis.
(B) A Charnley arthroplasty was used to replace the joint. (C) Twenty years later the patient was
asymptomatic and functional. He expired shortly afterwards from acute leukemia

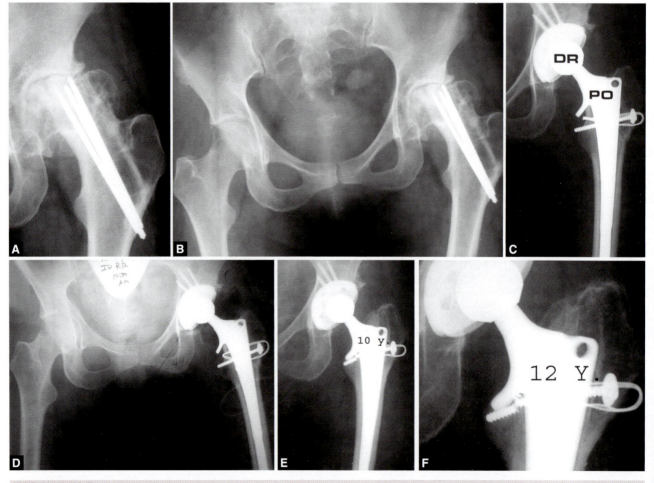

FIGS 39.5A TO F

(A) Radiograph of the arthritic hip of a 32-year-old woman who at the age of 14 had surgery for the treatment of slipped epiphysis. The femoral
head underwent avascular necrosis of the femoral head, painful limitation of motion and a rather grotesque limp. (B) Radiograph illustrating
the significant joint pathology and a pelvic obliquity. (C) Postoperative radiograph. A partial, short split of the femur produced during implantation
required the use of a transfixion screw. (D) Notice that the pre-existing pelvic obliquity was unchanged in the immediate postoperative film.
(E) Radiograph taken 10 years later showed the screw had broken. Though the patient had remained asymptomatic, I recommended its
removal. (F) Twelve years after surgery lytic lesions are developing around the proximal stem

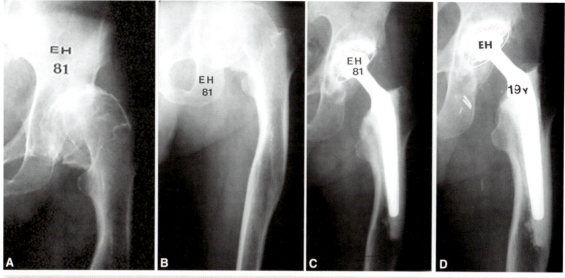

FIGS 39.6A TO D

(A and B) Radiographs of the left hip of a 60-year-old man who suffered a slipped capital epiphysis at the age of 12 years. He sustained a fracture of the femur at the age of 22 years. (C) Postoperative radiograph depicting the cemented titanium total hip arthroplasty. (D) Radiograph obtained 19 years postoperatively. The varus attitude of the femoral component did not result in loosening, probably due to the fact that a thick medial column of cement was preserved

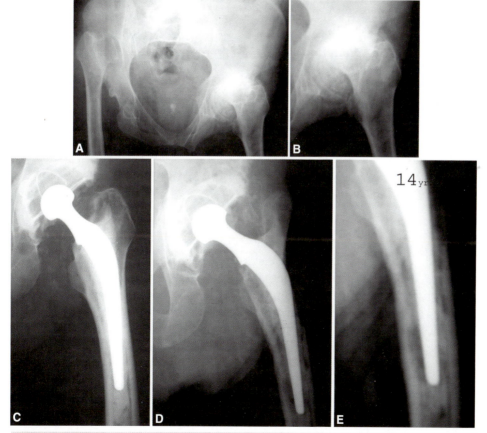

FIGS 39.7A TO E

(A and B) Radiographs of both hips of a 63-year-old man who suffered from congenital hip disease on the right side. According to the patient his right hip never received treatment. Though it made hip limp, it never caused him pain. He stated that at the age of twelve he suffered slipped capital epiphysis of the left hip that was treated by manipulation and cast immobilization. (C) A cemented titanium total hip arthroplasty was performed. (D and E) Radiographs obtained 14 years postoperatively shows lytic changes in the distal femur. The patient was reluctant to have surgery and died 3 years later

Section 2

rotation in the internal plane. It behooves the surgeon to determine to what extent the limitation is due to long-standing structural changes in the surrounding soft tissue, and how much secondary to bony impingement from inferior acetabular osteophytes. In the latter case, their removal is required; in the former case additional generous capsulectomy.

Ignacio Ponseti, from Iowa, one of the true great orthopedist of the twentieth century, speculated that Perthes disease and slipped capital epiphysis were the same condition that happened to develop at different ages. He had recognized that the younger child—the one who suffers Perthes disease—has a proximal physis directed in a rather transverse manner: the epiphysis sits on it in a mechanically stable mode. In the older child—the one that suffers slipped epiphysis—the physis has changed to a more vertical direction, therefore, the epiphysis sits on a sloping surface that makes slippage more likely. If the physis undergoes "softening" due to some inflammatory process, the head could undergo collapse and not slip if the inflammation occurs in the younger child. In the older child, the head under similar circumstances, would slip.

Very often in the practice of the profession we find it impossible, upon reading the X-rays of severely arthritic hip joints, to accurately determine the primary pathology that led to arthritic changes in later years. There are no consistent findings to precisely confirm the diagnosis. The deformities that we ordinarily see are so severe as to preclude such accuracy. However, if a patient has complete absence of internal rotation, and an accompanying fixed external rotation that has been present since adolescence, the chances are that he, or she, suffered slipped capital epiphysis.

When the time comes for replacement arthroplasty to overcome painful symptoms, several features must be kept in mind. First of all is the ubiquitous external rotation deformity of the hip. In addition, there often is significant shortening of the extremity and structural rotational abnormalities in the femur.

If the surgery is to be performed through a posterior approach, the necessary internal rotation of the hip for exposure of the femoral neck is not there. The space

between the head of the femur and the greater trochanter is too small to make the osteotomy uncomplicated. *A dislocation by means of flexion, adduction and internal rotation may be impossible.*

This problem can be overcome either by ostetomizing the greater trochanter or by amputating the femoral head in situ. Since good exposure is not always possible, it may be necessary to create the cut in the bone through the femoral head. Then the head is removed. Once the hip is flexed to 90 degrees and internally rotated, the neck of the femur is shortened with additional cuts of bone. In this manner, the desirable exposure of the neck of the femur can be achieved.

A severe preoperative shortening of the extremity requires careful consideration. Trying to gain too much length may result in sciatic nerve palsy. In orthopedics circles little is said about femoral nerve palsy, probably because it is rare. However, it does occur from time-to-time and its prognosis is quite unsatisfactory in many instances (See *Length Discrepancy*).

It is not uncommon to see patients with arthritic pathology in the femoral head, demonstrating a severe adduction contracture that makes more difficult the appropriate determination of the degree of shortening of the extremity. It is best, prior to surgery, to measure the length of both legs from the two anterior superior spines to the medial malleoli, as well as obtaining measurements from the umbilicus to the malleoli. *Matters are further complicated when an associated pelvic obliquity has reached a rigid status. In this instance, the pelvic obliquity does not improve with the passage of time. Other times, when the pelvic obliquity is not a rigid, structural one, it improves rather rapidly from activity an abduction exercises.* I have seen a few instances when scoliosis further complicated the problem.

I have seen a number of patients who along with painful symptoms secondary the arthritic disease complain of major leg length discrepancy. They usually accuse the surgeon who performed the arthroplasty of failing to equalize the length of the extremity, when in actuality the apparent length discrepancy is due, not the shortening of the leg but to an existing scoliosis, which is frequently progressive in the osteoporotic elderly.

40

Protrusio Acetabulum

I am not sufficiently knowledgeable on the subject of protrusio acetabulum, which is the classical idiopathic condition where the acetabulum covers too much of the femoral head, a fact that seems to lead to degenerative joint disease. The etiology of the disease has been thought to be an arrest in the growth of the segments that form the physis of the acetabulum. Whether or not this has been documented is not known to me.

I suspect that in most instances the pathology I was facing prior to surgery is secondary to either osteoarthritis or secondary to osteomalacia. To the best of my recollection most of my patients were females whose main complaint, in addition to pain, *was progressive limitation of hip abduction*. Radiologically, the depth of the acetabulum is disproportional to the smaller diameter of the femoral head. Clinically, the most striking features are the limitation of abduction, the presence of a flexion contracture and a loss of rotation of the hip. In my small series the condition was bilateral in most instances.

The indications for total hip arthroplasty, which I think is the only therapeutic modality available at this time, do not differ from those used for other degenerative conditions of the hip. *If the flexion contracture of the hip is bilateral, the need for simultaneous bilateral surgery becomes a serious consideration. Unilateral surgery may result in a recurrence of the flexion contracture, since the range of flexion of the operated hip will be dictated by the degree of flexion possible in the nonoperated hip.* The sitting position forces the hip to flex to the usual 90 degrees. However, if at the time of completion of surgery full flexion can be obtained, the nonoperated hip, having a 45 degree flexion contracture will keep the operated hip from flexing during the sitting position beyond 45 degrees. If the procedure cannot,

or should not be performed bilaterally, it is important to concentrate on maintaining the surgically achieved flexion of the hip through appropriate physical therapy modalities.

Bilateral adductor tenotomies are usually necessary if the adduction contracture is severe. This surgical step is best performed just prior to the making of the incision for the prosthetic replacement. Some times it is possible to gain some motion following the tenotomies; a gain that makes easier the arthroplasty. Testing the degree of improvement from the tenotomies must be conducted carefully in order to avoid fracturing the femur or the femoral neck. The chances of gaining much from the tenotomies alone are limited because of the associated capsular contractures.

Since I have performed the vast majority of hip arthroplasties through a posterior approach I have found it difficult to dislocate the hip in order to expose the femoral neck and carry out its osteotomy. *The lack of rotation of the hip makes it impossible to dislocate the hip, requiring therefore the severance of the neck in situ.* This is the same obstacle frequently observed during the replacement of a hip for the sequella of slipped capital femoral epiphysis, since this condition almost always presents itself with a fixed external rotation of the hip.

In order to lateralize the prosthetic head, and to avoid postoperative femoral neck impingement against the pelvic bone, it necessary to use femoral stems with low-offset. Other times it is sufficient to remove small portions of the rim of the acetabulum. I have serious reservations regarding the packing of bone in the acetabular cavity, which nonetheless is necessary in many instances. Some surgeons recommend this procedure and fill the entire cavity with bone graft (Figs 40.1 and 40.2). I think is best to limit the packing to the very bottom of the

Hip Surgery

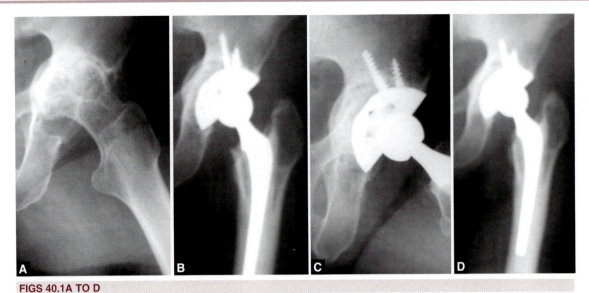

FIGS 40.1A TO D

(A) Radiograph of unilateral protrusio acetabulum. (B and C) Postoperative radiograph showing the hybrid arthroplasty, and the presence of bone graft firmly packed at the bottom of the acetabulum. (D) Radiograph obtained five years after surgery. Notice the apparent incorporation of the bone graft with the pelvic bone and the rounding of the calcar

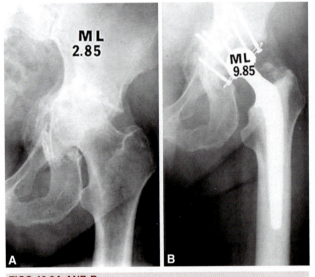

FIGS 40.2A AND B

(A) Protrusio acetabulum that developed within a few months in the absence of trauma or rheumatoid arthritis. (B) Radiograph obtained seven months postoperatively. The patient expired a few months later. In this instance a large bulk-graft was placed at the bottom of the acetabulum and stabilized with screws

acetabulum, to permit a large surface of the porous cup to be in direct contact with normal pelvic bone. The addition of a new interface between the porous metal and the normal bone appears to me to be unnecessary. Though there is some early evidence suggesting that the graft eventually grows into the porous material, I question the wisdom of relying on late bone ingrowth

for the attainment of permanent stability. I think is best to obtain early bone ingrowth by having immediate contact between the porous surface and the normal, vascularized pelvic bone, while waiting for the bone to become an integral part of the composite. As I indicated earlier, prevention of post-operative impingement of the neck against the pelvis is best accomplished by the use of longer prosthetic necks with a low-offset.

I am not aware of a higher incidence of damaged acetabular labrum in patients with idiopathic or acquired protrusio acetabulum. I raise the point, simply out of curiosity. If Ganz is correct in his theory of "impingement", the incidence of the condition in this group category should be higher, since contact between the neck of the femur and the labrum takes place sooner than in a valgus neck. In my experience, poorly documented from this point of view, has suggested that damage to the labrum is more likely to be seen in patients with long femoral necks, not with short ones.

Adding to my reservations about Ganz theory is the fact that the incidence of osteoarthritis of the hip is much lower in the oriental races. They sit on their knees for praying and other activities, forcing their hips to flex to extreme degrees, and therefore, provoking the impingement phenomenon. Such practices are not common among western races, who are the ones who suffer from hip osteoarthritis with greater frequency.

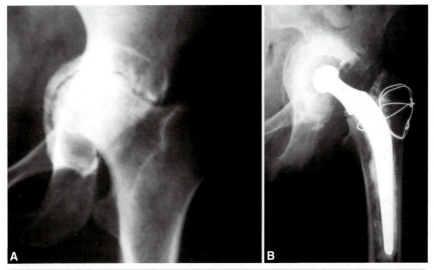

FIGS 40.3A AND B

(A) Idiopathic protrusio acetabulum. (B) The prosthetic head was lateralized using acrylic cement

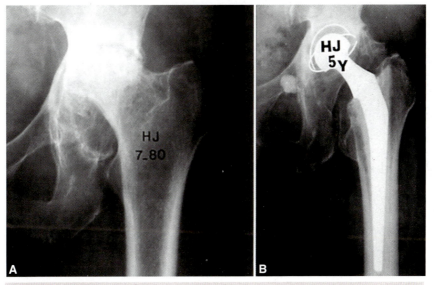

FIGS 40.4A AND B

(A) Radiograph of protrusion acetabulum of unknown etiology. Rheumatoid arthritis was ruled out. (B) Radiograph obtained five years postoperatively. *The prosthetic head had been lateralized using acrylic cement*

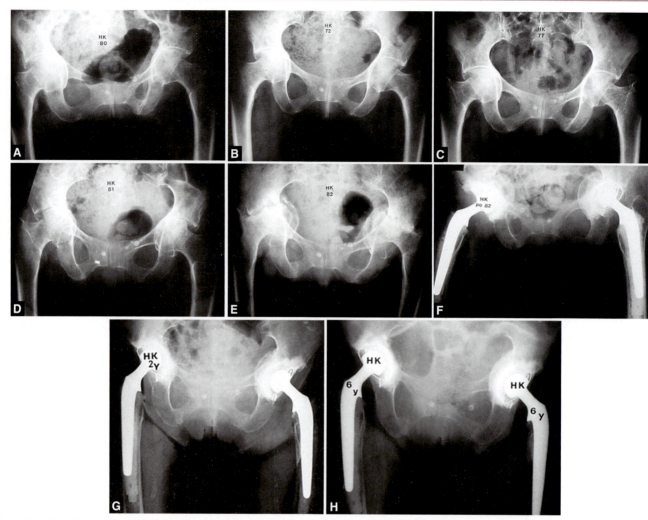

FIGS 40.5A TO H

(A to E) Radiographs sequentially obtained over a 10 years period demonstrating progressive protrusio acetabulum eventually *diagnoses as being secondary to osteomalacia.* Rheumatoid arthritis was ruled out. (F to H) Radiographs taken postoperatively over a 6 years period. The patient expired a few months after the last film; she was asymptomatic. The lateralization of the prosthetic heads was accomplished with acrylic cement

41

Prosthetic Replacement for Neoplasms

As progress in the care of malignant disease continues to expand, the role of surgery decreases. A number of malignant tumors of the musculoskeletal system, which were until relatively recently treated with amputation, at this time many of them respond to radiation therapy and/or chemotherapy. Major surgery, such as segmental bone resection accompanied with internal prosthetic replacement, is often possible and beneficial.

Questions of a philosophical nature come to my mind whenever I listen to reports on results from surgical treatments that required multiple major surgical procedures carried out over a long period of time. The sight of those people functioning with artificial internal implants generates, particularly in the case of children, enormous enthusiasm. It is only logical to get that kind of a reaction, however that enthusiasm must be tempered with a strong dose realism and objectivity. *There are many instances when an amputation is preferable to multiple surgeries.* I have seen a number of patients with malignant tumors below the knee, who after having undergone multiple major surgeries *end up end up with disability greater than the one a below-the-knee amputation would have produced.*

I have vivid recollection of the day when a 40-year-old surgeon from Lima, Peru, presented to me with a lesion on the neck of his femur. A biopsy showed chondrosarcoma. This happened in the mid-sixties, long before we had available techniques of extensive reconstructive surgery. In those days an amputation, in the form of hip disarticulation was the accepted approach. Accordingly, I made plans to carryout the procedure the following day. The night before the event I visited the doctor for the purpose of reassuring him that the amputation was very likely to "cure" the malignancy. He, once again asked me if I was certain that no other approach was available. The answer was a negative one. He inquired if an Austin Moore prosthesis should not be tried. The answer to this question was another negative one because the tumor extended beyond the bone that the endoprosthesis could replaced. The doctor, with tears in his eyes, said that as an amputee in his country his entire professional career was over and begged me to try the prosthetic approach. I acquiesced. The next day I performed the prosthetic replacement. Though grossly it appeared that the entire tumor had been completely excised, I knew better. His recovery was rapid and successful. He went home walking with assistance in anticipation of eventually doing so without a cane. I had an opportunity to visit with him in his native city of Lima six years later. He had continued his surgical practice, and was a very happy man. Two years later he developed lung metastasis and died quickly (Figs 41.1 to 41.3).

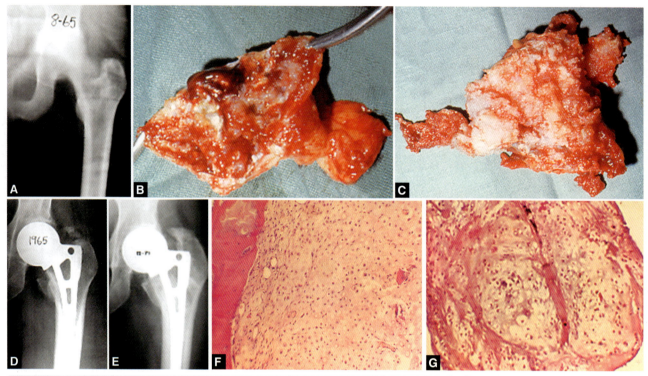

FIGS 41.1A TO G

(A) Radiograph of chondrosarcoma I treated in 1965 with removal of the femoral head and endoprosthetic replacement. (B and C) Pictures of portions of the specimen removed from the surrounding capsular tissue. (D) Radiograph taken shortly after surgery. (E) *Radiograph obtained six years after surgery demonstrating the mild sinking of the prosthesis into the femoral canal.* The hip had been asymptomatic all this time. The patient expired two years later from metastatic disease to the lungs. (F and G) Microscopic slides demonstrating malignant changes

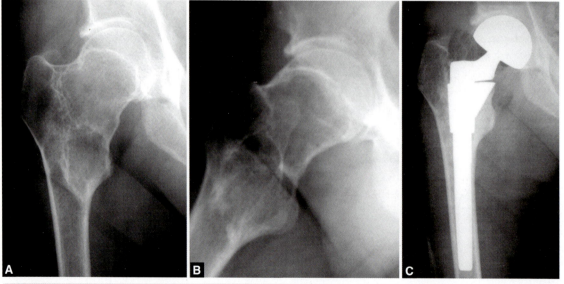

FIGS 41.2A TO C

(A and B) Radiographs of a proximal femur demonstrating a lytic lesion that extended into the femoral head. (C) Postopeartive radiograph shown the noncemented implant

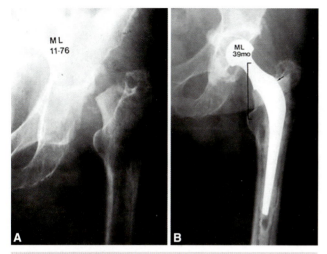

FIGS 41.3A AND B

(A) Radiograph of what was called a "disappearing head". Apparently a spontaneous lysis of the femoral head took place within a very short time. The surface of the neck of the femur suggests a surgical procedure. *The patient was not diabetic or suffered from any identifiable metabolic or neurological condition.* (B) A cemented titanium alloy prosthesis was used but showed extensive lysis thirty-nine months postoperatively

Paget's disease is not a very common disease. However, I have had the opportunity to perform total hip arthroplasty in 19 patients so afflicted. I have not found any specific reason to suspect that their behavior was different from that observed in patients with other types of osteoarthritis. The surgery is in most instances a bit more difficult when the osteoblastic changes are greater than the osteoclastic ones. Identifying the medullary canal and enlarging it is time consuming.

Though a common finding, rarely mentioned in the literature, is that patients suffering from Paget's disease often experience pain over a bony lesion, *preceding the development of a fracture at that level within a few days.* The lesson I learned from that information was the need to take appropriate precautions, such as closer observation and the use of external support. Currently, the MRI and CT scan can facilitate matters. A nondisplaced fracture can be identified before plain X-rays show the fracture (Figs 41.4 to 41.8).

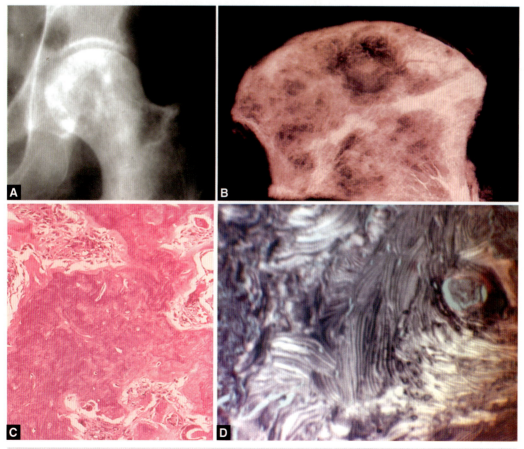

FIGS 41.4A TO D

(A) Radiograph of a hip showing Paget's disease. Usually when the head of the femur shows pathological involvement, the adjacent pelvic bone appears for quite some time normal. The reverse is also true: when the pelvis is involved the femoral head remains normal, or show pathological changes at very late date. (B) Photo of a sectioned femoral head. (C and D) Microscopic slides showing the mosaic pattern, so characteristic of Paget's disease

Section 2

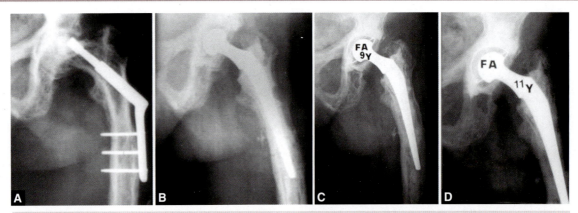

FIGS 41.5A TO D

(A and B) Radiographs of a painful hip on a patient suffering from Paget's disease showing the abnormal bone and a sliding nail used to stabilize a nondisplaced fracture of the femoral neck. (C) Radiograph obtained nine years after prosthetic replacement. (D) Radiograph taken 11 years after surgery. It is not uncommon for patients with Paget's disease to experience pain for several days prior to suffering a fracture

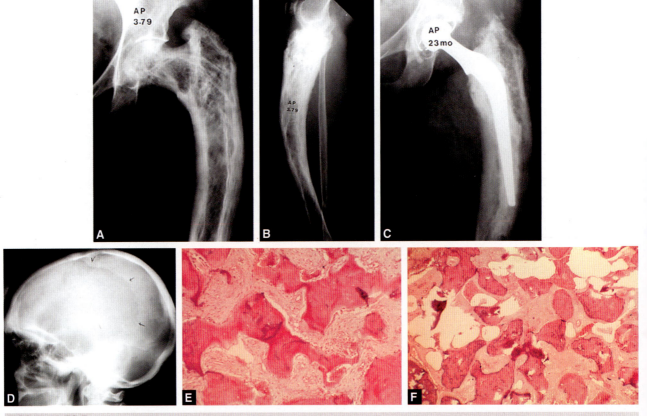

FIGS 41.6A TO F

(A) Paget's disease involving the proximal femur. Notice the apparent absence of the disease on the pelvic side of the hip. (B) Tibia demonstrates similar pathological changes. (C) Radiograph obtained 22 months after prosthetic replacement. It is suspected that the patient died shortly afterwards. (D) Radiograph of the patient's skull demonstrating the thickness of the outer table. (E and F) Microscopic slides depicting the typical Paget's disease changes

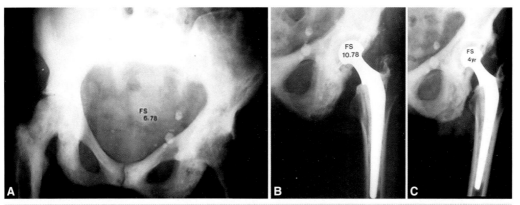

FIGS 41.7A TO C

(A) Radiograph of Paget's disease involving both femurs and pelvis. (B) Radiograph obtained shortly after surgery.
(C) Radiograph obtained four years later

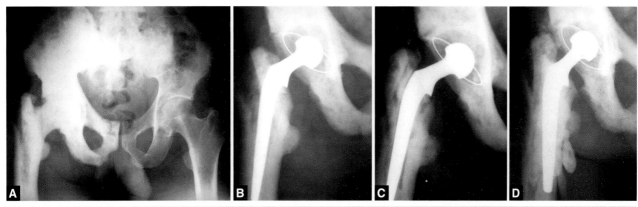

FIGS 41.8A TO D

(A) Radiograph of the pelvis showing the extensive involvement of Paget's disease. Notice the unilateral involvement in the pelvis and femurs.
(B) Radiograph obtained following total hip arthroplasty. (C) Within three years there was evidence of loosening of the femoral component.
(D) Revision was difficult and the femur was inadvertently perforated in the process of removing the cement. The bone was extremely hard.
This radiograph was obtained three years after revision. The patient expired one year later

*References**

11, 54, 103

Section 2

___
* References provided at the end of the book after annexures.

42

Synovial Chondromatosis

Synovial chondromatosis is not as common in the hip joints as it is in the knee. At least it is the universally accepted belief. *The fact that during surgery for idiopathic osteoarthritis one runs, with some frequency, into multiple loose bodies, have made me wondered if it is possible that the arthritic process had begun with chondromatosis that eventually damaged the joint in the typical osteoarthritic manner.* These loose bodies are frequently attached to the femoral neck or acetabulum. Where do they come from? Are they the result of synovial metaplasia or fragmentation? And why is it that in many instances they are entirely cartilaginous and in other instances bony bodies with a cartilaginous cap? *The bodies that are osteochondromas must have a vascular connection, or had one that was somehow lost.* Ossification must have a source of blood supply, while calcification does not require it. I suspect that free floating osteocartilagenous bodies are either fragments of bone that at one time were part of the femur or acetabulum but became free at a later date. Those made entirely of cartilage are most likely the product of synovial metaplasia.

My experience with total hip replacement performed for synovial chondromatosis is limited. I do not believe I have performed the procedure under those circumstances in more than a dozen patients. Nonetheless, *I have drawn the conclusion that surgical excision of loose bodies in the hip joint is not always a gratifying procedure.* There is some relief of symptoms but the relief is not long-lasting. Ultimately, arthritic changes develop. I suspect that the loose bodies are only a "symptom" rather than a disease *per se.*

This observation can be compared with the arthroscopic removal or repair of the acetabular labrum. *If at the time of the arthroscopic procedure early signs of arthritis are identified, the changes are that the improvement obtained is minimal or nonexistent.* This is an observation I have acquired vicariously since I have never held an arthroscope in my hands.

The two illustrated clinical cases (Figs 42.1 and 42.2) illustrate the point:

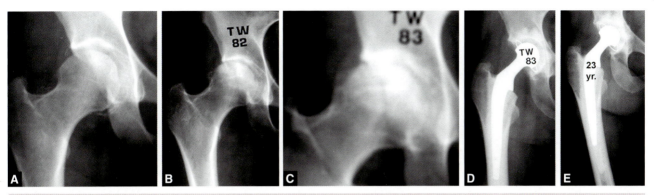

FIGS 42.1A TO E

(A) Radiograph of a hip diagnosed clinically and microscopically as synovial chondromatosis. The patient was 38 years of age at that time. At the time of surgery multiple loose bodies were removed. *The articular cartilage of the femoral head had early sign of arthritis.* (B) Twelve months painful symptoms had increased. (C) A year later the symptoms had become incapacitating. (D) Postoperative radiograph. A total hip arthroplasty was performed using a cemented titanium alloy implant. (E) Radiograph obtained 10 years postoperatively. (F) The most recent radiograph taken 23 years after surgery. The patient has been totally asymptomatic, and the radiographs have not shown evidence of wear or signs of loosening

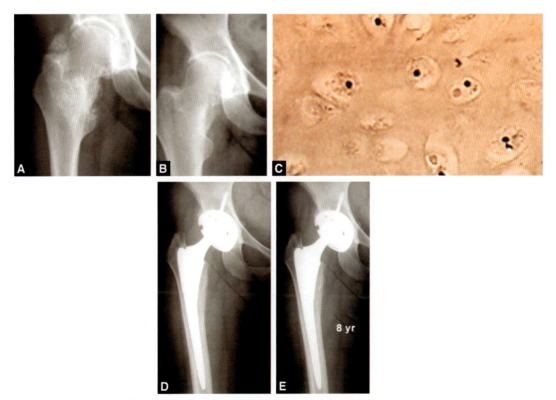

FIGS 42.2A TO E

(A) Radiograph of painful hip diagnosed with synovial chondromatosis. (B) Radiograph appearance of the hip following resection of osteocartilaginous tissues. (C) Radiograph taken shortly after surgery. (D) Postoperative radiograph shown the noncemented implant should apply. (E) Radiograph obtained three years postoperatively.

Addendum: Shortly after these films were obtained, the patient began to experience pain in the groin and the presence of a mass at that level. I then refereed her to Thomas Temple, MD, the distinguished oncologist at the University of Miami, who diagnosed an aggressive type of chondrosarcoma. The tumor extended into the ischium and proximal femur. He revised the implant with a large oncology prosthesis

*Reference**

* Reference provided at the end of the book after annexures.

Section 2

43

Neuropathic Hip Joints

I have no data regarding my experiences with neuropathic hip joints. I suspect that unknowingly I must have replaced a fair number. I base this comment under the assumption that several patients with advanced diabetes probably had neurological changes which I did not bother to look for in any serious manner. The patient, whose X-rays I illustrate in Figures 43.1A to C had been treated for syphilis during her youth. When I examined her I noticed that the relative benign symptoms did not parallel the advanced radiological findings. It was not until after I had performed surgery that I began to suspect she was suffering from a Charcot joint. *The bony fragments seeing throughout were suggestive of the neurological impairment.*

The patient recovered quickly and became totally asymptomatic within a very short time. However, in less than one year after surgery, signs of loosening had appeared. Under someone else's care she had the hip aspirated because of the possibility of an infection explaining the lysis and loosening. The aspiration was negative. She remained minimally symptomatic for a number of years when she died of chronic heart disease (Figs 43.1A to C).

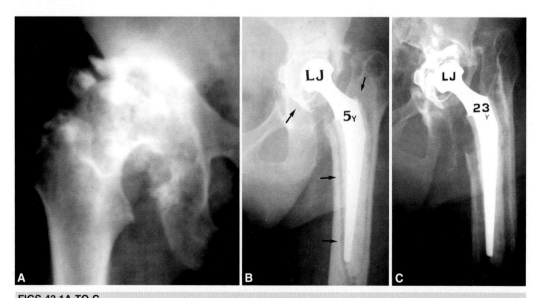

FIGS 43.1A TO C

(A) Preoperative radiograph demonstrating loose bodies suggestive of a Charcot joint. (B) Loosening of both components and lysis of the acetabulum and femur five years postoperatively. Despite the massive changes, pain was not a major problem. Patient refused surgery. (C) Radiograph obtained 23 years after surgery

I have tried to learn more about neuropathic hip joints treated with total arthroplasty but with little benefit. All authors simply emphasize the risk of dislocation because of the lack of proprioception.

On a different occasion, I treated a man in his late 40s who had had a severe injury to his groin many years earlier. The injury had resulted in a severance of the quadriceps and a permanent damage to the femoral nerve. The sensory territory of the femoral nerve was impaired. The quadriceps remained paralyzed. The radiographs showed partial disappearance of the femoral head and the presence of loose bodies throughout (Figs 43.2A to C).

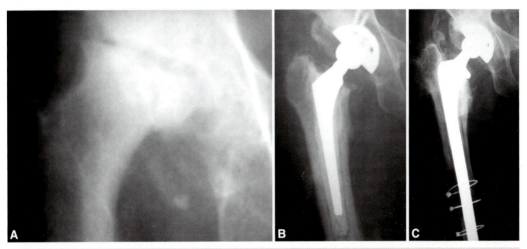

FIGS 43.2A TO C

(A) Radiograph of a neuropathic hip joint following a blunt injury that severed the quadriceps and permanently injured the femoral nerve. (B) After I performed total hip arthroplasty using the hybrid system, the hip dislocated a few days after surgery. A brace was applied but signs of loosening of the femoral component progressed rapidly and the hip became painful. The arthroplasty was then revised. Nothing unusual was detected during the surgical procedure. The hip was revised using a long-stem cemented prosthesis. (C) The arthroplasty failed and required revision with a noncemented prosthesis. Radiograph taken four years later

Section 2

44

The Infected Hip

One of the most dreadful complications associated with hip replacement is infection (See *Endoprostheses*). Over the years this problem has become less frequent and today we have assumed a rather cavalier attitude that one day we might regret. Our heavy reliance on the power of antibiotics is partly responsible for that attitude.

As far as I know, most, if not all surgeons, performing endoprosthetic replacement or during primary and revision total hip arthroplasty use prophylactic antibiotics in different ways and amounts. It is of great interest to realize that Charnley, did not use prophylactic antibiotics of any kind, and depended on the clean air system for the prevention of infection. He stated that infections had an exogenous origin. Furthermore, he did not irrigate the wound. With such a protocol, his infection rate was extremely low. Food for thought, particularly at this time when we are confronting a near catastrophe as a result of the almost epidemic increase of metacyllin-resistant organisms (mersa), which the pharmaceutical industry may not be able to respond effectively. We must take some responsibility for the impending debacle, since for too long we have abuse antibiotics, either prophylactically or therapeutically.

There seems to be ample evidence to indicate that intravenous antibiotics must be given immediately preceding surgery in order for them to be truly effective. Also, that one day of antibiotic prophylaxis is all that is needed. In spite of that evidence, I have not been able to discontinue the administration of IV antibiotics for three postoperative days. This is the protocol I have used for the past three decades. If surgery of any kind had been performed earlier in the hip, I withhold the administration of the drug until I have obtained a sample of fluid from the joint and have sent it to the laboratory for gram stain studies and permanent cultures. I am afraid that the prior administration of antibiotics might give a false reading. I also profusely irrigate the wound with an antibiotic solution throughout the entire surgical procedure.

In the very recent past new techniques have been developed to enhance the detachment of pathogenic organisms from acrylic cement and metallic surfaces: Vortexing and Sonification. These two technique will very likely improve the care of infected arthroplasties.

If the synovial fluid is clear and the patient had no previous surgery, I proceed to request the IV injection of antibiotics. For the past few years I have used one gram of Ancef, which I give for three additional days, four times a day. Other use different antibiotics with greater spectrum.

It is possible that the amount of antibiotics I give is unnecessary high. I continue to do it based on reasons that may not be scientific or logical. I do it because I think that the prolonged administration might be good in preventing possible infection associated with the epidural and/or Foley catheter. I leave the Foley catheter in place for 24 hours. I, no longer leave the epidural catheter in place longer then 24 hours. I gave up the old practice upon noticing a high incidence of hypotensive episodes upon initiation of ambulation on the first postoperative day.

For many years I have insisted that *replacement of the dressing applied in surgery should not be done too soon after surgery, unless an unexpected amount of drainage is present. I often wait as long as three or four days before I change the dressing.* There is nothing to be gained from the early exchange; quite the contrary, it may be potentially harmful due to the possibility of contamination with organisms carried out by the different nursing personnel in the hospital wards. If one waits a few days before exposing the wound to the environment, the changes are that the initial biological "seal" that forms at the suture line would prevent the penetration of organisms into the deep tissues.

We have submitted for publication a manuscript summarizing my personal experiences with infection in over two thousand total hip arthroplasty. Doctor Anukul Goswami, from the United Kingdom, who served as a reconstruction surgery fellow in our department in Los Angeles ten years ago, conducted the study.

When he first showed me his preliminary findings indicating that the number of infected primary total hips was very low, I reacted by saying that, to the best of recollection, I have had more infections that the small number he had presented to me. I mentioned by name several patients I could readily remember. It turned out that most of these patients had had secondary rather than primary surgery. A previous procedure such as nailing of a fracture, an osteotomy or partial joint replacement had been performed earlier.

Doctor Goswami divided the data into three categories:

a. Primary arthroplasties, made of the truly "virgin hips";
b. Secondary arthroplasties, consisting of patients who had previous surgeries, excluding total hip replacements; and
c. Revision surgery that included only those patients who had had a previous total hip arthroplasty.

The results were very interesting: The deep infection rate for the first group (group a) was 0.8 percent; for the secondary group (group b) was 1.5 percent; and for the revision group (group c) 2.5 percent. The findings suggested that if the protocol described above is carefully followed the infection rate in total hip surgery could be very low.

Surprised by the small difference in the incidence of infection between revision of total hips and replacement for failed internal fixation of femoral neck fractures, I came to the conclusion that the rather cavalier attitude we take in the debridement of the area between the two conditions may offer an explanation. In the case of the revised total hip, we pay a great deal of attention to the removal of all tissues that do not appear to be normal and resect membranes from the acetabulum an femoral canal. In the case of the failed multiple pin nailing, the debridement is not as thorough. In one occasion we took cultures in surgery after debridement of the area that were reported as negative. However, new culture of

tissues coming from the reaming of holes in the bone left by the pins were positive.

I have been pleasantly surprised to see the success rate recently obtained with antibiotic management of infected total hips. In earlier years I saw a number of infected total hips, which in spite of removal of all foreign material and thorough debridement of the area, continued to drain. Oftentimes, a second or third debridement was necessary. At this time, prolonged IV antibiotic therapy following thorough debridement has made the prognosis much better.

A couple of years ago I was asked to care for a rheumatoid woman in her early sixties who had an infected total hip prosthesis that drained profusely. *Staph. aureus* coagulase positive was the identified organism. She refused my recommendation to remove the implant.

Because of her adamant plea for the preservation of the implant, I acquiesced. I opened the hip widely and debrided as much as I could. The cemented metallic and plastic components were bathed in pus and the quality of the soft tissues was poor, as is often the case in patients with subacute chronic infections, particularly in the rheumatoid patient. I left draining systems in place and I closed the skin loosely. Then I asked the infectious disease specialist to prescribe the appropriate antibiotics. She received intravenous antibiotics for six weeks. The wound never drained again and the hip became asymptomatic. Two years later she suffered a major stroke that left her operated side markedly spastic. The prosthesis dislocated but her treating physician did not recognize the dislocation for nearly two months.

Under the new painful circumstances she agreed to the removal of the implant. No signs of infection were found, and all cultures taken at the time of surgery were negative. I think such success was made possible by better antibiotics.

As I look at my personal experiences with infected arthroplasties and at the role new antibiotics have had in their management, I have concluded that the old precept of thorough debridement is the single most important element in their management. *In the absence of a good debridement no antibiotic, no mater how powerful it might be, is not going cure a deep, well established infection.*

Although I do not have the data to accurately confirm my suspicion, I feel that the very late failure of total hips replacements is more likely to occur in the acetabulum rather than in the femur. Migration of the cup into the pelvis is a common finding. Such migration is likely to be the result of low-grade infection that goes unrecognized.

The debate that raged some years ago concerning the issue as to whether or not primary exchange of an infected total hip was appropriate has lost momentum. Most orthopedists believe that one-stage reimplantation is not a safe procedure, and that a two-stage surgery is the most appropriate approach. It makes sense and it is probably the safest method of care. Nonetheless, I admit that in a few instances I have done and will probably do primary exchange surgery. I qualify my statement by saying that such an approach may be safe only if other features are kept clearly into consideration. It the patient is a good health, the sedimentation rate is elevated only minimally, the c-reactive protein is not significantly elevated or normal, the bone scan (the ones used to identify infection) is negative, and upon the opening of the joint the appearance of the tissues is benign, I seriously believe that a thorough debridement and reimplantation could render good results. Sustained prolonged intravenous administration of antibiotics is then implemented. I have had no occasion to regret this approach. The use of Vortexing and Sonification has given stimulus to some to carryout primary reimplantation. Whether the early results from Switzerland can be duplicated in the future remains unknown.

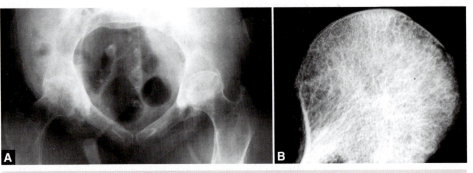

FIGS 44.1A AND B

(A) Bilateral septic arthritis depicting the rapid narrowing of the joint space. (B) The microradiograph of the femoral head shows the disappearance of the articular cartilage

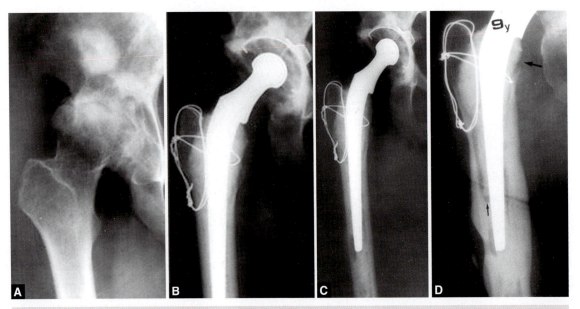

FIGS 44.2A TO D

(A) Radiograph of an osteoarthritic hip joint obtained 30 years after the onset of hematogenous septic arthritis at the age of three. The hip had been surgically drained a few times but after a few months no further drainage occurred. (B) Radiograph obtained five years after surgery. The hip had been replaced 30 years after the initial episode. Though no bacteria were identified in surgery, the patient was instructed to remain on antibiotics for a "long time". (C) *Nine years after surgery, in the absence of symptoms, the antibiotics were discontinued. A few months later pain appeared over the lateral-distal aspect of the femur.* (D) Antibiotics were reinstituted but to no avail. Gross changes were identified throughout the entire proximal half of the femur. The prosthesis was removed at another institution and I finally lost her to follow-up

I was never convinced that the use of antibiotic-impregnated cement beads was a miracle drug. A good debridement and intravenous antibiotics is better.

Once an infected prosthesis is removed, it is inevitable that the extremity would significantly shorten. The degree of shortening is greater than the one usually seeing following a Girdlestone procedure carried out for other conditions. This problem is being effectively offset by replacing the removed prosthesis with an endoprosthesis made of acrylic cement. At a later date, when the definitive procedure is performed a new implant is introduced.

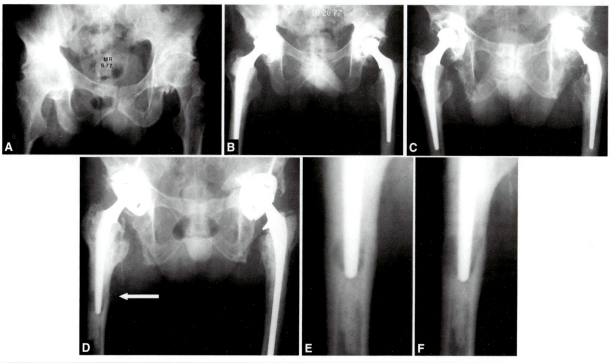

FIGS 44.3A TO F

(A) Ankylosing spondylitis affecting both hips. (B) The hips were replaced with cemented total hips. (C) Twenty years later the replacement failed requiring revision surgery. (D to F) Three years after revision of the right hip pain ensued at the level of the tip end of the prosthesis. *Infection was identified during surgery. I chose not to remove the implant but simply to curettage the area and packed it with bone graft.* (I had learned this procedure from Austin Moore, who often treated chronic osteomyelitis in long bone through curettage and packing of "morselized" bone into the defect. Currently, the term used to describe the prepared bone is "morselized". Three years later the patient is asymptomatic

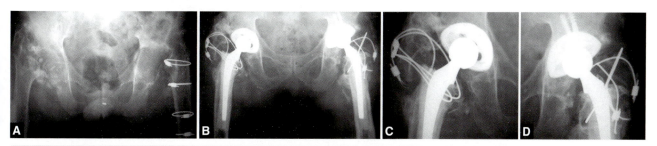

FIGS 44.4A TO D

(A) Radiograph obtained after resection of infected total hip arthroplasties. (B) Radiographs obtained after replacement of joint with hybrid arthroplasties. Notice the nonunion of the greater trochanters. (C and D) Close-up views of ununited trochanters. His became asymptomatic and stable. There was residual power of abduction but the patient, though of an advanced age, was able to walk without external support

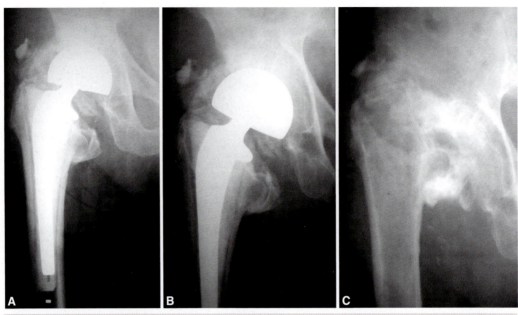

FIGS 44.5A TO C

Bipolar endoprosthesis became painful shortly after surgery. The joint space disappeared in a very short time, and heterotopic bone formed. These three features, when combined, are pathognomonic of infection

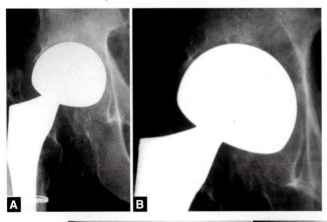

FIGS 44.6A AND B

(A) Bipolar endoprosthesis inserted as treatment for an acute fracture of the femoral neck. The hip became painful beginning a few days after surgery, and the joint space virtually disappeared within a couple of weeks. (B) Pain continued and the prosthetic head migrated superiorly into the pelvic bone. An infection was confirmed

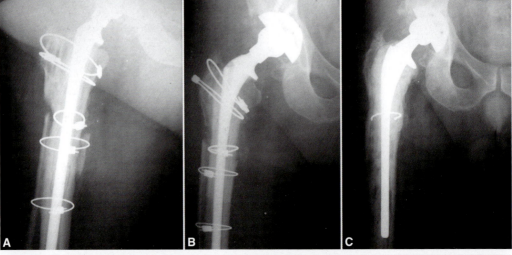

FIGS 44.7A TO C

(A) Total hip replacement performed three months after excision of infected total hip arthroplasty that presented with severe lysis of the femoral cortex. Bone graft was used to reinforce the weakened bone. (B) The graft healed and the hip remained asymptomatic. (C) The wires irritating the soft tissues were removed

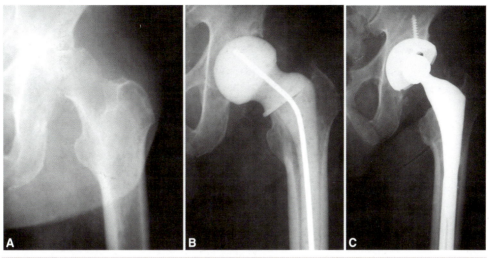

FIGS 44.8A TO C

(A) Hematogenous septic arthritis shows the disappearance of the join space, the flattening of the femoral head and the superior subluxation of the hip. (B) The hip was debrided, the femoral head was removed, and an acrylic endoprosthesis was inserted in order to prevent shortening of the extremity. (C) Three weeks later the permanent metallic prosthesis replaced the temporary acrylic implant. (*Courtesy:* Jack Cooper, MD)

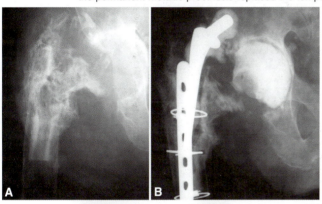

FIGS 44.9A AND B

(A) Radiograph taken after removal of infected total hip arthroplasty. The infection was allegedly produced by *Staph. aureus*. The debridement does not appear to have been adequate. (B) Apparently at the time the femur was fractured, requiring metallic plate fixation. Attempts were apparently made to create a temporary implant. However, the components dislocated

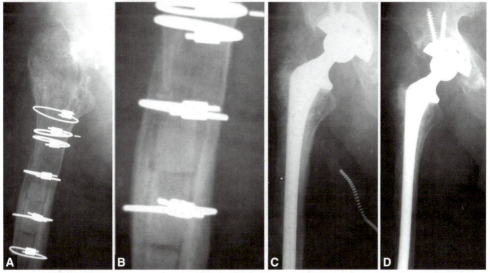

FIGS 44.10A TO D

(A) Resection arthroplasty performed for the care of a deep infection in diabetic patient. Apparently a fracture occurred and circular wires were used to stabilize the fracture. The infection subsided. (B) Notice the remnants of acrylic cement in the medullary canal that should have been removed at the time of the resection arthroplasty. (C) The patient's leg was kept under wire traction for 6 weeks and then a cemented arthroplasty was performed. During the period in traction the patient received intravenous antibiotics. (D) Two years later the hip was only minimally symptomatic and without signs of infection

Section 2

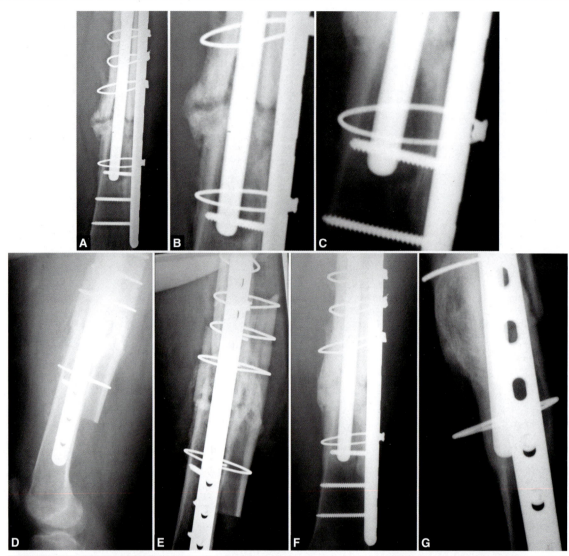

FIGS 44.11A TO G

(A) Radiograph of total hip arthroplasty with an alleged fracture that developed a few months after surgery. The facture was then stabilized with a plate (B) Notice the lytic defect just below the end of the prosthesis. (C) Closer view of the lytic defect representing an infection. produced by *Staph. aureus*. (D) *I enlarged the lytic defect, and the cavity curetted, irrigated with antibiotics and packed with cancellous bone.* (E) A large strut of cortical bone was then fastened to the femur, over the packed defect. Intravenous antibiotics were started and continued for six weeks. (F) A closer view of the graft. The nail obscures the plate. The graft incorporated with the femoral cortex. The fracture healed and the infection did not recur. (G) A final radiograph obtained one year postsurgery. Patient was asymptomatic

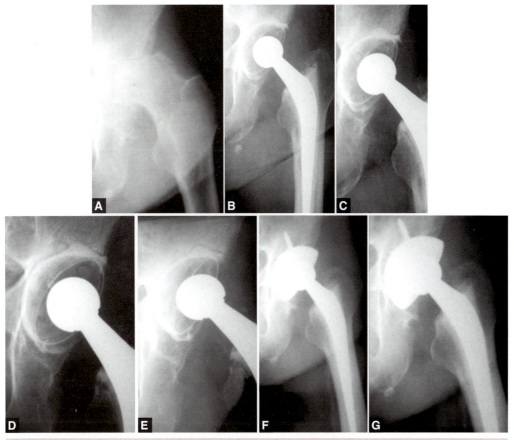

FIGS 44.12A TO G

(A) Avascular necrosis of the femoral head following radiation therapy for carcinoma of the intestines. At the time of the replacement arthroplasty, the bone was significantly osteoporotic and cultures were negative for infection. Microscopic examination of the femoral head showed what the pathologist called *"infection cysts"*. The specimen could not be cultured because it already had been placed in formaldehyde. (B) The joint was replaced with a totally cemented arthroplasty. (C to E) Over a period of three months, consecutive radiographs demonstrated progressive loosening of the acetabular component. (F) The acetabular component was replaced with a non-porous implant. Cultures were negative. (G) Six months later the hip was only minimally symptomatic. Six months later, while traveling to another distant city she developed septic shock and had the implant removed. She died a few days later

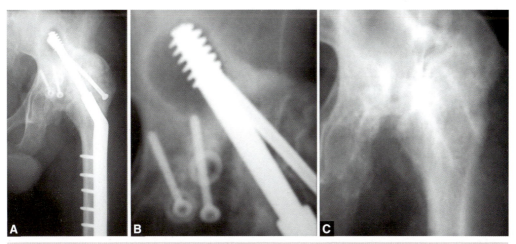

FIGS 44.13A TO C

(A) Infected hip following a hip nailing procedure. Notice lytic/septic defect proximally. (B) Closer view of lytic defect. (C) A resection arthroplasty was performed. Plans to replace the joint were cancelled because of the patient's extreme lack of cooperation

Section 2

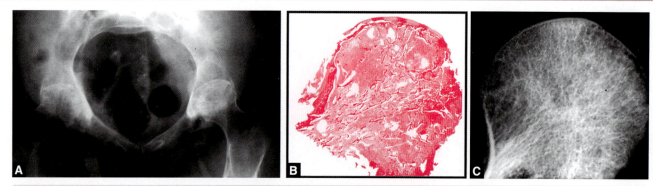

FIGS 44.14A TO C

(A) Radiograph of hematogenous septic arthritis. (B and C) Microscopic section of femoral head and correspondent radiograph

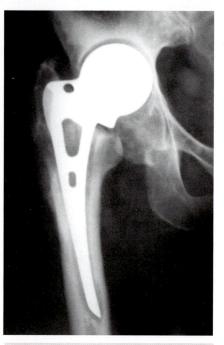

FIG. 44.15

Radiograph of infected endoprosthesis. There is lysis present in the acetabulum as well as in the distal femur

*Reference**

80

45

Conversion of Osteotomized Femurs

For several generations osteotomy of the femur was perhaps the most popular procedure performed for the treatment of the arthritic hip. Osteotomy of the acetabulum, perhaps because it was more difficult to perform, did not have the popularity or the femoral one. This lack of popularity did not preclude the design and performance of at least ten different procedures that attempted to create a bony roof over the arthritic femoral head. Some type of bone graft was their most common denominator. The Chiari osteotomy achieved the desired coverage without the use of a bone graft. One must speculate that success was attained in many instances; otherwise the procedure would have been abandoned earlier. Fusion indeed was also a frequently performed procedure that was not abandoned until recent years when arthroplasties of various types became possible. The same applied to resection arthroplasties.

It is widely known that a common undesirable sequella of femoral osteotomy is osteoarthritis of the knee joint. The altered mechanics of gait is often dramatically changed leading to major abnormal stresses in the knee; a phenomenon even more common following hip fusion.

I suspect there are very few patients still alive in the United States who had femoral osteotomies performed. However, I had the opportunity to spend a couple of days with Renato Bombelli, form northern Italy, who was strong advocate of femoral osteotomies for number of years. Bombelli practiced in the region of Europe where the highest incidence of congenital hip

dysplasia is found. During my stay with him in the mid 1970s, I saw him perform several of his specially designed femoral osteotomies as well as several isoelastic total hip arthroplasties. He had learned and fell in love with Morscher's isoelastic implant and became its strongest supporter. Bombelli had been an admirer of Pawels, the famous German surgeon, who perhaps better than anyone else studied the mechanics and biomechanics of the hip joint. Bombelli, deviated somehow from some of Pawels teachings and modified the master's techniques. Only time will tell who of the two thinkers came closer to the correct answers.

Bombelli made available to me at that time his entire X-ray files of hundreds of patients, on a given day he brought to his out-patient clinic 75 patients who had either osteotomies or total hip replacements (Figs 45.1 to 45.8). I must admit that I was extremely impressed with what I saw that day. I returned home and performed approximately 70 isoelastic prosthetic replacements before I abandoned their usage. The complications rate had become unacceptable.

It would be foolish for me or anyone else at this time in history to suspect that osteotomies of the femur ever came close to providing the rather consistent good results that contemporary total hip arthroplasties do. However, the memory of the many of Bombelli's successful osteotomies lingers, and I wonder why so many of his patients did well. I suspect that, in general, femoral osteotomies seldom rendered excellent clinical results, because they were usually performed for advance osteoarthritis. At this time we are witnessing

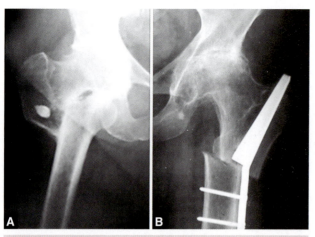

FIGS 45.1A AND B

(A) Femoral osteotomy designed to displace the distal fragment medially. The procedure altered weight bearing distribution and in that manner improve symptoms. Postoperatively required cast immobilization. (B) Osteotomy with the use of a nail-plate combination that eliminated the need for plaster immobilization

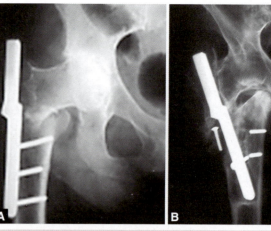

FIGS 45.2A AND B

(A) Varus femoral osteotomy stabilized with a nail-plate combination. (B) The stabilization of the osteotomy was lost and a nonunion took place

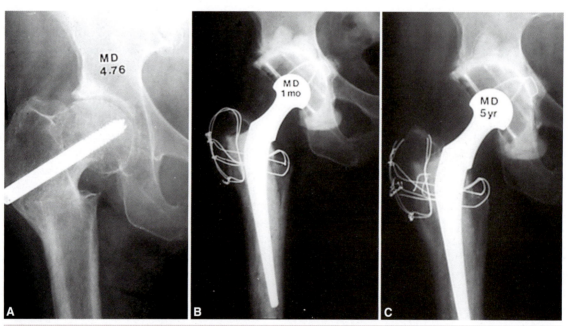

FIGS 45.3A TO C

(A) Radiograph of healed varus osteotomy. There is no history to explain the presence of the nail. (B) Postoperative radiograph of Charnley arthroplasty obtained one year postoperatively. (C) Last radiograph of Charnley arthroplasty 5 years later. Total hip replacement often requires additional precautions against dislocation, because of the soft tissue instability likely to be present at the completion of surgery

a renaissance of interest in periacetabular osteotomies and are impressed with the results reported by the likes of Ganz, Matta and Santore. We must keep in mind that those surgeons have made it very clear that success can be achieved only when the surgery is performed early and before even moderately advanced arthritis has developed. Can we speculate that comparable results with femoral osteotomies can be obtained if criterion similar to that of acetabular osteotomies were applied to acetabular osteotomies.

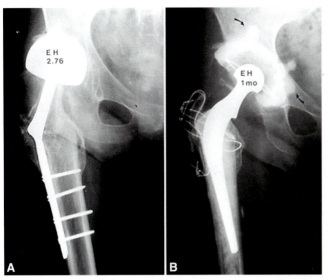

FIGS 45.4A AND B

(A) Radiograph of high subtrochanteric valgus osteotomy following a failed mold arthroplasty. (B) The failed procedure was treated with a Charnley arthroplasty

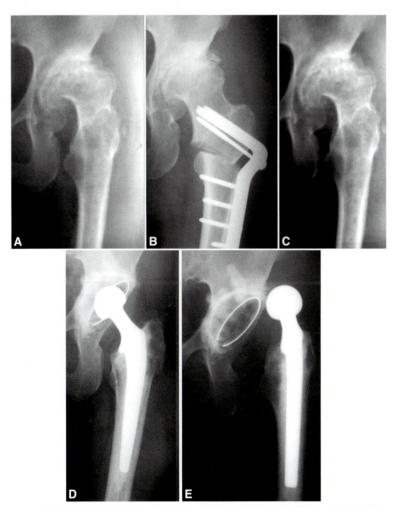

FIGS 45.5A TO E

(A) Osteoarthritic hip probably secondary to congenital hip dysplasia. (B) Apparently planning the angle of inclination of a proposed osteotomy, views were obtained with the hip in abduction well as in adduction. (C) Radiograph obtained shortly after the osteotomy was performed. (D) Radiograph prior to completion of healing of the subtrochanteric osteotomy. (E) The failed osteotomy was treated with a cemented total hip arthroplasty. The hip dislocated a few days later

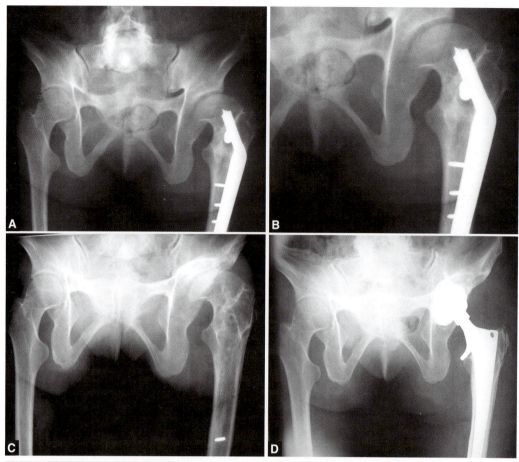

FIGS 45.6A TO D

(A and B) Radiographs of a 33-year-old woman who had congenital hip dysplasia treated with a subtrochanteric osteotomy 14 years earlier. Notice the pelvic deformity that can be described as severe anteversion. (C) Radiograph of the pelvis after removal of the trochanteric device. (D) Radiograph after noncemented total hip arthroplasty. It took extreme care to determine the appropriate position of the acetabular and femoral components in order to prevent later dislocation

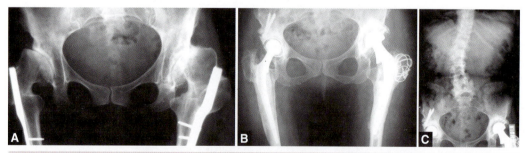

FIGS 45.7A TO C

Radiographs of bilateral subtrochanteric osteotomies performed for the care of osteoarthritis secondary to congenital hip dysplasia. Radiograph of bilateral cemented Bechtol prostheses. Radiograph of associated moderately severe scoliosis

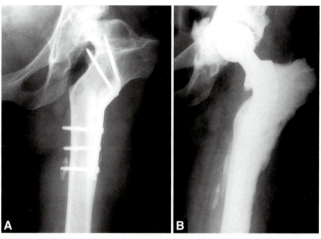

FIGS 45.8A AND B

(A) Radiograph of subtrochanteric osteotomy performed probably in an attempt to improve the symptoms associated with a congenitally dysplastic hip. (B) Radiograph of cemented arthroplasty performed without osteotomy of the greater trochanter or correction of the femoral deformity. The patient left the country and no further follow-up was possible

Section 2

46

Conversion of Girdlestone Arthroplasties

Most total hip arthroplasties currently performed for the salvage of flail hips are for patients who had previously had an infected implant that was surgically removed. Girdlestone, if I am not mistaken recommended the procedure for patients with tuberculosis. Later, others began to perform the procedure for the care of nonunion of the femoral head. I personally have treated a few patients with such nonunions with reasonably good results. The operations were performed before the advent of total hip arthroplasty. I also saw Newton McCollough Jr., from Orlando, present a series of elderly patients with acute, vertical and severely displaced femoral neck fractures who had the Girdlestone resection as the primary treatment. He did so upon realizing that internal fixation of those fractures had a very poor prognosis. As his resident I was deeply impressed with the clinical results. *Many of the patients were able to walk with the aid of crutches or canes without pain.* Subsequently, I personally treated in a few instances a displaced femoral neck fracture by skillful neglect. The patients were kept in balanced suspension for a few days until the acute symptoms subsided and began passive and active exercises as soon as possible. I learned that if there is no contact between the femoral and femoral neck fragments, pain disappears within a few weeks. Needless to say, such a therapeutic approach is not likely to present itself too frequently at this time. Having this approach as an option, however, is probably not a bad idea.

Patients who had the resection arthroplasty performed for the care of infections usually present themselves with a significantly shorter extremity and contractures. If the condition for which the operation was performed was an infected total hip arthroplasty there is usually a greater degree of shortening and the contractures and limitation of motion more apparent.

The use of a temporary acrylic prosthesis (spacer) following the removal of the components prevents the shortening (Fig. 46.1). There is not as yet extensive data to support the routine use of the procedure.

The implantation of a total hip prosthesis following a Girdlestone procedure is usually time consuming and technically demanding. *Because of the associated shortening, efforts to regain length must be carefully monitored primarily because to the risk of a nerve injury.* This is the most common reason used by surgeons to justify a trochanteric osteotomy. *However, I have learned that the osteotomy is rarely necessary providing an extensive soft tissue release is carried out.* The soft tissue release includes the severance of the iliopsoas muscle from the lesser trochanter, as well as the severance of the adductor muscles from the pubic area. *On occasion, subperiosteal stripping of the gluteal muscles from the pelvis further helps the bringing down the femoral shaft.* The distal transfer of the shaft to make possible the insertion of the acetabular component must be done gradually.

The greater the limitation of flexion of the hip prior to surgery the grater risk of nerve palsy and the more important it becomes to gradually strip the soft tissues

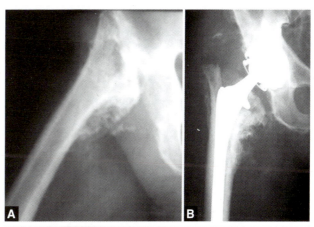

FIG. 46.1
An acrylic endoprosthesis used as a temporary "spacer" following the removal of an infected arthroplasty

from the surrounding osseous structures. Attempts to forcefully gain flexion by actively forcing the hip into flexion places tension on the sciatic nerve that has not been placed under tension for whatever time the hip has been in extension. *Translated into practical terms it means that the more the hip can flexed before surgery the greater the amount of length that can be gained surgically without damaging the sciatic nerve. The passive force the surgeon places on the hip trying to gain motion should be done with the knee in flexion because if the knee is in extension while the hip is flexed the tension on the nerve is significantly increased.* Oftentimes upon completion of the replacement arthroplasty the hip cannot be fully extended. I have observed that the remaining flexion contracture is temporary and that within a few days or weeks the contracture is overcome with appropriate extension exercises.

It is widely recognized that the sciatic nerve is the nerve must likely to be injured during attempts to gain length, however, I have witnessed two instances where the injured was limited to the femoral nerve. I can extrapolate that the injury to the nerve occurred when forceful attempts to gain hip extension was being made with the knee in extension.

This tedious and time consuming stripping of the soft tissues is the same that can and should be done during the performance of total hip surgery for the care of congenital hip dysplasia. This is why it is unwise for the surgeon to ascertain prior to surgery the amount of length that can be gained. It depends on how well and how successfully the soft tissues are released.

There are times when no amount of stripping makes possible the necessary distal displacement of the femur to allow the placement of the acetabular component into the old acetabulum. In these instances a trochanteric osteotomy and shortening of the femur is the best approach.

When the trochanter is osteotomized and reattached the incidence of nonunion is very high. However, in most instances the abductor mechanism works well enough to make unassisted ambulation possible. *However, the nonunion predisposes to dislocation and an external rotation of the femur becomes permanent.*

FIGS 46.2A AND B
(A) Radiograph of a hip following removal of prosthetic components after infection developed. (B) The attachment of the abductors muscles was preserved. This 69-year-old man had significant limitation of motion prior to surgery. One year later his hip flexed to 80 degrees. It *was chosen at the time of surgery to use a self-constrained acetabulum to prevent dislocation*

Section 2

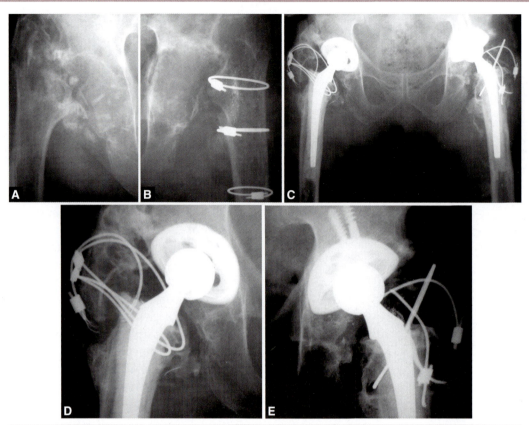

FIGS 46.3A TO E

(A and B) Radiographs obtained following removal of infected bilateral total hip arthroplasties. (C) Radiograph showing the bilateral total hip arthroplasties. Notice the nonunion of the greater trochanters. (D and E) Closer views of nonunited trochanters. Despite the failure of union this older gentleman managed to walk at home without external support and without pain. A external rotation deformity persisted. This is a very common sequella of trochanteric nonunion

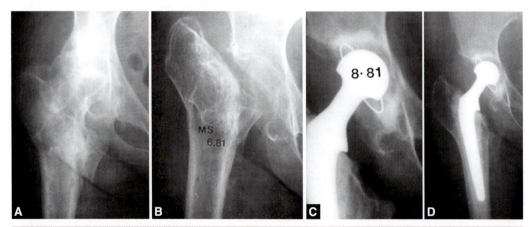

FIGS 46.4A TO D

(A) Radiograph of infected proximal femur following internal fixation of fracture. (B) Radiograph obtained six months after resection of the head and neck of the femur. (C) Radiograph obtained shortly after prosthetic replacement. (D) Radiograph obtained 14 years after surgery

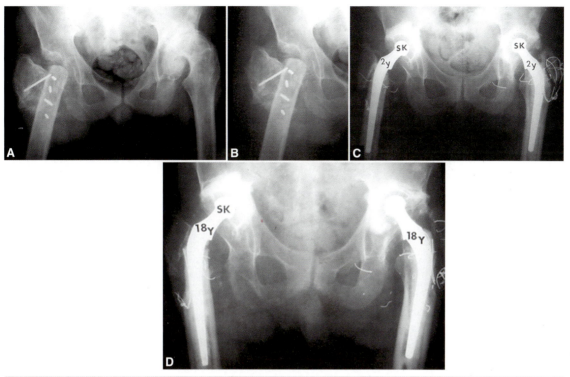

FIGS 46.5A TO D

(A) Preoperative radiographs showing the resected femoral head and the trochanter attachment to the femoral shaft on the right. (B) Closer view of right hip. (C) Radiograph obtained 2 years postbilateral total hip Charnley arthroplasties. (D) Radiograph demonstrating the appearance of the hips 18 years postoperatively

47

Conversion of the Fused Hip

Prior to the modern era of arthroplasty, fusion of the hip joint was a frequently performed surgical procedure in the management of a number of conditions. Fortunately, today such an operation is rarely necessary. Young trainees complete their residency without ever having seen the procedure performed.

Needless to say, a fused hip eliminates the pain produced by a septic or degenerative condition. *It makes possible painless ambulation and very frequently in a manner that approximates the normal gait.* I have seen a number of people with a fused hip where it was impossible to guess which hip was the fused one. Only when sitting down and asked to don or doff their shoes that their true condition was identified. They flexed the knee on the fused side and in that manner reach the shoe. For them to sit down without slouching back too much, they must flex the spine and bend the knee in an adducted position of the hip. They usually get used to the absence of motion of the hip and carry out the activities of normal living.

A debate concerning the "ideal" position for the fused hip raged for as long as the operation was part of the armamentarium of the orthopedic surgeon. I do not believe an agreement was reached. However, the most commonly recommended position was that of a 25 degrees flexion, 25 degrees of abduction and a few degrees of external rotation. This recommendation makes sense since it makes possible to assume the sitting position in a rather normal manner; of course, predicated on the presence of good spine motion to compensate for the lack of hip mobility. The slight abduction and external rotation of the leg also appeared to have functional and cosmetic benefits.

It was known to orthopedic surgeons, however, that many patients with fused hip developed back pain at a later date and that also many ended up with a progressively deformed valgus knee. The ensuing back and knee pain became a big problem. Osteotomies of the tibia and or femur were rarely the answer.

It is not difficult to guess as to why these complications were so common. Back pain was brought about by the abnormal stresses that the immobilized hip placed upon it. If the degree of flexion of the hip was excessive walking in an erect manner was impossible. If the degree of flexion of the hip was insufficient, then sitting straight became an impossibility. A hip fused in abduction creates a condition that forces the knee into a valgus attitude. No weight-bearing joint can tolerate for very long such stresses without eventually developing arthritic changes. *Even today, when total knee arthroplasty is readily available, the changes of its failure in the presence of a fused hip are almost guaranteed.*

If the hip is fused in adduction, as some have recommended, a varus deformity and subsequent arthritis of the knee frequently develop.

With a hip fused in adduction theoretically a more efficient gait results by virtue of the resulting narrow base; sitting and walking becomes more difficult. The hip fused in abduction produces the opposite response by creating a valgus arthritic knee. It is not uncommon either to see one knee with a valgus deformity and the opposite with a varus deformity (Figs 47.1A to C). At this time the recommended position for a fused hip is 25 degrees of flexion, 10 to 15 degrees of adduction and a few degrees of external rotation.

The surgical procedure is usually difficult to carry out. As a resident, I recall, I had to learn the various

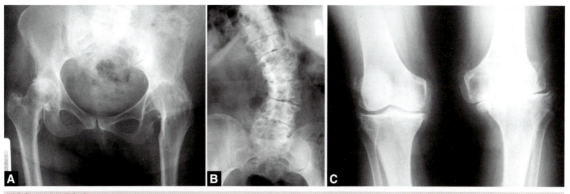

FIGS 47.1A TO C

(A) Radiograph of pelvis illustrating the arthritic changes in the right hip and a virtually fused left hip. The fusion took place in a neutral attitude of abduction. (B) A severe scoliosis developed. (C) Radiographs of both knees showing a varus deformity of the left knee

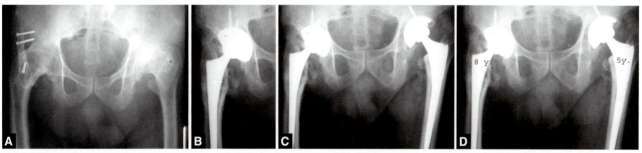

FIGS 47.2A TO D

(A) Radiograph of the pelvis of a 62-year-old man who had his right hip fused at the age of 28 years allegedly for the treatment of osteoarthritis secondary to bilateral Perthes disease. (B) Radiograph obtained postoperatively. (C and D) Radiographs taken five years postsurgery on the lefts and 8 years on the right. The patient sits straight and walks without external support. His low back has become painful but the symptoms are readily controlled with exercise and analgesics

techniques, as well as the names of the surgeons who had first described them. *An orthopedic Fellow was recently surprised when I made reference to the fact that many fusion procedures were carried out without the surgical removal of the articular cartilage.* He was under the impression that without removal of the diseased cartilage a fusion could not take place. I then made him aware that the Trumble, Britain as well as many other procedures were carried out extra-articularly. I am not sure that I am correct in stating that the Charnley technique necessarily called for removal of cartilage. Charnley created a defect on the medial wall of the acetabulum into which he pushed the femoral head. He wanted to shorten the medial lever arm and in that manner improve the efficiency of the gait. A concept he later applied to his total hip arthroplasty. I performed one of his fusions without destroying the cartilage.

That day I told the fellow that I once I had fused an ankle, inserting two screws from the tibia into the talus without opening the joint. The fusion that ensued

was painless and the function of the foot very good. He had readily compensated with motion in other joints in a most effective way. William Wagner, the famed foot surgeon from California, had both his ankles fused when he already was a grown-up man. His gait was normal and no one could have guessed the condition of his feet.

Today is possible to take down fused hips that have developed arthritic changes in the spine and/or knees (Figs 47.2 to 47.5). Technically, the revision is possible and not necessarily very difficult. There are, however, several matters that must be very seriously considered before carrying out the procedure. *One of them is the possibility of injuring the sciatic and or femoral nerves as motion is introduced into the previously fused joint.*

I have long believed that during the performance of hip arthroplasty in situations when gaining additional length is desirable, *the gain in length is primarily determined by the degree of flexion the hip had prior to the surgical intervention.* If the hip can be flexed to normal or near normal degrees it means that the

Section 2

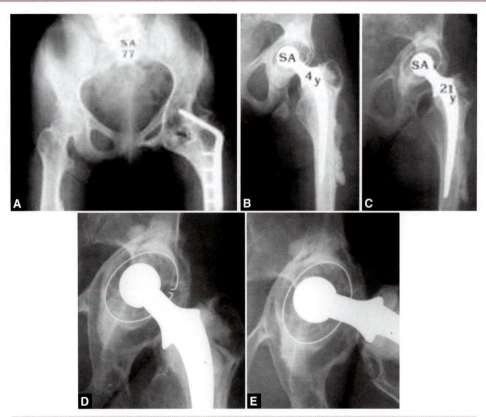

FIGS 47.3A TO E

(A) Radiography of spontaneously fused hip of a 16-year-old girl following a head injury. She also had sustained an intertrochanteric fracture. The lumbosacral spine had been surgically fused. The combination of a fused lumbosacral spine and hip made it impossible for her to assume the sitting position. (B) A Charnley arthroplasty was performed. Four years later there was no evidence of pathology associated with the arthroplasty and the patient, though severely spastic and requiring a walker for ambulation did not have pain. (C) Twenty one years later, despite the appearance of radiolucent lines in the acetabulum the hip has remained painless and functional. (D and E) Radiograph obtained 28 years after surgery. The patient lives in a facility for the mentally impaired but remains as functional as she was ten years earlier

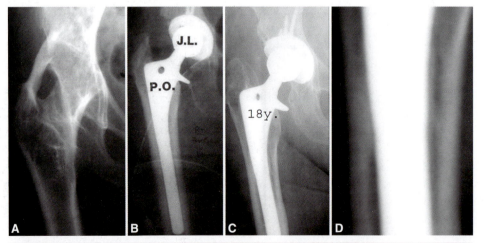

FIGS 47.4A TO D

(A) Radiograph of the right hip of a 50-year-old woman who had her hip fused at the age of 25, allegedly for the treatment of bone tuberculosis. (B) Radiograph obtained postoperatively. (C and D) Radiographs obtained 18 years postoperatively. The patient regained almost complete flexion of the hip but continued to be limited in rotation. Notice then "welding point" indicating bone ingrowth at the level of the distal end of the porous surface

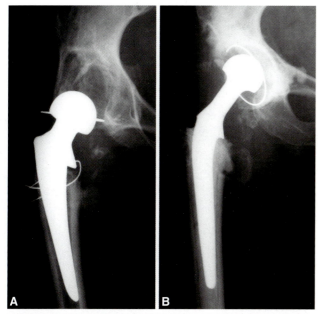

FIGS 47.5A AND B

(A) Radiograph of a hip previously fused and subsequently replaced with a total hip arthroplasty. *I had advised the 45-year-old patient not to have the procedure performed because it was obvious that at the time of surgery the inferior gluteal nerve had been permanently damaged. The minimal limp she had with her fused hip was changed into a severe gluteus medius limp.* (B) Because of repeated dislocations and pain I performed a revision arthroplasty. The hip never dislocated again but the limp, obviously, persisted

major nerves crossing the joint had been subjected to normal stretching to their fibers. If little or no motion existed in the hip, one can surmise that the normal gliding and stretching of the nerves had not taken place for a long time. *Therefore, the sudden flexion of the hip in the operating room, following the reduction in the newly inserted prosthesis can easily produce an excessive stretching of the nerves and a resulting palsy that usually has a poor prognosis.*

In those instances where gaining length is desirable but the little or no motion in the joint was possible prior to surgery, it is best not to attempt major flexion of the hip in surgery. Assuming the tension on the sciatic nerve is minimal, it is best to allow a spontaneous stretching to take place during the following weeks or months. This consideration obviously is of a greater importance in the case of the fused hip.

Another important feature that must be kept in mind prior to the conversion of a fused hip into a total hip is the condition of the musculature around the hip. I am referring to their innervation. *If the inferior gluteal nerve had been damaged at the time of the fusion procedure—a nonuncommon fact—the patient will display a greater limp after surgery.* The chances of spontaneous dislocation are increased due to the absence of the tethering effect this muscle normally provides.

During the "taking down" of a fused hip, I deliberately release soft tissue from the femur to the greatest possible degree. This stripping of tissues from their attachment facilitates the gaining of motion and the avoidance of sudden stretching of nerves.

One should not expect immediate restoration of motion to the newly operated joint. Several months are usually necessary before a satisfactory degree of motion is attained. The back and or knee pain, for which the procedure was performed, improves in most instances. However, there are times when the improvement is only moderate and not necessarily long-lasting.

I have come to the conclusion that a patient with a fused hip who begins to experience knee pain many years after the fusion, but not as yet demonstrating obvious pathology in the knee, is probably better served if the hip is "taken down" at that time. To wait for the knee to become arthritic and unstable before performing the reconstructive procedure sound a bit impractical. This consideration also applies to patients with arthritic hips that demonstrate progressive loss of motion and experience early signs of knee pathology.

48

Revision of the Failed Femoral Components

It was not until relatively recently that most surgeons began to realize that revision surgery for failed total hip prostheses could be safely performed without trochanteric osteotomy in most instances. For a number of years, even those who used the posterior approach in primary arthroplasty felt that in revision surgery the trochanter had to be osteotomized in order to obtain adequate exposure of the acetabulum. This is not necessarily true. Very good exposure of the proximal femur and acetabulum can be achieved without trochanteric osteotomy.

By this time we all have recognized that failure of union of the reattached greater trochanter in revision surgery is very high. In revision surgery, one is likely to find the greater trochanter very osteoporotic. Bringing it down against the femoral shaft and holding it with wires or other devices very often result in their fracture, displacement of the trochanter, nonunion of the fragment and an increase in the degree of rotation of the hip joint, which predisposes to dislocation. If filiform cables are used the seriousness of the problem is magnifies manifold (See *Broken Wires*).

Revision of one component without revision of the other is possible without osteotomy of the greater trochanter in most instances. *The secret behind the success is sufficient dissection of soft tissues from the bone, particularly from the proximal femur.* Severance of the insertion of the iliopsoas muscle is a necessary step in instances when a significant amount of shortening of the extremity needs to be overcome. This also applies to primary surgery, such as arthroplasty performed for congenital dislocation of the hip with major shortening of the leg.

Detachment of the insertion of the gluteus maximus from the proximal femur is essential for good exposure in most revision cases. On the other hand, severance of the gluteus medius and minimus is, in my opinion, unnecessary. It is better to osteotomize the trochanter than to section the muscles and then repair them. Under this latter circumstance the repair that takes place under tension frequently breaks lose. Lengthening of these muscles can be best achieved by stripping their insertion from the wing of the ileum. Care, however, must be exercised to avoid injury to major vessels and the inferior gluteal nerve.

Attempts to remove a failed femoral component without trochanteric osteotomy may result in fracture of the trochanter. Therefore, it is important to expose well the proximal-lateral aspect of the femur. If the failed implant was cemented, the proximal-lateral cement mantle must be removed prior to any attempts to "hammer" the implant out of the canal, and the medial wall of the greater trochanter thoroughly rasped. Otherwise as the broader section of the proximal prosthesis exists from the canal, it can easily break the osteoporotic trochanter (Fig. 48.1).

Upon completion of the procedure the severed insertion of the gluteus maximus on the shaft of the femur should be repaired. For a number of years I considered this step unnecessary until I realized that some patients had a deformity of the buttock as a result of the superior displacement of muscle belly, as well

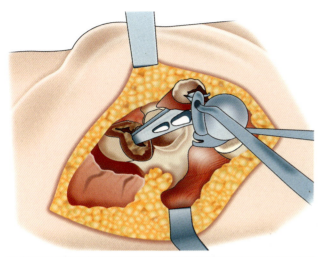

FIG. 48.1

Removal of cemented or uncemented prostheses without trochanteric osteotomy may produce a fracture of the greater trochanter unless great care is exercised

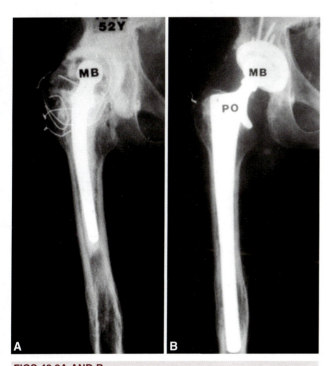

FIGS 48.2A AND B

(A) Radiograph of failed total hip arthroplasty. (B) Radiograph obtained after revision arthroplasty using a noncemented prosthesis

as mild weakness of the muscle. In order to successfully perform revision surgery without trochanteric osteotomy the incision must be a generous one.

It is a common mistake to hold the hip in flexion and internal rotation during the exposure and preparation of the acetabulum. Such positioning does nothing but make the surgery more difficult. The hip should be held in a neutral position or only in a few degrees of flexion. The knee is also held in extension.

The extended position of the hip and knee not only facilitates exposure, but also precludes possible damage to the major vessels of the leg; damage that probably sets the stage for the development of thromboembolic disease because of the kinking of the vessels at the time of surgery (See *Thromboembolic Disease*).

Significant flexion of the hip and knee should be maintained only during the preparation of the proximal femur and only for the shortest possible time. There is no need for the assistant to hold the leg in that position while the cement is being mixed. This period of waiting should be utilized by carrying out passive exercises of the hip, knee and ankle. Exercises, I suspect, are more valuable than any chemical or mechanical prophylactic measure against thromboembolic disease (See *Thromboembolic Disease*).

When revision surgery is performed in instances where extensive lysis of the lateral aspect of the femur is present, the danger of fracturing the femur at that level, during the flexion position of the femur, are significant. *As the hip is flexed and internally rotated, the greater trochanter may abut against the pelvis producing forces that can easily fracture the weakened bone.* In order to prevent fracture it is often best to perform the splitting procedure of Wagner, which consists of separating the entire lateral wall of the femur, including the greater trochanter, and retracting it until completion of the work that needs to be done on the femur. Then the bony wall can be reattached to the main femoral shaft.

Section 2

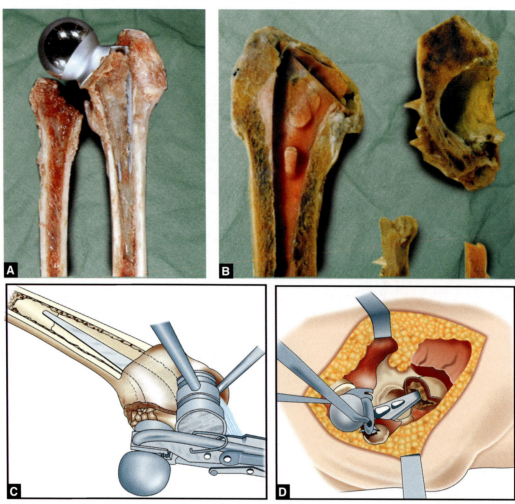

FIGS 48.3A TO D

(A) Illustration of a coronal section of a femur where an Austin Moore prosthesis had been inserted 48 hours earlier. (B) Illustration of a coronally sectioned femur after removal of Austin Moore prosthesis. (C) Illustration of the removal of a femoral stem placed in varus. The risk of fracturing the greater trochanter is high, often requiring its osteotomy. (D) *Illustration of the trochanter being fractured during the removal of the femoral stem*

Section 2

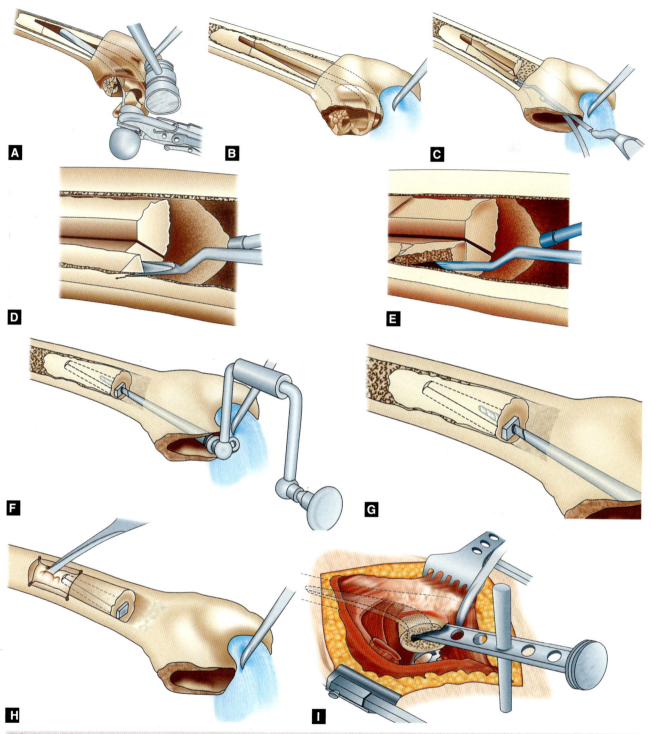

FIG. 48.4A TO I

Steps taken during removal of failed femoral components. These steps, however are not sufficient to remove some stems where access to the distal column of cement is not possible, requiring the performance of a window distally. Other times a long splitting of the lateral cortex of the femur is necessary. The Wagner technique is ideal

Section 2

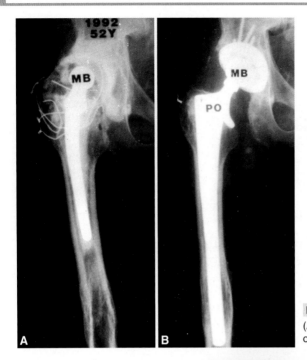

FIGS 48.5A AND B

(A) Failed Charnley arthroplasty. (B) Revised without the need for trochanteric osteotomy

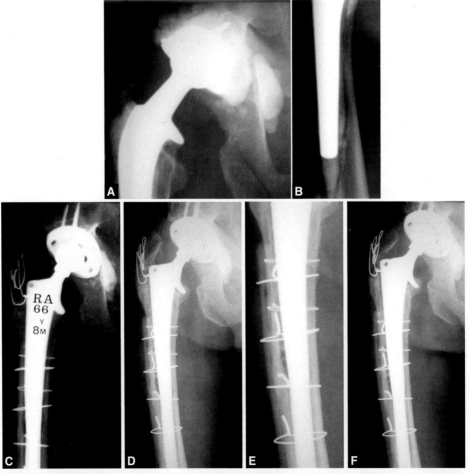

FIGS 48.6A TO F

(A and B) Radiographs of the acetabulum and distal femur respectively demonstrating loosening of the components. (C) Radiograph obtained eight months postoperatively. (D to F) Radiographs obtained two, eight and nineteen years postoperatively

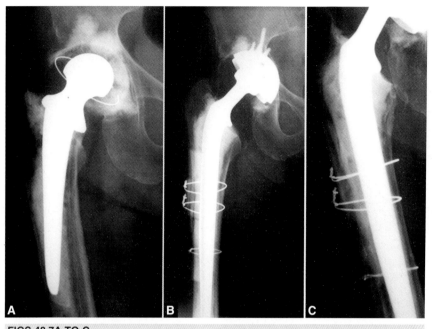

FIGS 48.7A TO C

(A) Radiograph of failed Muller prosthesis. (B) Radiograph obtained six months after revision surgery, which included a lateral bone graft. (C) Radiograph taken 13 years postoperatively. Notice the resorption of the femoral graft

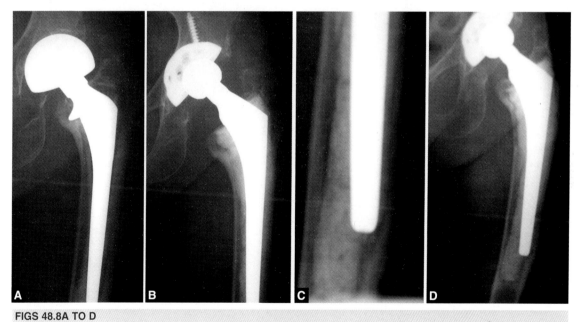

FIGS 48.8A TO D

(A) Radiograph of failed cemented bipolar prosthesis. (B) First postoperative radiograph. Notice the imperfect cementation technique. (C and D) Radiographs taken eight years after surgery. The hip is painful, the stem has shifted into varus, and the bone-cement radiolucent lines have widened

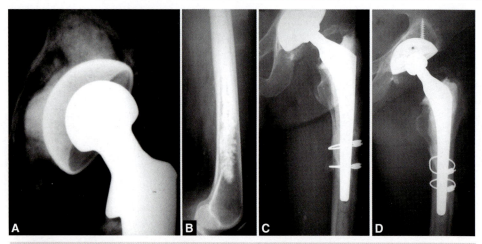

FIGS 48.9A TO D

(A) Radiograph of failed cemented total hip arthroplasty. (B) Radiograph showing the extension of the cement column into the distal femur. Apparently a plug was not used. (C) Radiograph obtained following revision. A window was created in the femur to make possible removal of cement. (D) Radiograph taken seven years postoperatively

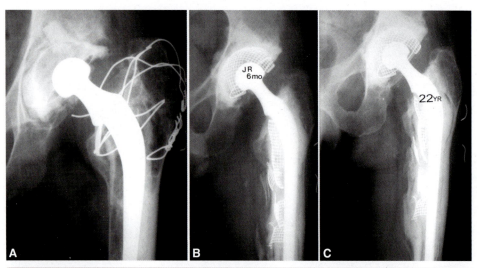

FIGS 48.10A TO C

(A) Radiograph of failed cemented prosthesis. (B and C) Radiographs obtained five years after revision surgery. Radiograph taken 22 years after revision. Notice the incorporation of the bone graft

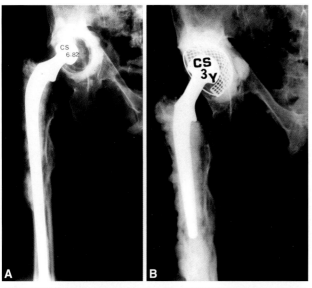

FIGS 48.11A AND B

(A) Failed femoral and acetabular components associated with lysis.
(B) Radiograph taken three years after revision of both components
using cement. *A shorter stem was thought to be appropriate*

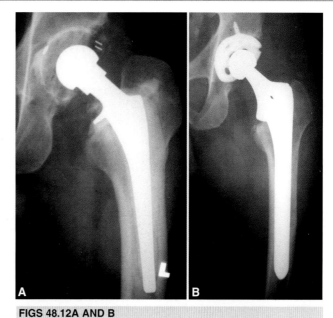

FIGS 48.12A AND B

(A) Failed femoral and acetabular cemented components. (B) Both
components were revised with noncemented appliances

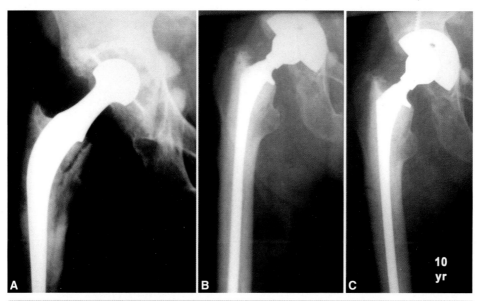

FIGS 48.13A TO C

(A) Failed femoral component 14 years after surgery. The acetabulum shows some wear but no signs of
loosening. (B) Radiograph taken after revision of the femoral component using acrylic cement. The
acetabular component was not revised. (C) Radiograph obtained ten years after revision surgery. Notice
what appears to be no further evidence of wear

Section 2

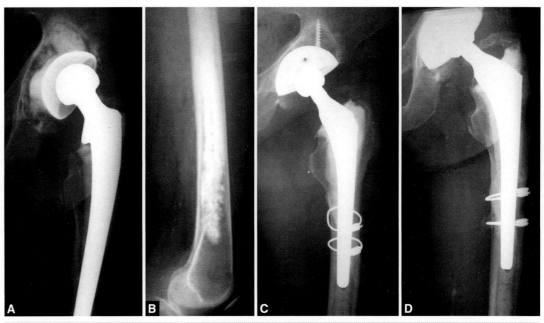

FIGS 48.14A TO D

(A) Radiograph of failed cemented femoral and acetabular components. (B) Notice the long column of cement that extends almost down to the knee joint. (C and D) Radiographs obtained two and nine years postrevision surgery. A window was necessary for removal of cement

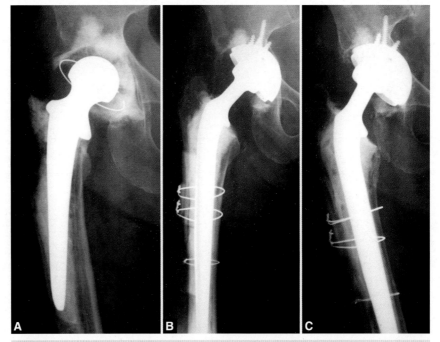

FIGS 48.15A TO C

(A) Radiograph of failed cemented Muller prosthesis in a 69-year-old woman. The acetabular component does not appear to be loose. (B) Radiograph obtained after revision of both components. The acetabular polyethylene was found to be loose at the time of surgery. A bone graft was used to reinforce the femoral cortex. (C) Radiograph taken 11 years post-revision surgery. Though there are radiolucent lines around the stem, the patient has remained asymptomatic

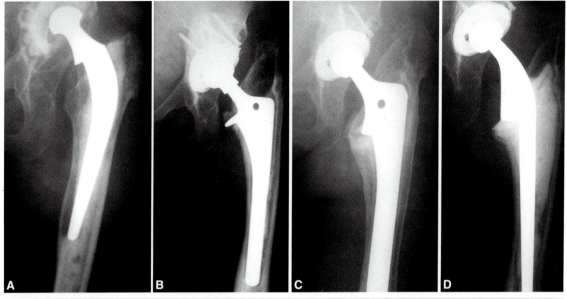

FIGS 48.16A TO D

(A) Radiograph of failed cemented Bechtol prosthesis. (B) The acetabulum was replaced with a noncemented component and a bone graft, and the femur with a cemented implant that promptly failed and migrated distally into the femoral canal. (C) A second revision of the femoral component was carried out using a platform type implant in order to regain length. This implant also failed and the prosthesis one again sank in the canal. (D) A third revision was performed using cement and a longer platform implant. This arthroplasty also failed and was treated at another institution using a noncemented implant. It is my understanding that after a period of relief of symptoms the implant has shown signs of loosening

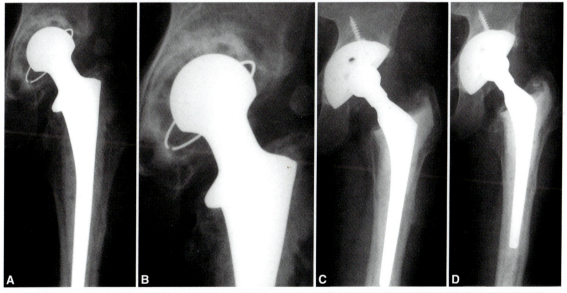

FIGS 48.17A TO D

(A) Radiograph of failed cemented total hip arthroplasty. (B) Notice the degree of polyethylene wear six years after surgery. (C) Radiograph obtained one year after revision with a hybrid implant. (D) Radiograph taken eight years postrevision

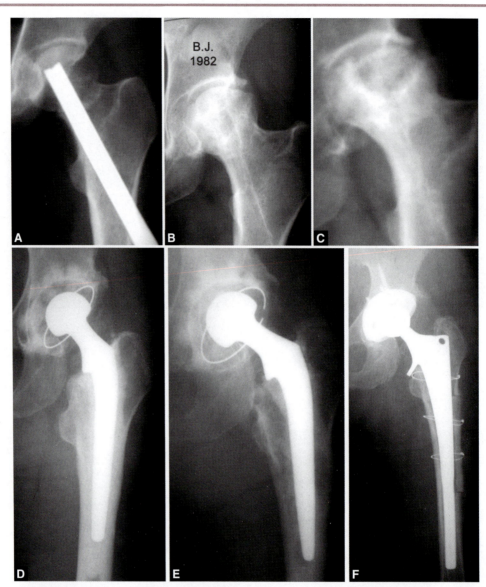

FIGS 48.18A TO F

(A) Radiograph of healed fracture of the femoral neck in a 34-year-old woman. (B) Radiograph taken 2 years after the initial injury demonstrating avascular necrosis of the femoral head. (C) One year later the avascular necrosis shows a large defect. (D) The condition was treated with cemented titanium (STH) components. (E) Seven years later there were signs of lysis in the neck of the femur and significant wear of the polyethylene. (F) One year later (eight yeas postoperatively) the lysis had extended and both components were loose. A noncemented arthroplasty was performed. Radiograph obtained three years postrevision surgery. Radiograph taken three years later demonstrating early signs of loosening

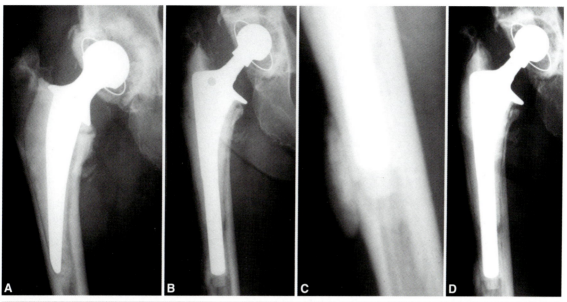

FIGS 48.19A TO D

(A) Radiograph of failed cemented total hip prosthesis. The acetabulum (A 32 size prosthetic head) did not appear to be loose. (B and C) Closer view of the distal end of the prosthesis showing the lateral migration of the stem against the femoral cortex. (D) The femoral component was revised with a cemented long stem. Radiograph showing the leak of cement distally. This was not noticed immediately after surgery. Apparently the cortex of the femur, already weakened by the shifted stem was further damaged during the removal of the cement. Radiograph obtained four years after revision. The patient had remained asymptomatic, but the radiograph shows early signs of loosening. The patient expired five years later after developing septicemia secondary to spontaneous hematogenous infection in the operated hip

*References**

19, 20, 34, 35, 45, 60, 61, 81

---

* References provided at the end of the book after annexures.

49

Revision of the Failed Acetabular Components

Revision of failed acetabular components often is a challenging and time-consuming enterprise. When the component is of the porous type, the difficulties are greater if bone ingrowth has already taken place. In this instance the risk of perforating the pelvic wall increases manifold. Fortunately, the success from primary total hip arthroplasty using porous coated components has been remarkable. Currently, most failures occur on the femoral side (Figs 49.1 to 49.13).

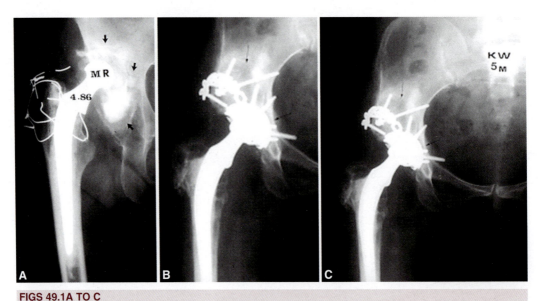

FIGS 49.1A TO C

(A) Failed cemented total hip arthroplasty with damage to the roof of the acetabulum and fracture of the plastic socket. (B) The large defect in the acetabulum was replaced with a noncemented porous cup and reinforced with a femoral head. Plates were used to stabilize the femoral graft. (C) Five years later the graft appears to have incorporated with the acetabular floor

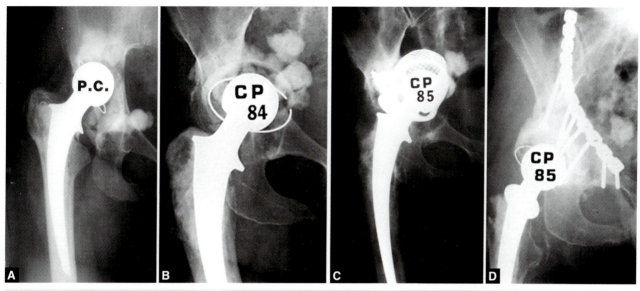

FIGS 49.2A TO D

(A) Failed acetabular component. (B) It was, apparently, treated with another cemented acetabular component that also failed rapidly. (C) A third procedure, consisting apparently of the addition of a metallic ring also failed. (D) The lost bone in the pelvis was replaced with bone graft held in place with plates and screws. Patient was lost to follow-up. If grafts held in place with metallic implants and accompanied with bone grafting are not protected from weight bearing, failure is likely to take place. The bone graft maintains most of its mechanical properties until its revascularization begins. Then it becomes softer and may collapse or reabsorbs. The revision surgery was performed by my associate Joel Matta, MD

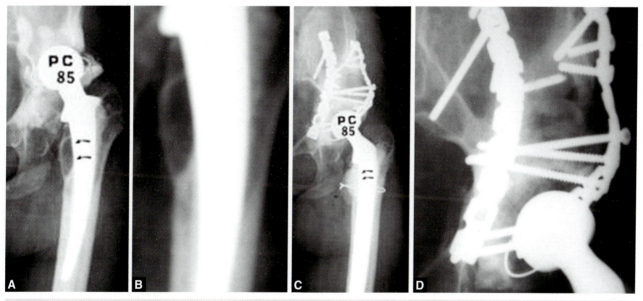

FIGS 49.3A TO D

(A) Failed acetabular component. The prosthesis migrated into the pelvis and destroyed the roof of the socket. A large lytic lesion developed at the level of the lesser trochanter. (B) Closer view of the lytic lesion. (C) Reconstruction was carried out using a large femoral bone graft stabilized with two plates and screws. (D) Radiograph obtained seven years later. The mechanical fixation has been apparently maintained without visible changes in the bone graft. The surgery was performed by my associate Joel M Latta, MD

Section 2

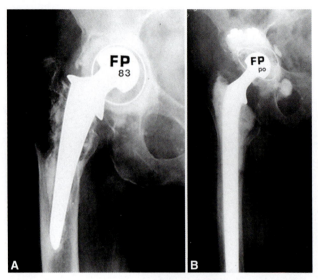

FIGS 49.4A AND B

(A) Failed acetabular and femoral components. The acetabular component has migrated superiorly, and the femur shows extensive lysis. (B) The defect in the superior acetabulum was filled with acrylic cement and a long stem was cemented in the femur

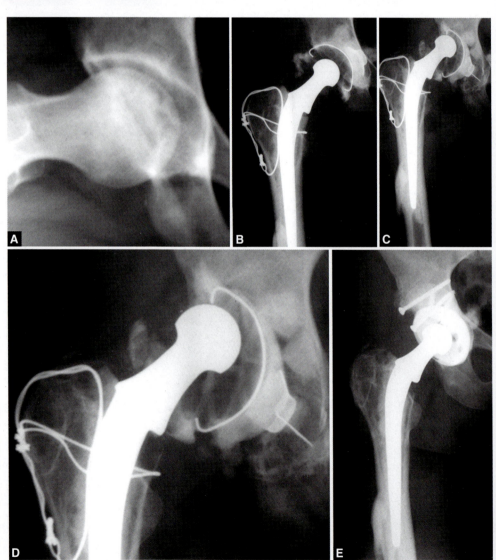

FIGS 49.5A TO E

(A) Radiograph of avascular necrosis secondary to sickle cell anemia. (B) Radiograph of Charnley arthroplasty performed 25 years earlier. (C) The acetabular component spontaneously became loose. (D) Closer view of loose acetabular component. (E) The revision consisted of bone grafting of the acetabulum and addition of a porous ring

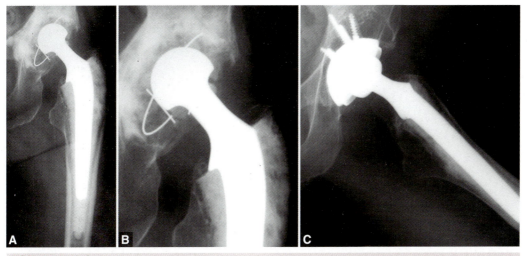

FIGS 49.6A TO C

(A) Radiograph of a 18-year-old titanium total hip. (B) Radiograph obtained 22 years after surgery, following gradual development of pain and the sensation of "clicking" during certain motions of the hip. Notice the fracture of the identifying peripheral wire. (C) In surgery the acetabular component was loose but the polyethylene cup was intact, showing, however evidence of wear

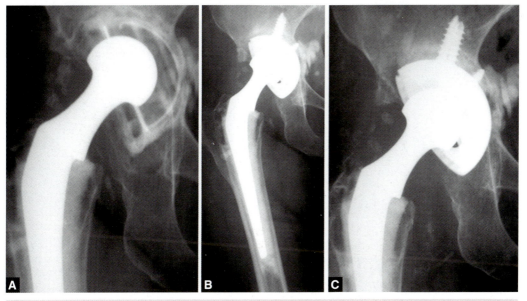

FIGS 49.7A TO C

(A) Failed acetabular component in a titanium arthroplasty performed 25 years earlier. Notice the superomedial migration of the polyethylene socket. (B) Severe damage to the floor of the acetabulum was documented in surgery. The floor of the acetabulum was packed with cancellous bone and a porous cup was anchored with metallic screws. *Notice the exaggerated valgus of the socket.* (C) The cup was revised and placed in a more horizontal plane. The acetabular component tolerates some exaggerated valgus, however a more transverse position is desirable

Section 2

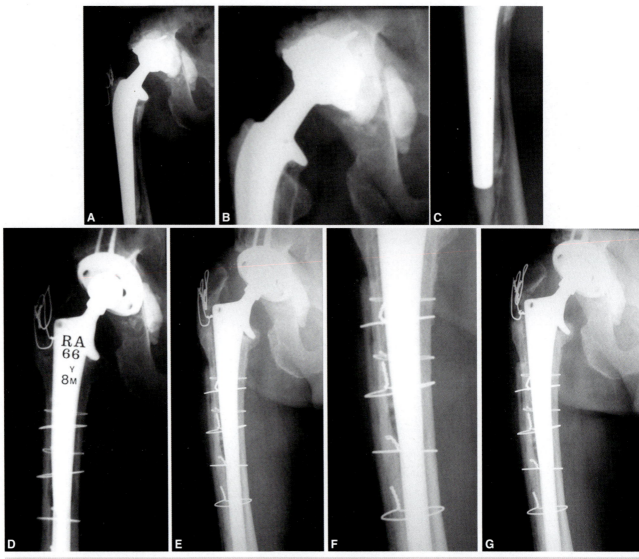

FIGS 49.8A TO G

(A to C) Radiographs illustrating failed acetabular and femoral components in a 63-year-old man. Notice the lateral shift of the femoral stem. (D to G) Radiographs obtained following revision surgery that consisted of a noncemented acetabular component and a cemented femoral stem. The surgery required the placement of a cortical graft on the lateral aspect of the femur. The last radiograph (F) was taken 13 years post-revision. The patient has remained minimally symptomatic

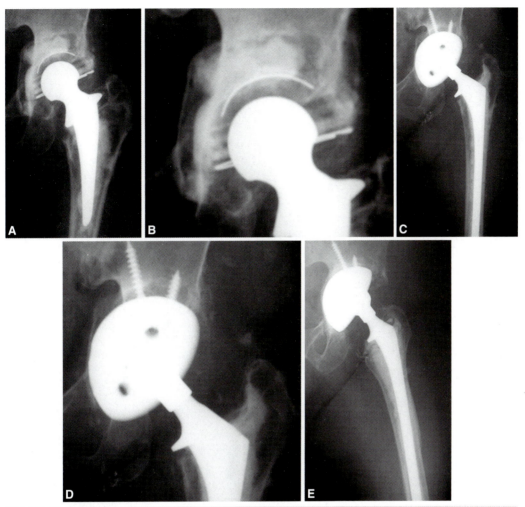

FIGS 49.9A TO E

(A and B) Radiographs of a failed cemented total hip arthroplasty in a 66-year-old woman diagnosed at the time of having a nonmetastasized breast carcinoma. (C) Radiograph showing the revised hip. A noncemented acetabulum and a cemented femoral component were used. The acetabular cup appears to be in an exaggerated valgus position. (D and E) Radiographs taken two years later showing maintenance of fixation of the components. The hip never dislocated. The patient expired a few months later from metastatic carcinoma

Section 2

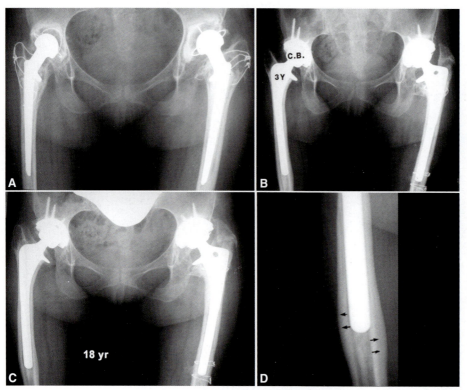

FIGS 49.10A TO D

(A) Radiograph of failed bilateral total hip cemented arthroplasties in a woman 26-year-old. The surgery had been performed six years earlier, allegedly for the care of osteoarthritis secondary to congeal familiar chondrodystrophy. (B to D) Radiographs taken three, eight and eighteen years postrevision arthroplasty. Closer view of the distal left femur showing a healthy femoral hypertrophy. The patient had remained relatively asymptomatic all those years. However, she has notified (Twenty years postrevision) that she is scheduled for surgery in her home town for failure of her right arthroplasty. I was unable to obtain the radiographs and have not received a response from the operating surgeon regarding the outcome from surgery

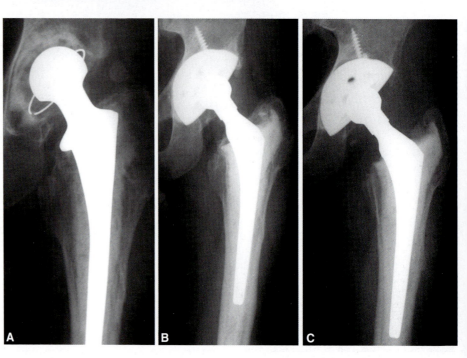

FIGS 49.11A TO C

(A) Radiograph of failed cemented total hip in a 51-year-old man. (B) Radiograph taken postoperatively following revision with hybrid components. (C) Radiograph obtained 10 years postoperatively

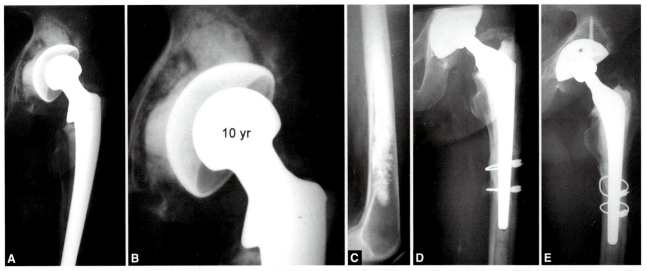

FIGS 49.12A TO E

(A and B) Radiographs of failed femoral and acetabular cemented components. (C) Illustration of column of cement driven too far distally into the femoral canal. (D) Postoperative radiograph. After windowing the femur in order to remove the cement, a long-stem prosthesis was cemented in place. (E) Radiograph obtained twelve years postoperatively

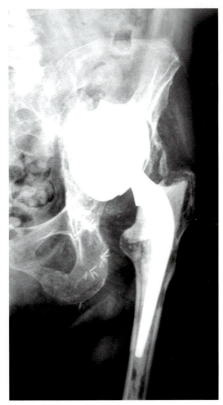

FIG. 49.13

Radiograph of failed acetabular component. The initial surgery was preformed 35 years earlier. A Girdlestone procedure was performed in preference to reconstruction. The patient's age and general condition dictated that choice

*References**

24, 31, 33, 50, 54, 57, 64, 79, 81, 104, 111

---

* References provided at the end of the book after annexures.

Section 2

50

Surface Replacement

The concept of a total hip replacement that preserved a large segment of the femoral head and did not violate the femoral canal was first described in the literature in the late 1970s by an Italian surgeon, whose name I regret having forgotten. The idea was received with enthusiasm in the United Kingdom as well as in America since it represented a significant theoretical advantage over traditional arthroplasties. Michael Freeman, in England, embraced the concept. With enthusiasm he performed the procedure numerous times. Similarly in the United States, William Capello, from Indiana, delved into the study of the new technique. Unfortunately, the two British and American surgeons soon ran into complications and reported their high failure rate. Avascular changes in the femoral head and loosening of the implants were among the most common complications. Harlan Amstutz, from Los Angeles, was among the American surgeons who first expressed interest in the system and studied its possible applications. Contrary to the attitude of the other above-mentioned surgeons, Amstutz persevered and thought the complications could be avoided by strict adherence to specific surgical details. To this date he has continued to report on his results with enthusiasm. It is yet too early to tell if his commitment to find a permanent place for surface replacement in the armamentarium of the orthopedic surgeon will prove correct. To abandon efforts to solve the current problems at this time would be unfair and perhaps regrettable, if nothing else because its rationale is sound. More recently, the Birmingham surface replacement has received a great deal of publicity. Reports indicate and unexpected high degree of success. Nonetheless, some investigators have been disappointed with their results, due to a

higher incidence of fractures of the femoral neck and revision surgery. I remain skeptical about the system and think it popularity is primarily due to a very effective marketing onslaught. The cavalier disregard for the potentially harmful of metallic debris into the lymphatic and bloodstream might one day come to haunt the orthopedic community.

My personal experience with the procedure is minimal when it comes to its performance, though moderately rich when it comes to observing and revising failed surface replacements. As I look back at the revised procedures, I feel that many of the failures could be readily traced to improperly performed surgery. The wrong attitude of the femoral cup over the femoral neck, the insufficient depth of the acetabulum and the orientation of the acetabular cup seem to have been the most common errors that led to their ultimate failure. It is very likely that loosening of the femoral component was due in some instances to avascular necrosis of the femoral head.

The following examples (Figs 50.1 to 50.8) of successful, as well as unsuccessful surface replacements simply have allowed me to speculate on the reasons for the success or failure of the implants.

This 75-year-old man was referred to me by another orthopedist with the diagnosis of failed hip surface replacement. He had had the replacement performed five years earlier, and his hip had remained asymptomatic until very recently. Though the symptoms pointed toward the operated hip, and passive motion of the hip was painful, I was never convinced they clearly fit into hip pathology. The pain had failed to respond to conservative methods, so much that I eventually accepted the patient's pleas to have his hip replaced. I went as far as scheduling him

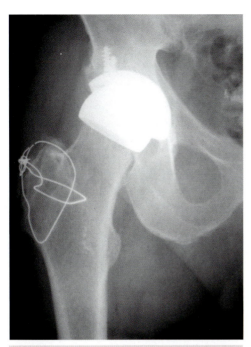

FIG. 50.1

A five-year-old asymptomatic surface replacement that suddenly became painful. The pain subsided spontaneously within a few weeks without finding an explanation for the localized symptoms

for surgery, which I cancelled the morning of the scheduled day. I could not bring myself to carrying out a surgical procedure I did not think it was justified, since clear evidence of pathology had not been clearly documented.

I turned out to be correct in my "gut feelings". Three weeks later his hip had decreased significantly, and a few weeks later the symptoms had completely disappeared. I never knew what had caused the pain and its subsidence. All laboratory work for gout and other conditions was negative. It turned out that the patient was having pain as a result of "shingles".

Having had the personal experience of experiencing the "shingles" myself a few months ago, I can testify of the many ways in which this condition can manifest itself. Almost overnight I began to feel pain in my cervical spine and felt it was due to perhaps having twisted it the night before. I also experienced what I thought could have been the symptoms of a common cold: malaise and low-grade temperature. Within a couple of days the neck pain extended into my right shoulder making it difficult to use. The pain, however, never extended down my arm. Concerned that I had developed disk problems I had an MRI study. It shows minimal arthritic changes at the 3 to 4 level and even a mild bulging disk. Neither rest, heat nor cold

applications helped the situation. One week after the onset of symptoms I finally made the diagnosis when I noticed 2 small red spots just above the anterior aspect of the elbow. Three additional spots had formed within the next 24 hours along the tract of the ulnar nerve in the forearm. The infectious disease specialist confirmed my diagnosis and prescribed an antibiotic, which made me deadly sick. For several days I took the medication until I came to the conclusion that the treatment was worse than the disease. By that time, fortunately, the medication had done the job.

I wonder how many times we have made the mistake of diagnosing osteoarthritis and blamed it for the presence of suddenly appeared symptoms, simply because an X-ray had shown arthritic changes. The fact that we have become so subspecialized has made us unaware of a number of basic findings responsible for the presence of joint pain of unexplained etiology. In at least ten times in the last ten years I have seen patients referred to me with hip pain who also had significant back pain. Several of them had their spines operated upon to alleviate the condition but to no avail. The hip was the culprit. I am sure that the other side of the coin is also revealing, since patients whose basic pathology is in the spine end up having hip surgery that does not help their disabling back condition. In a very recent instance, a very competent back surgeon insisted that the pain the patient was experiencing was coming from the spine despite the presence of arthritic changes in the hip because of moderately severe atrophy of the quadriceps. It took me a while to convince him that *I had never seen a patient with a painful hip disease that did not develop quadriceps atrophy within a relatively short-time.*

At first glance is difficult to understand the confusion. The two entities have very different symptoms and behavior. I tell my secretary not to accept patients who point at their buttocks as the location of their pain, since almost without exception their problems are related to the spine not to the hip. I simplify matters by telling her, as well as the patients that pain in the buttocks does not come from the hip. Hip pain is almost always, with a few exceptions, such as trochanteric bursitis, located in the groin. Needless to say, this is an oversimplification of a more complex issue, but has kept me from being inundated with obese patients with back pain.

My loss of follow-up following of patients after replacement arthroplasty has been discouragingly high despite a deliberate effort to reach all patients on a

Section 2

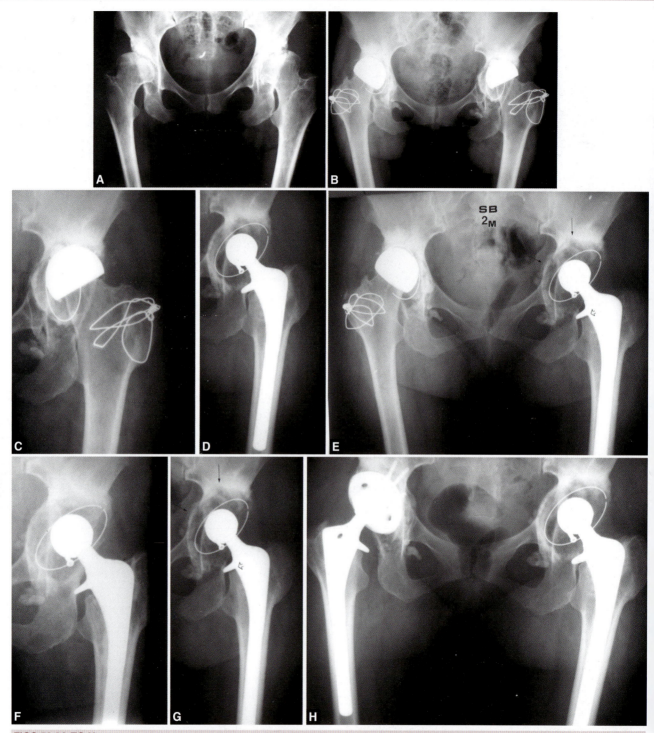

FIGS 50.2A TO H

(A) Radiograph of bilateral osteoarthritis in a 36-year-old woman, probably secondary to congenital hip dysplasia. (B) Bilateral surface replacement was performed. (C) The left hip became painful and radiographs showed loosening of the acetabulum and its superior migration. (D and E) The left implant was replaced with an isoelastic acetabulum. (F and G) The newly replaced left hip began to show early changes in the acetabulum, manifested by loss of the sclerotic line at the plastic-bone interface. As the right hip began to become painful the (H) Radiograph showing virtual disappearance of the sclerotic line at the interface. The right surface replacement was replaced with a noncemented Harris-Galante implant. The patient was lost to follow-up shortly afterward. It is very likely that the isoelastic necessitated revision within a few months or years, based on our observed fate of those implants. The Harris-Galante prosthesis may have suffered the same fate

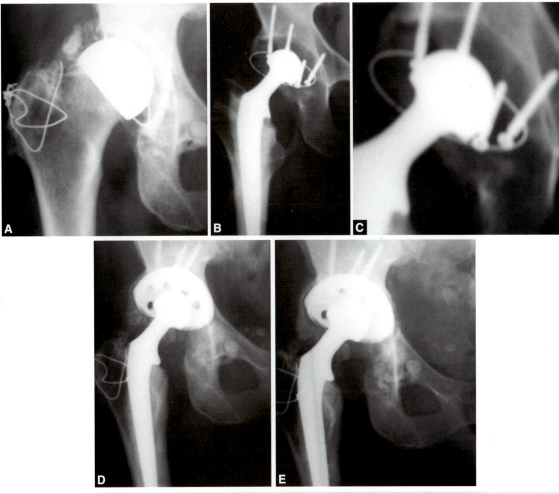

FIGS 50.3A TO E

(A) Radiograph of a painful surface replacement performed approximately seven years earlier for the treatment of avascular necrosis. At the time of revision, the acetabulum was found to be loose and the femoral neck with lytic defects. (B) The failed hip was revised with an isoelastic socket and a cemented titanium stem. (C) Within four years the acetabulum began to show the loss of the sclerotic line at the plastic-bone interface. The hip was painful. (D) The failed acetabulum was then replaced with a noncemented porous cup. (E) The hip has remained painless and functional for an additional 14 years

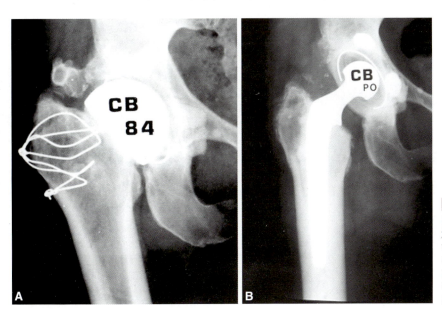

FIGS 50.4A AND B

(A) Failed surface replacement performed for the treatment of osteoarthritis in a 50-year-old woman. (B) The failed implant was revised with a cemented titanium stem and a cemented polyethylene socket. Allegedly, the hip is asymptomatic 15 years later. However, the patient refuses to have another X-ray of her hip

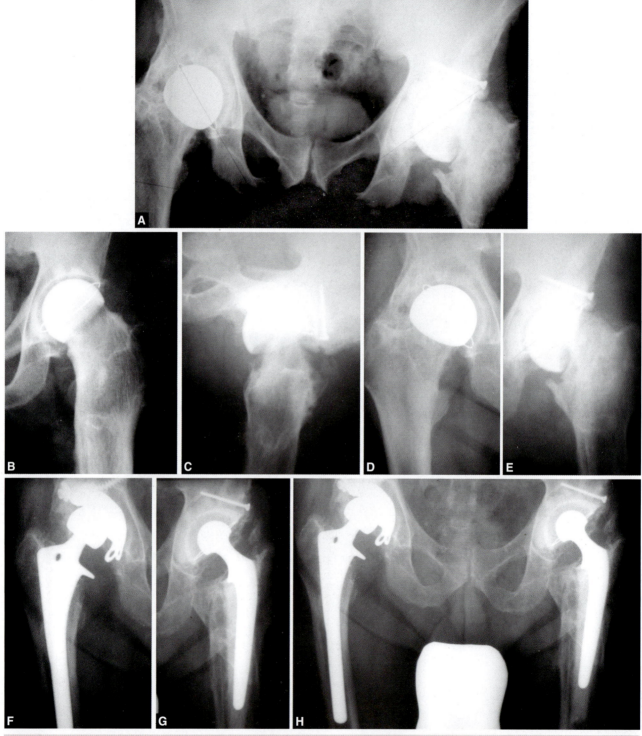

FIGS 50.5A TO H

(A) Bilateral surface replacement arthroplasties performed in a 55-year-old man for the treatment of osteoarthritis seven years earlier. The hips were painful and had moderate limitation of motion. (B) Closer view of the left hip showing what appears to be a stable implant. (C) The lateral view of the hip is suggestive of loosening of the femoral component. (D) Films taken 6 months after show no changes in the right hip but complete dislocation of the femoral component in the left hip. (E) The right hip was revised with non cemented components. The left hip was revised with a cemented titanium implant and a cemented polyethylene acetabulum. (F to H) Follow-up radiographs obtained three years after surgery at which time there was still limited but improved range of motion of the hips and no evidence of wear or loosening of the components. The patient was contacted 3 yeas later and stated that the condition had not changed since the last examination but refused to have additional X-rays taken

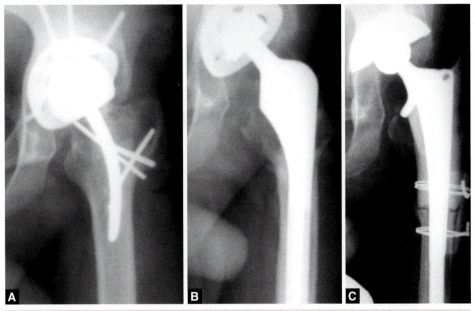

FIGS 50.6A TO C

(A) Radiograph of surface replacement in a 22-year-old boy allegedly performed for arthritis secondary to slipped epiphysis. (B) The surface replacement was revised by another surgeon with a noncemented arthroplasty that became painful three years later. Notice lysis on Zone I. (C) The failed hip was revised with a cemented stem and noncemented acetabulum. The young man's weight was 260 pounds and rather irresponsible in his behavior

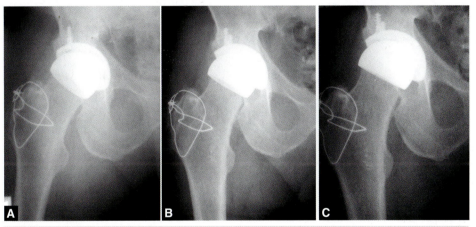

FIGS 50.7A TO C

Radiographs of a surface arthroplasty obtained at five years interval. There are no radiological signs of pathology, other than wear

regular basis. I have always sent to every patient a "form" letter every year to which I added a personal note. This practice allowed me to develop a good relationship with most of them. However, many patients stopped corresponding for reasons I do not always understood. Sometimes, it is logical to assume that the many had expired or became mentally incapacitated. Other times they probably established a relationship with their local doctor and did not see a reason to continue writing and sending me X-rays.

What troubles me is the fact that several orthopedists who publish their results, claim a very high rate of successful follow-up of their patients. I suspect that surgeons who deal for the most part with local patients in cities or states with stable populations are in a position to ensure a higher rate of follow-up success. However, in institutions, where the vast majority of patients come from other states or countries, the loss to follow-up has to be very high. Their publications do not reflect that factor.

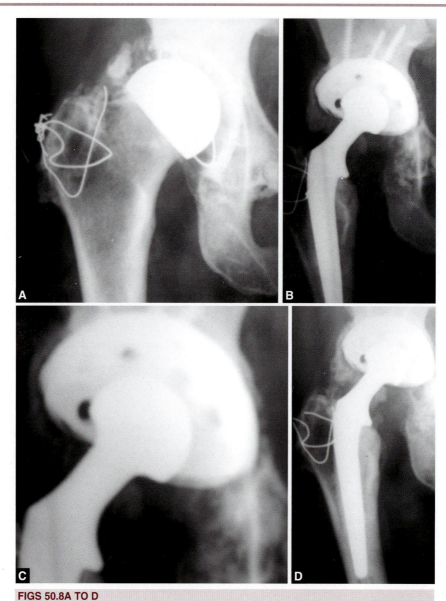

FIGS 50.8A TO D

(A) Radiograph of a painful surface replacement arthroplasty, which was revised into a hybrid titanium arthroplasty. At the time of revision loosening of the cup was identified. (B and C) Radiographs obtained postoperatively. (D) Radiograph obtained 18 years postoperatively demonstrating no evidence of complications. No measurable wear is evident

In more recent years a strong marketing effort has been devoted to newer types of surface replacement arthroplasties, particularly the Birmingham arthroplasty. Reports are published on a regular basis indicating a high success rate over a relatively short period of time. It is possible that this implant will prove to be a major improvement over earlier ones.

My concern with this and similar metal on metal prostheses is the unknown ill-effects metal debris will have in a long-run. The fact that people with the high reputation of Patrick Case, from Bristol, England, have identified chromosomal abnormalities in areas of metalosis is something that I find worrisome. To ignore this finding, as it seems to be the case today, may prove to have been a fatal mistake. In a very recent article the authors reported on "tumors" under the metallic shell. There was no clear definition of the type of the lesions and their histological diagnosis. In any event, it is something to keep in mind.

51

Isoelastic Total Hip Prostheses

In the early 1980s, when the noncemented total hip prosthesis was first introduced on the market, an isoelastic prosthesis was strongly heralded as the answer to the alleged problems arising from the "cement disease". I joined the crowd and began to look for the best noncemented implant. Different ones became available within a few months. Somewhat skeptical at that time about porous implants, I took advantage of a trip to Europe to visit some of the individuals heavily involved in the development and use of the new implants.

Erwin Morscher, from Basle, Switzerland, advanced the concept of isoelastic prosthesis. The idea made a lot of sense to me. He had proposed an implant that had mechanical properties closer to those of bone and made of a material with a low modulus of elasticity. Loosening, therefore, should be lower. I visited with Morscher, learned about his technique and philosophy and observed him perform the procedure. I was very impressed with his early results. Then I went to Italy, where I visited with Renato Bombeli. He had a wealth of experience with the method and had capitalized on the huge northern Italian population suffering from osteoarthritis secondary to congenital hip dysplasia.

It was during my visit to northern Italy that I learned about the frequency of congenital hip disease in that part of the world. A high frequency shared by the southern Germans, particularly those from Bavaria. I later learned that there are only three other racial groups in the world with an even higher incidence of

congenital hip disease: the Eskimos, Navajos and the Indians of Ecuador. The theory frequently expressed that congenital hip dislocation is due to the practice of wrapping the infants in a mummy-like garments that hold the legs in adduction loses credibility. Neither the Germans nor the Italians dress their infants in that manner. The Eskimos and Ecuadorian Indians do.

Bombelli gave me the opportunity to see him perform surgery in a large number of patients and allowed me to look at the pre and postoperative X-rays of all of his patients. The European experience with the two surgeons, who later were to become good personal friends, convinced me that the Isoelastic prosthesis was "the way to go". Upon my return to America, I began to perform the procedure. The early results were most gratifying clinically and radiographically. I must admit, however, that I never used the femoral component of the ssoelastic implant, only the acetabulum. I had been using a titanium alloy implant with a low modulus of elasticity and therefore I did not see a reason to use the isoelastic femoral component.

Shortly afterwards Morscher came to Los Angeles as my guest for a postgraduate course on total hip surgery. I performed surgery and he assisted me. I wanted to be sure that I was performing the procedure well. A couple of years later I received a telephone call from him informing me that the most recent review of his isoelastic prostheses had indicated an unexpected high incidence of complication. Loosening and lysis were seen with disturbing frequency. I argued with him that my experiences did not support

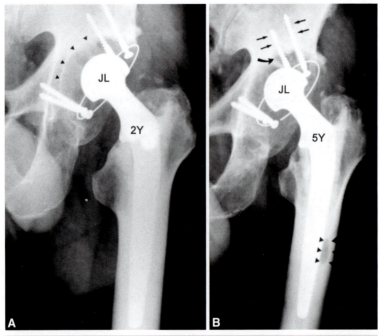

FIGS 51.1A AND B

(A) Isoelastic acetabulum demonstrating at two years the desirable sclerotic line at the bone-plastic interface. (B) Three years later the line has disappeared and lytic lesions developed at the level of the calcar and on zones 2-3 of the femur

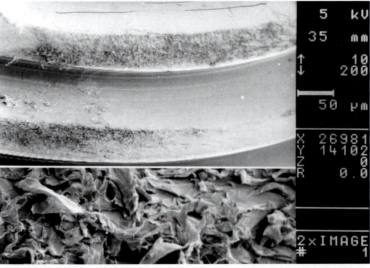

FIG. 51.2

Under high magnification this unused isoelastic acetabulum component shows serious manufacturing defects, which probably result in the rapid production of debris

his; that my better results could be explained by the fact that I had not used the isoelastic femoral component.

I began to look more carefully at the X-rays of my patients. Lo and behold, in a short time I identified the same problems Morscher had seen. Within the very short follow-up of seven years I saw more than 70 per cent of my patients developing sufficient pathology to require revision surgery. *At the time of the revision surgery we demonstrated massive amount of plastic debris separating the plastic cup from the underlying bone.* Doctor Adolfo Llinas, a surgeon from Bogota, Colombia, then serving a fellowship with us undertook the task of carefully analyzing the material and studying the microscopic findings.

He discovered a very interesting feature: *brand-new, unused isoelastic cups were often found to have manufacturing defects consisting of rough, unpolished surfaces that under repeated motion could fragment and break off.* We surmised that such a defect was one of the reasons for the high failure. Obviously, micro or macro-motion between the cup and the acetabular bone was producing the harmful plastic debris. The findings were published at a later date.

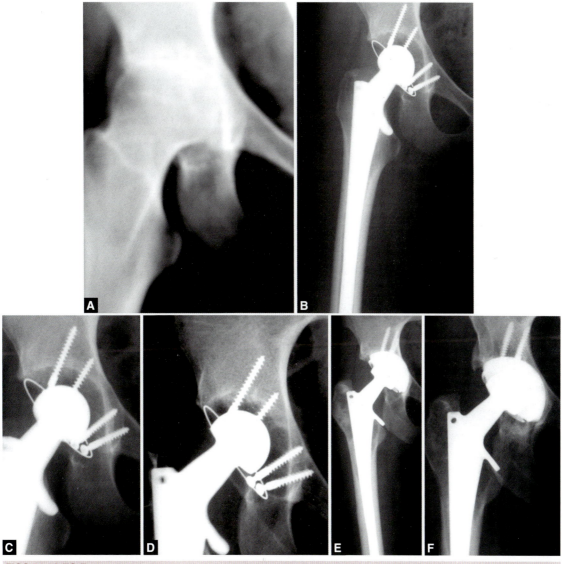

FIGS 51.3A TO F

(A) Radiograph of a hip in a 27-year-old woman suffering from rheumatoid arthritis. (B) Radiograph obtained shortly after surgery. (C) Radiograph showing the desirable demarcation at the plastic-bone interface two years after surgery. (D) Radiograph taken four years after surgery showing the loss of demarcation in the acetabulum. The hip was becoming painful. (E) The failed arthroplasty was revised with a noncemented bias prosthesis. (F) Three years later the films showed trochanteric lysis that required revision surgery. The procedure was performed by another surgeon in a distant city. I am not aware of the final outcome

Section 2

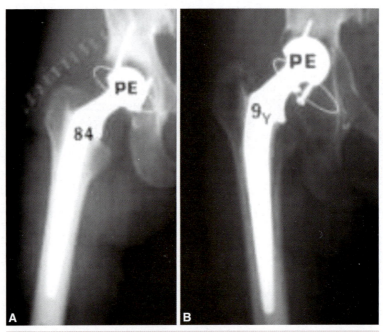

FIGS 51.4A AND B

(A) Radiograph of a isoelastic prosthesis obtained immediately after surgery in a 44-year-old woman. (B) Radiograph taken nine years later demonstrating penetration of the prosthetic head into the plastic acetabulum. The patient had been lost to follow-up after three months postsurgically. Inspection of the plastic material at the time of revision suggested that gradual wear had taken place over the previous years

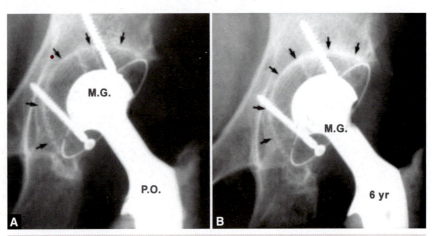

FIGS 51.5A AND B

(A) Postoperative radiograph of an isoelastic prosthesis performed in a 64-year-old woman suffering from osteoarthritis of the hip. (B) Radiograph taken six years after surgery showing the desirable clear demarcation between the bony acetabulum and the plastic socket

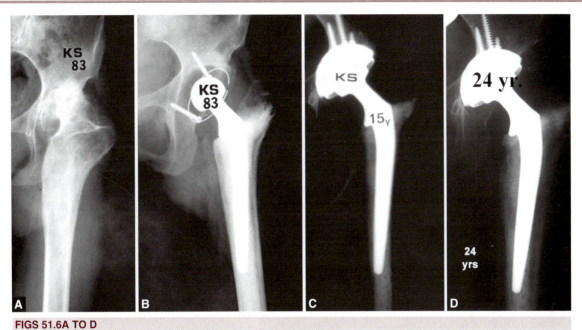

FIGS 51.6A TO D

(A) Radiograph of arthritic hip probably secondary to surgery performed in infancy for the treatment of a congenital problem not yet identified. It is likely that the growth of the proximal femoral epiphysis was arrested. (B) The hip was reconstructed with a cemented titanium monoblock prosthesis and an isoelastic acetabulum. (C) Within a short period the acetabulum became loose requiring additional surgery. A noncemented acetabulum was used. Radiograph obtained 15 years after the first arthroplasty. (D) Radiograph taken 24 years after the revision of the isoelastic acetabulum. The patient has remained asymptomatic

I began to look more carefully at the X-rays of my patients. Lo and behold, in a short time I identified the same problems Morscher had seen. Within the very short follow-up of seven years I saw more than 70 per cent of my patients developing sufficient pathology to require revision surgery. At the time of the revision surgery we demonstrated massive amount of plastic debris separating the plastic cup from the underlying bone.

I have always admired the intellectual honesty Morscher displayed when he called to inform me of the problems he was having with his prosthesis, and to advice me to abandon its use. Not many people do that. This is depicted by the fact that a number of prostheses have disappeared from the market because of failure, but without the developers or manufacturers letting the orthopedic community know about the failure and the reasons for discontinuing their usage. Worse than that, several of those implants continue to be marketed and sold. I was not surprised when I found out that some implants that have been discredited in the United States were being heavily marketed in Latin America. I surmise that the distributors of the implants were hoping to get rid of whatever inventory still existed. A very dishonest practice.

*Rererences**

63, 81

Section 2

---

* References provided at the end of the book after annexures.

52

Metal-on-Metal, Ceramics and Bigger Prosthetic Heads

Despite the fact that it has been rather obvious that wear debris is the major culprit in the failure of many total hip implants, a major effort to address in earnest the source of the debris and find a resolution to the problems it generates was not undertaking until relatively recently.

Though the articulating surfaces are likely to be the main producers of harmful debris, the issue is more complex than that. Debris is also generated from modular components, from screws use to anchor acetabular implants, from porous surfaces and from the stems themselves. At this time, the greatest attention is being paid to the joint components through modifications of the polyethylenes, the use of metal-on-metal surfaces or ceramic components.

The most talked about system is the use of metal-on-metal implants. Will they work or will they prove to have been another "flash in the pan" that quickly disappeared from the scene? It is hard to tell. The concept is not new. Marshall Urist, from California, reported in the 1950's his experiences with a metallic endoprosthesis used in combination with a Smith Petersen-like acetabular metallic cup. The procedure never gained wide acceptance and I have surmised it was because of unsatisfactory results. A few years later McKee and Farrar, in England, described their metal-on-metal total hip arthroplasty (Figs 52.1A to D). Their prosthesis was widely used throughout the world with mixed results. Peter Ring, also from England, used his own concept of an Austin Moore prosthesis and a metal socket that fixed in the pelvic bone with a long and thick screw. I spent a few days with Mr. Ring and was impressed with his dexterity and early results. Upon my return to the States I performed a moderately large number of Ring prostheses (See *Chapter Ring Prostheses*). *However, the failure rate was high as the acetabular screw became loose and produced pain.* The Charnley approach to total hip arthroplasty won the day and it became the preferred method eclipsing the contribution of the other three British surgeons.

Contributing to the demise of the MacKee-Farrar arthroplasty was the presence of an annoying increased friction between the components, and the finding of severe metallosis in a number of instances. In spite of that, many MacKee-Farrar arthroplasties did very well and currently some still exist in patients who are functioning perfectly well 40 to 50 years after implantation. At this time, I personally follow several such implants where surgery was performed between 40 and 50 years ago.

Webber from Switzerland, an honest reporter, was a strong proponent of metal-on-metal arthroplasty. His results were most encouraging, suggesting that a successful return to the concept was around the corner. He, as well as others, claimed that the McKee-Farrar implants failed because of poor matching of the two components and a poor design of the contact areas. They may be right. *Unfortunately, as it is frequently the case, the manufacturing industry has marketed the implant by all possible means before adequate follow-up had been obtained.*

Reasonable arguments have been given regarding the advantages and disadvantages that various

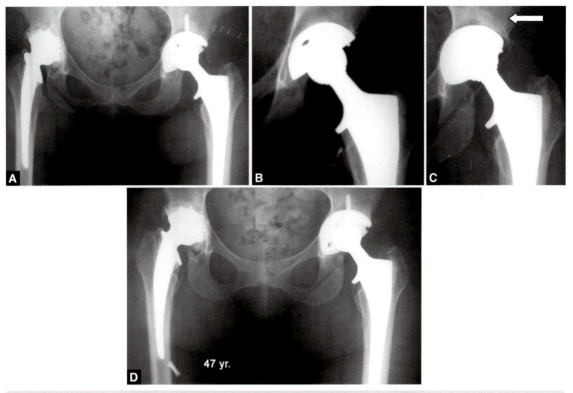

FIGS 52.1A TO D

(A) Radiograph of a McKee-Farrar metal-on-metal total hip prosthesis on the right and a cemented hybrid total hip on the left. The McKee-Farrar prosthesis was asymptomatic and had been in place for 40 years. The hybrid implant on the left was painful and had been performed five years earlier. (B and C) The painful hybrid hip showing the gradual migration into the pelvic bone. (D) The left hip was revised with a hybrid arthroplasty. No infection was encountered. Radiograph of the bilateral hips obtained 47 years after the performance of surgery on the right, and seven years after surgery on the left

Section 2

material have when used as opposing articulating surfaces. *Stainless steel against stainless steel, for example appears to be the worst combination, while cobalt/chrome against cobalt/chrome performs better.* Ceramics against ceramics offers the lowest friction and therefore, at least theoretically, should be the best method. The same appears to apply to ceramics articulating with metal.

The problem is that results from laboratory studies are not always reproduced *in vivo*. Vivid in my mind is my own experience with titanium alloys. When we tested the performance of a titanium alloy head against polyethylene, we found out that its wear behavior was as good if not better than other materials. It was not until many years of implantation in the body of hundreds of such implants that we discovered that the softer nature of the alloy could become scratched by a foreign body resulting in severe wear. John Charnley's experience with Teflon can be considered to be a confirmation of my argument.

At this time, it is believed that the manner in which the two opposing surfaces of the metal-on-metal prostheses is important. Among the three types

available, polar, mid-polar and equatorial, the mid-polar seems to be the best. Not enough time has elapsed as yet in order to be able to categorically state that a certain combination of metals or type of contact among them is ideal.

There are, however, other serious considerations that should not be ignored. Though there is laboratory data to indicate that friction between metal surfaces is less than that present between metal against polyethylene, *wear still takes place.* I am not certain that we have enough data to know how the opposing metal will respond in the long run to the three types of wear with which we are familiar: abrasive, adhesive and third-body. Metallic debris is inevitable. Will this debris be harmful? Can it be a source of malignant changes? Several reports in recent literature have documented several instances of significant metal debris in metal-on-metal total hips of contemporary designs. It should be noted that patients who had McKee-Farrar prostheses implanted many years ago have shown elevated amounts of metal in their urine and serum in highly significant degrees. There is abundant evidence that metal debris can travel to major organs, such as the heart and brain. Shall we cavalierly dismiss the possible long-term effect of such a development?

Of greater concern, in my opinion, should be the reported finding of chromosomal abnormalities around areas of metallosis in patients with hip implants. Professor Patrick Case from Bristol, England, has illustrated his findings in a very serious manner. The degree of chromosomal abnormalities in these instances is higher than that found in the normal population. Professor Case and his associates recently published a most comprehensive summary of the issue at hand, and clearly reviewed the pertinent literature, The evidence they presented should make any thinking surgeons about the serious potential complications that may follow from the increase of metal ions in various vital organs. Others like Jonathan Black, in Philadelphia, Joshua Jacobs, in Chicago, and the group at McGill University in Montreal have shed further light into the issue. This latter finding makes one have second thoughts as to whether metallic implants likely to generate debris should be used in women during their reproductive years or in young people with an anticipated long residual life span.

Prompted by the reading of an article on the subjects, published in the British Edition of the Journal of Bone and Joint Surgery, I wrote following Letter to the editor:

"I had looked with anticipation the reading of the article, *Transplacental transfer of cobalt and chromium in patients with metal-on-metal hip arthroplasty*, published in the March issue of the Journal. However, I am concerned over my inability to understand why the authors, after acknowledging a significantly increased level of metal in their studied patients, as well as in research done by others, insist on recommending the continued use of metal-on-metal hip implants, as if in their absence from the market the successful surgical replacement of the hip joint will come to an end.

The use of polyethylene and ceramics, and more recently cross-linked polyethylene has proven to render long-term satisfactory results, without the real and potential dangers associated with high quantity of metal debris. If the possibility of carcinogenic effects or chromosomal abnormalities does not represent a serious concern, what do we need to see before the trend is brought to an end? Dismissing the increased presence of metal in the blood in patients with metal-on-metal implants, simply on the basis that the increase is not statistically significant, does not stand to reason.

Nonstatistically significant differences oftentimes eloquently describe trends.

The fact that metal-on-metal prostheses are more expensive and new and hopefully better polyethylene sockets have been introduced in the market, casts doubts on the future of the more expensive metallic implants. It is deeply disturbing that some surgeons, financially interested in the success of the system, have chosen to use the media to market their product and to claim the method to be the ultimate solution to the problems surrounding total hip replacement. They make these claims despite the fact that their own clinical data is based on a few years of follow-up. They are acting as unprofessionally as those who claim, also in the absence of any clinical data, that new polyethylenes justify the performance of total hip surgery on patients of any age. The manufactures of the implants are equally as guilty of unprofessional conduct by advertising implants as "guaranteed for life".

The more I read about the heavily marketed metal-on-metal total hips, me more convinced I have become that we are playing with fire. In light of the good and more promising results from ceramics and cross-liked polyethylenes, it is almost impossible to find a single redeeming feature to justify the continued use of metal-against metal. I predict metal-on-metal will soon disappear from the scene, despite the major financial investment made by the implant manufacturing industry, and that some of the surgeons emotionally and economically involved in the issue will have to accept defeat. There is nothing wrong with that scenario. I have personally suffered a number of comparable defeats, which in the final analysis only benefited me, as well as the patients who otherwise would have been harmed by my continued use of imperfect metals or techniques.

I read the abstracts of the papers presented at the 2010 meeting of the British Hic Society, and was appalled to see the huge number of presentations dealing with surface metal-on-metal arthroplasties. I could not understand the interest on the subject. The only possible explanation I can extrapolate is the almost unprecedented deep marketing commitment the surgical implant industry has made to ensure the success of these new implants. If my suspicion is correct, it must be concluded that such an avenue is unprofessional if not outright unethical.

Recent reports in the literature suggest that ceramic components, because of their low friction will replace other combinations of metals and polyethylenes. Some of the reporters are individuals of known professional integrity; therefore their findings must be taken seriously. However, in even more recent literature, occasional reports have appeared indication that lyric lesions have been identified with ceramic components, as well as fractures of the rim of the acetabular component, associated with wear. Impingent or "less than ideal" positioning of the cup are identified as the culprits.

However, a major concern with ceramic components is the alleged frequency of "squeaking" of the joint during frequently required motions of the hip. Otherwise, wear has been reported to be minimal. The onset of the "squeaking" has been reported to be of 14 months. Cross-linked polyethylenes have been used for the past years with great enthusiasm. Their performance under laboratory conditions is superior to the traditional high density polyethylene. Questions still remain as to their long-term performance. The possibility of late fracture of the material is becoming a reality.

Claims that the clinical and radiological results from any of the three systems have unequivocally proven to be superior are inappropriate.

I am still puzzled by the remarkable performance of the original polyethylene we used in the 1970s while performing the traditional, unmodified Charnley arthroplasties. As I illustrated in the Chapter Long-term Follow-up of Charnley Arthroplasties, I have reported on 134 successful unrevised Charnley arthroplasties with follow-ups ranging between 15 and 36 years. In many instances there was no evidence of wear or lysis (See Chapter 9).

I have surmised, without being able to scientifically prove my conclusion, that the monoblock structure of the implant and the quality of the cement, the metal and the polyethylene used in those days are the ingredient that made such results possible. Among them, I suspect, the most important feature is the absence of modularity.

During the past few years an effort has been made to convince the orthopedic community that bigger prosthetic heads are superior to smaller ones. Evidence has been presented to indicate that the rate of dislocation is lower. This is a logical observation, but ignores the fact that there is a downside to increased diameter of the head, particularly the higher production of debris. To ignore this point is a dangerous attitude, for it is very likely that sooner or later it will be proven that long-term adverse effects will manifest themselves. Recently, a European report stated a higher incidence of complication with their use.

Increased confidence in the durability of implants resulting from better wear properties of the articulating materials has brought about a resurgence of interest in the use of bigger prosthetic heads. The claim is based on the argument that larger prosthetic heads allow for greater motion of the hip joint while reducing the incidence of dislocations. Though from the pure mechanical point of view, it is true that larger heads allow for greater range of motion, the question must be raised as to whether or not the range of motion that currently smaller heads provide is really responsible for the occasional dislocations; or if patients are complaining of limitation of motion that is clearly attributable to the size of the head.

I believe that dislocations are rarely the result of prosthetic heads that are too small. Charnley demonstrated quite well that his 22 mm prosthetic heads allowed for normal range of motion. Others, including myself can testify to the accuracy of his observation. We have seen dislocations from with all different prosthetic head sizes. The Austin Moore prosthesis, with heads as large as 65 or 70 mm occasionally dislocates. To blame the occasional dislocations on poor femoral neck design is rather simplistic, since millions of such prostheses have been implanted for the past 55 years with reported very low incidence of dislocation. Many surgeons believe that the posterior approach to the hip is the main culprit, and that the use of other surgical approaches, not the size of the head, is the answer to the occasional problem.

Despite nearly half century of hip surgical experience with thousands of arthroplasties, I do not recall a single instance when a patient complained of limitation of motion that I could trace to the size of the prosthetic head. Those who had less than adequate range of motion of the operated hip experience the limitation due to fixed soft-tissue contractures that had not been corrected, or were impossible to correct in surgery, as in the case of some previously fused hips. The limitation of motion can also be the result of attempts to gain significant length that precludes the attainment of satisfactory motion even at the time of surgery. Though the limitation of motion in some instances improves with time, there are occasions when the limitation of motion is permanent.

The above-mentioned instances have occurred while using small prosthetic heads. To believe that larger heads would prevent the problem of limitation of

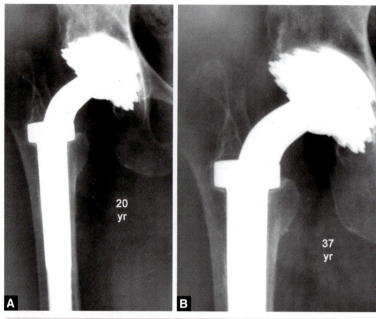

FIGS 52.2A AND B

Radiographs of a Zivash total hip prosthesis developed by the Russian surgeon in the 1970s taken 20 and 35 years postoperatively. The implant is a unit that precludes separation of the femoral from the acetabular component—a self-constraint implant. It is made of titanium. Notice the lack of evidence of loosening or wear. I had an opportunity to see several patients who had the prosthesis implanted. Most of them had been failures

motion is rather naïve. Quite the contrary, bigger heads would make the problem even more severe.

From my experience, I have concluded that the vast majority of dislocations following total hip replacement occur because of soft tissue imbalance, regardless of the size of the prosthetic head. A 40 mm prosthetic head would dislocate, probably as easily as a 22 mm head, if upon completion of the surgical procedure there is a significant degree of soft tissue imbalance. Other times the dislocation is the product of improper alignment of the components. In this instance, I must agree, the larger heads have an advantage. However, the avoidance of this surgical error is preventable. To allow this single factor to accept the disadvantages of bigger heads is difficult to justify.

From basic mechanics we have long-known that the bigger the head in any ball and socket arrangement, the greater the volumetric wear. This was the basis of Charnley selection of a small 22 mm head. He was willing to accept a greater degree of penetration in order to reduce the volume of polyethylene debris. Despite the improvements made in recent years regarding the wear properties of prosthetic components, wear has not been eliminated. The enthusiasm for larger heads is inevitably increasing volumetric wear. Whether this feature is important is still being discussed. I have chosen to remain reluctant to look at the "problem" with too much complacency, and suggest that the smaller heads be used until long-term sufficient evidence becomes available.

53

Ring Total Hip Prostheses

Metal-on-metal total hip prostheses, which at this time are generating interest in the orthopedic community were used extensively in the 1960s and 70s. Metal against polyethylene articulations did not appear on the screen until several years later. McKee and Farrar, from England designed a total hip implant where both surfaces were made of metal.

The popularity of their prosthesis was diminished when John Charnley reported on his experiences with his lowfriction arthroplasty using a 22 mm femoral head articulating with a polyethylene acetabular cup, both fixed with acrylic cement. Marshall Urist, in the United States had previously experimented clinically with metal-on-metal hip joint using a Cobalt-chrome Smith-Peterson cup, without additional mechanical fixation, and a Thompson endoprosthesis in the femur. His results were never reported in peer-reviewed journals and its use was promptly discontinued.

Among others trying various systems of arthroplasty was Peter Ring, from England, who designed a metal acetabulum that would be fixed in place with a long screw that penetrated deep into the acetabulum and an Austin Moore femoral component. I had an opportunity to spend a couple of days observing and listening to Mr Ring in his institution. I was highly impressed with his inquisitive mind, his logic and his technical skills. For me it was not difficult to respond favorably to his system since I had been Austin Moore's student and had performed Moore's prosthetic replacement at least 1,000 times. Previous to my visit to Ring's hospital I had already performed his procedure approximately 75 times with less than ideal results.

Although my visit to Mr Ring had been a worthy experience, upon my return to the United States I never again performed his procedure and became a strong advocate of Charnley's arthroplasty.

My experience with the Ring prosthesis taught me a great deal about the behavior of hip arthroplasties. I had already lived through the enthusiasm and later disappointment with the Austin Moore prosthesis. His belief that bone would grow into the fenestrations of the implant was deeply ingrained in his mind. He had repeatedly said that when the graft in the fenestration matures, the implant becomes "part of the living body". *It did not take me very long to conclude that even if the bone graft grows and matures to the point of becoming a bridge with thick cortical walls, there is, almost in all instances, a residual motion of the stem around the graft.* The motion is not readily detected by push and pull of the implant or by moving it in an anteroposterior direction. *The mode of failure of endoprosthesis as well as total hip prostheses usually is in a rotary mode.*

But the question for which I still do not have an answer has to do with the importance of motion of the prosthesis in the medullary canal. Instinctively we sense that rigidity of fixation is essential for success. However, in many instances we see radiographs that without doubt depict motion but the patient is asymptomatic. Other times pain is present when everything suggests firm fixation.

With the Ring prosthesis we see a rather consistent radiological phenomenon (Figs 53.1A and B): sclerosis at the tip end of the acetabular screw often associated with radiolucent lines parallel to it. These lines we interpret as signs of loosening, and this can be conformed at the time of surgery. I revised many of my Ring prostheses and do not recall a single instance when removal of the implant was difficult. *No matter how firm the fixation of the implant was upon completion*

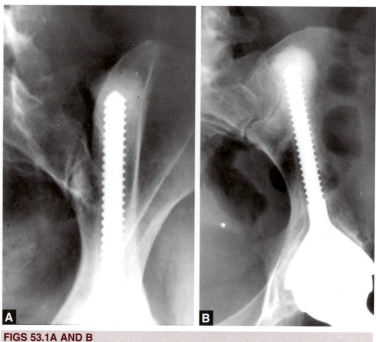

FIGS 53.1A AND B

(A) Radiograph showing the typical sclerosis that forms at the distal end of the screw, suggesting increased concentration of forces, and (B) The radiolucent lines around the shaft of the screw and the cup itself, indicating motion between the bone and the metal

of the original procedure the fixation does not last. The loss is most likely due to the fact that the modulus of elasticity of the screw compared to that of the pelvic bone is enormous. With every step taken the bone is subjected to bending forces that the softer bone can not prevent.

This motion of the stem in the pelvic bone is found every time we introduce any stiff material in the body. The intramedullary nail in the femur is a good example. It is said that Kuntscher, following the development of the IM nail, was called several times by some agitated surgeons, who in the process of nailing a femur had discovered that the nail could not be driven further into the canal or extracted in order to use a smaller diameter nail. He responded by saying that the appropriate thing to do was to wrap the exposed nail in sterile dressings and to send the patient to his hospital. Upon the patient's arrival to his hospital, Kuntscher did not rush the patient to surgery, rather kept him in bed an additional period of time. Then, with one single blow of the hammer the nail came out. Cold flow as well as resorption of the bone had loosened the nail.

When I first learned Kuntscher story I had the opportunity to confirm the thesis by removing, during an autopsy performed 24 hours after surgery; it was an Austin Moore prosthesis that I had driven in the canal with great difficulty because the fit was very tight. When I tried to remove the implant 24 hours later, the procedure was carried out without difficulty. I am certain the same could be said about noncemented contemporary prostheses that we implant with so much force that producing fractures of the femur is not an uncommon development.

When I reviewed the films of the Ring prostheses I had performed and became aware of the presence of the sclerotic and radiolucent lines, I asked myself if those features were the result of poor surgical technique in many instances or an avoidable phenomenon. I think the answer is the latter because even in those instances when the clinical results appeared satisfactory the lines were there.

From the relatively small number of Ring prostheses that I inserted there is only one patient I have been able to follow for a long period of time. She is a lady whose left hip I replaced with a Ring prosthesis 37 years ago. Her right hip I replaced 25 years ago with a cemented titanium alloy prosthesis. The ring prosthesis—side is totally asymptomatic, however the titanium—side is painful and the radiographs show loosening of the acetabular component (Figs 53.2A and B). The majority of the remaining patients had their implants revised, in some instances by me, in others by others surgeons.

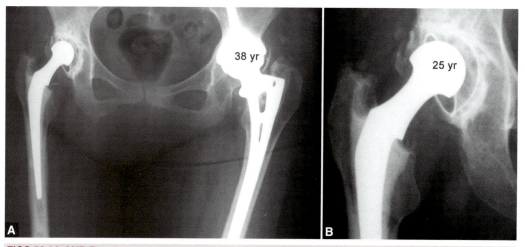

FIGS 53.2A AND B

(A) Radiograph obtained 12 and 38 years after their respective surgeries. (B) Radiograph showing the loosening and wear of the cemented titanium prosthesis 25 years postoperatively and the still intact and painless *Ring prosthesis inserted 38 years ago*

I saw in many instances darkening of the tissues, clearly depicting metal debris. At that time the orthopedic community had taken very cavalierly the presence of metal in the surrounding soft tissues. I was no exception.

In retrospect, one might speculate that the loosening of these prostheses was not necessarily due to differences in modulus of elasticity, but also the tissues reaction to the metal debris.

Recently I learned that a shoulder arthroplasty has been introduced on the market, which is designed in a manner similar to that of the Ring prosthesis. *A suspect that the procedure will provide very good initial results, but ultimately it will loose as a result of the profound difference in the modulus of elasticity between the two components.*

One cannot complete a discussion on the Ring prosthesis without making reference to Mittlemier's experiences with his own prosthesis. *As it was 30 years ago, and still is today, orthopedic surgeons place undue emphasis on mechanics to explain success as well as failure of implants.* Mittlemier, from Germany, described an acetabular component that should virtually guarantee its permanent stability. His acetabulum was designed to function as a screw with deep grooves and was inserted into the bony cavity in that manner. Once the cup "hit bottom" and pressed firmly against the floor of the socket its stability was unquestionable.

Mittlemier was a bright and innovative orthopedist endowed with tremendous physical strength. I saw him perform his operation with great skill. Upon finishing the "screwing" of the cup into the acetabulum, he literally was able to lift the patient's buttocks off the operating table.

Despite the initial fixation of the implant, loosening of the acetabulum was noticed in a number of instances. I suspect the mechanism of failure was similar to that observed with the Ring prosthesis. The difference in the modulus of elasticity between the material that makes the implant and that of the cancellous acetabulum is great, perpetuating stresses that lead to bone resorption at the interface.

Section 2

54

Modular Components

The concept of modularity was a novel and logical concept. Charnley, McKee-Farrar and the other pioneers in hip replacements used monopolar prostheses, which obviously have serious limitations, among them the inability to overcome major shortening of the operated extremity. The available Charnley implants came only in two shapes, straight and curved stems. One could, if the discrepancy was too great, build a longer neck with acrylic cement. Oftentimes, patients ended up with residual significant shortening of the leg, which only a lift in the shoe could overcome. John Charnley made it very obvious that a residual shortening was not a problem. Needless to say, his complacent attitude did not fit very well with the more demanding American audience.

As it is true for most technical innovations, the concept of modular heads—longer or shorter necks, as well as bigger and smaller heads—the new concept ran into obstacles. Concern was expressed over the possibility of corrosion at the level of the Morse taper articulation, due to imperfect fit of the articulating surfaces (Figs 54.1A and B).

The same applies to the modular noncemented, more specifically porous acetabular shells, in relation to the polyethylene liner. *A liner not firmly held in place would be subjected to forces that bring about motion between the two components and the eventual creation of plastic debris that ultimately produces lysis in the acetabulum and or femoral canal. The screws that are used to further stabilize the porous cup, and which are not deeply buried into the metal cup, scratch the convexity of the liner, leading to the production of plastic debris. Motion—even micro-motion—between the screws and the holes in the metallic cup can produce metallic debris.*

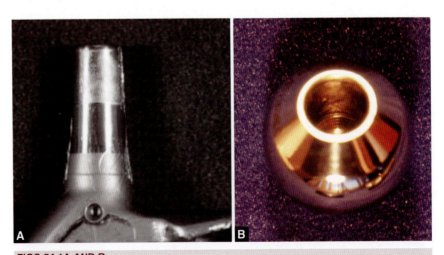

FIGS 54.1A AND B
(A) Photograph of corrosion on the Morse taper surface of a prosthesis. (B) Corrosion visible in the inner surface of a prosthetic head

Improvements of modular components have been made, resulting in a very low incidence of lysis secondary to modularity. Today virtually all total hips are modular.

Upon learning that on the femoral side of the prosthesis *bone ingrowth takes place most consistently at the distal end of a porous patch* that, in some instances, is no longer than a couple of inches, I realized that in many instances there was no contact between that porous area and the cortical bone, since the rasping of the canal frequently leaves behind a cavity much larger than the width of the prosthesis. This is particularly true in the case of revision arthroplasty. The development of a "weld spot" suggesting bony ingrowth at that level is probably due to the fact that when a prosthesis is driven into the canal, the most distal end of the porous patch is the only part likely to be in contact with the femoral cortex. The proximal portion of the patch does not always touch the cortex and remains either in contact only with cancellous bone or simply without contacting with any bony structures.

We then thought that a modular prosthesis could be made to ensure the maximum contact of the porous surface with the surrounding femoral cortex. We approached the engineers at Zimmer, who found the idea appealing and offered to finance the project. *The innovation consisted of the making of removable wedges of various sizes that had their outer surface covered with porous material, while the inner smooth surface would fit into a slot in the body of the stem and locked permanently in place.* The fit of the wedge and its stability had to be as perfect as possible to ensure that corrosion was prevented. The wedges were to come in different sizes to accommodate the size of the canal proximally. Trial

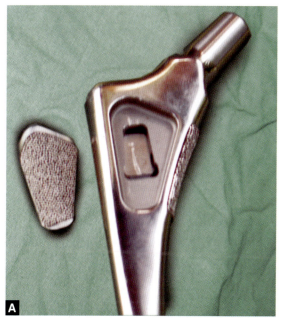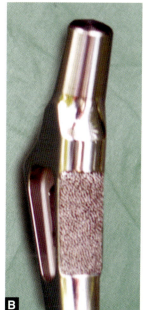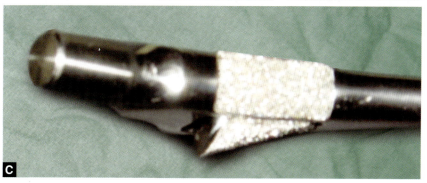

FIGS 54.2A TO C
Photographs of a modular prosthesis that used wedges of different sizes with a porous surface that attempted to obtain maximum contact between the femoral cortex and the porous implant

wedges were to be available in order to determine the size of the permanent wedges.

The engineers at our Research Laboratory worked diligently with the engineers at Zimmer and made considerable progress in a relatively short period of time. The stability that could be gained from the wedges was documented as well as the stability of the wedges. Zimmer was ready to proceed with manufacturing of the commercial device (Figs 54.2A to C).

At that time I attended the meeting of SICOT in Munich, Germany, where to my great disappointment I saw an exhibit from Italy that demonstrated an implant based on the same ideas we were developing. In retrospect we had reinvented the wheel! Though disappointed we continued our work. Suddenly, the vice-president for research at Zimmer notified us that the project had been discontinued because of concerns regarding the stability of the wedges. Not only that, he felt that modularity was not an area they were interested in pursuing. His reasoning was sound and I soon became convinced that his caution was justified. All I can do at this time is to ponder on "what if" we had implanted the new prosthesis in the human. At times I think that the concern of the Zimmer engineers was out of proportion, and the concern over modularity was exaggerated. Modularity has become a well-accepted concept in total joint surgery, and more recently has gained acceptance in trauma implants.

It is interesting to note that the engineer from Zimmer, who had been put in charge of the study and to sustain the cooperative effort with our engineers at the USC/Orthopedic Hospital of Los Angeles, suddenly left the organization and went to work at another competitive orthopedic manufacturing firm. He took with him all the data from the study, and convinced his new superiors to pick-up the project. They indeed accepted the idea and eventually came out with an implant. I found out about the completion of the study when I attended a continuing education meeting in Palm Beach, Florida. A former resident of ours, and subsequently a member of our full-time faculty, described from the podium the new implant and illustrated with slides the greatness of the prosthesis. However, nothing did he say about clinical experiences. He made the whole idea sound as being his own. I wonder what happened to the new prosthesis. I assume it never got off the ground.

The photos of the prosthesis shown above are of the implant produced by the second company, not Zimmer, simply because ours never reached the photographing stage (Figs 54.2A to C).

Now that modularity has been introduced in trauma products such as interlocking nails, early reports of lytic changes in the surrounding tissues are appearing in the literature. Nails broken at the site of modularity have shown corrosion. I am certain that if blood and urine tests were conducted in these patients, as it has been done in patients with failed total hip prostheses, the presence of metal would be identified. This may not be of great concern at this time but it could eventually become a problem particularly in light of the fact that most victims of trauma are young people in their reproductive years (See *Lysis*).

Due to major advances in the surgical management of malignant bone tumors in growing children, emphasis has been placed in the development of modular prostheses that allow incremental gain of length to the operated extremity by percutaneously, or otherwise, manipulating the modular components. The concept is fascinating; however, serious consideration must be given to the still unknown ill-effects that the modular components might have. Corrosion and the release of meal debris into the surrounding tissues may become a problem.

References*

66, 72

55

Wear of Total Hip Components

At the time of this writing, wear in total hip arthroplasty is the topic getting the greatest attention, simply because we finally realized that it constitutes the seminal and most important issue that will determine if the procedure will ever becomes one whose success can be guaranteed to last the remaining of the patient life regardless of his or her age.

As soon as Charnley was able to demonstrate that his operation was accompanied with a high rate of success imitations of his prosthesis and surgical technique exploded throughout the land. Neither the orthopedic community nor the manufacturing industry was willing to wait a reasonable period of time to see if his results could be reproduced. The imitations and changes made dealt, to a great extent, with matters that eventually proved to be of relatively minimal importance.

The changes dealt with the length of the implants, the size of the prosthetic head, the shape of the neck of the prosthesis, the cement technique, the speed of cement polymerization, the reinforcement of acetabular fixation, etc. The realization that bone lysis had become a real and frequent problem attention was focused on the acrylic cement. The "cement disease" was identified and a war against it was declared.

It would be wrong to dismiss the many changes that were made in an attempt to improve the clinical results from the operation, however, the orthopedic community ended up squandering a great deal of time and effort by ignoring the prophetic warnings that Charnley himself had made, when

he repeatedly stated that wear was the problem that needed the greatest attention. He had gone through the deeply disturbing fiasco with the use of Teflon as the material to fabricate an acetabulum. As it is well known, he performed several hundred arthroplasties using Teflon in the acetabular side. He had concluded that Teflon was a good material, since among other things it had wear properties that appeared to be good. *All the arthroplasties he performed failed within a relatively short period of time necessitating their removal.* Massive lysis developed in the femur as well as in the acetabulum. Large granulomas formed to a degree that they could be seen protruding under the skin of the abdomen and thigh (Figs 55.1 to 55.3).

I had an opportunity to see the alleged last patient to have the Teflon socket removed by Sir John Charnley. The patient came to Wrightington while I was there. The lysis to the pelvis and femur was massive and granulomata had formed in large masses that could be easily seen and palpated under the skin of the thigh and abdomen.

Charnley was not only a great and brilliant thinker but also a man of impeccable professional integrity. Undeterred by the disastrous experience with Teflon, he began to experiment with other materials until he found out high-density polyethylene, the material that half a century later has proven to have excellent wear properties and still is the preferred one.

Charnley, despite his success with high-density polyethylene, warned us that it would not last the life

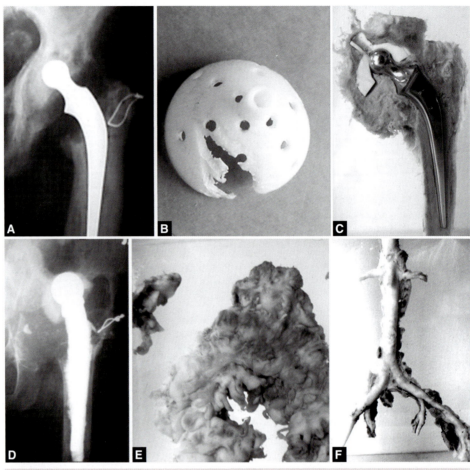

FIGS 55.1A TO F

(A) Radiograph of the original Charnley arthroplasty using a Teflon acetabulum. Notice the penetration of the metal head into the plastic acetabulum and the lysis in the proximal femur. (B) A Teflon socket showing wear and mechanical failure. (C) Coronal section of a proximal femur and pelvis showing the boring of the metallic head into the Teflon acetabulum. (D) Radiograph of hip with Teflon acetabulum demonstrating massive wear and lysis. (E) Granuloma produced by plastic debris. (F) Teflon granuloma seen in the lymphatic chain in the abdomen

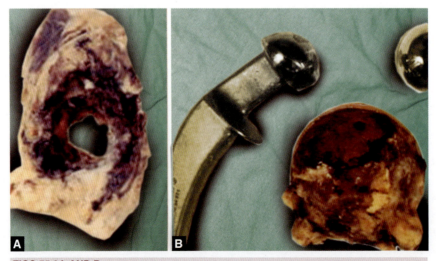

FIGS 55.2A AND B

(A) The floor of the acetabulum recovered from a failed titanium alloy prosthesis that had been reinforced with a metal-backed acetabulum. (B) Notice the worn-out prosthetic head and the darkly stained surrounding tissues

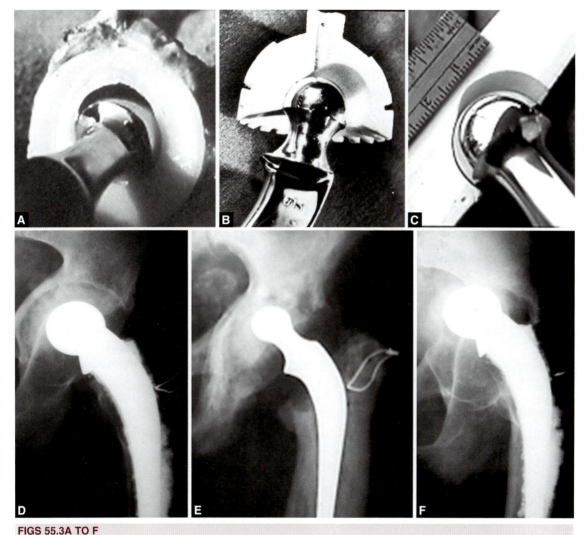

FIGS 55.3A TO F

(A to C) Wooden replica of the plastic acetabulum that underwent major wear. (D to F) Radiographs illustrating the progression of wear of a Teflon acetabulum. Notice the massive wear and lysis

span of a young, active individual. He actually said that in such a patient the implant would not last 30 years. He urged further investigations.

Despite his prophetic remarks, he was wrong to some extent. Many patients who had the procedure performed 30 to 40 years ago *are still functioning well and their radiographs have not shown evidence of wear.* Nonetheless, the fact remains that wear is seen in many patients requiring revision surgery (See *Long-term Follow-up of Charnley Prostheses*).

It is of great interest to observe the long-term results of those components implanted 30 to 40 years ago that have shown no signs of complications and then compare them with other series of patients who had the same procedure using modified Charnley implants. To the best of my knowledge, no other cemented implant has demonstrated comparable clinical results. The Charnley

prosthesis remains the "gold standard" against which all other hip arthroplasty must be measured.

One cannot help to wonder why is that the best results with the Charnley prosthesis were obtained with the original "model", indicating that many of the alleged improvements made over the years did not improved the operation, but made it less successful. It is possible that the different metals and alloys used by the modifiers of the implants did not represent progress. The same can be said about the various acrylic cements, the sterilization methods, the use of modular implants, and others.

I am not qualified to scientifically discuss the issue at hand. All I can do is to record my personal observations and those I have vicariously acquired.

Though we no longer witness massive lysis with the frequency and intensity Charnley observed with his original Teflon prosthesis, the problem has not disappeared. It is seen with totally cemented implants as well as with hybrid operations and with non-cemented prosthesis. Its incidence is decreasing.

To the best of my knowledge, I assisted in the development of the first titanium alloy total hip prosthesis in the United States. I was then unaware that Pierre Boutin, from Pau, France, had been working also in the making of a titanium alloy implant. *He, however, was using a ceramic head. This explains why his results were better than mine.* Despite the fact that for several years our results with the titanium prosthesis were quite good, longer follow-up showed an increasing number of failures, many of them due to lysis. *Apparently the titanium, being a softer metal, is subjected to scratching, which in turn generates metal particles that eventually damage the plastic acetabulum. The resulting plastic debris seeps into the medullary canal and then produces bone lysis* (See *Titanium Prostheses*).

Even though the use of titanium heads cannot any longer be justified, the fact remains that hundreds of Monoblock titanium prosthesis have done well for periods of time between 15 and 30 years (See *Titanium Prostheses*).

The etiology of wear is not as simply as I have described it. Quite the contrary is very complex. Metal or plastic debris can be produced by modular components, such as a "Morse taper" due to corrosion arising from unexpected motion between the two surfaces (Figs 55.4A and B).

The relationship between wear and lysis is not as yet totally clear. No one questions the fact that debris is found in areas of lysis, *but significant wear is not always associated with lysis.* Attempts have been made to explain this phenomenon on chemical basis with convincing evidence. Quite often we see patients with bilateral replacements demonstrating similar degrees of polyethylene wear but marked difference in the degree of lysis (Figs 55.5A and B).

It is commonly agreed that the degree of wear of polyethylene is related to the age, weight and activity of the patient. The argument in relation to activity is not difficult to accept; however, the data concerning the patients' weight and age is not necessarily valid. Our own studies suggest that the elderly does not necessary experiences less wear (Fig. 55.6).

Wear of polyethylene is found also with noncemented arthroplasties (Figs 55.7 and 55.8). The etiology under this circumstance is probably the same as suspected with cemented arthroplasties, except for the presence of cement that falls in the articulation that initiates a third body wear process.

A few years after the introduction of cemented total hip arthroplasty it was noted that the incidence of lysis was greater with the new implants. Over the years the picture has improved, so much that at this time several series

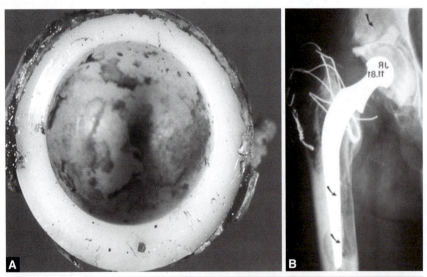

FIGS 55.4A AND B

(A) A worn-out polyethylene socket showing the changes on its concavity, and remnant of acrylic cement particles, which once caught between the metallic had and the polyethylene surface might initiate a third-body wear process. (B) Radiograph of a Bechtol total hip arthroplasty showing severe lysis of the femur and loosening of the acetabular component. It is possible that small pieces of broken wires might have traveled to the joint and initiated the third-body wear process

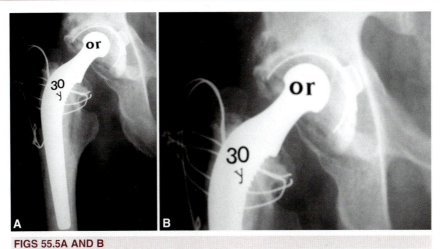

FIGS 55.5A AND B

Two views of a 30 years follow-up of a Charnley arthroplasty in a very active man who plays tennis twice a week. The wear shown in the X-ray has not as yet reached a critical level

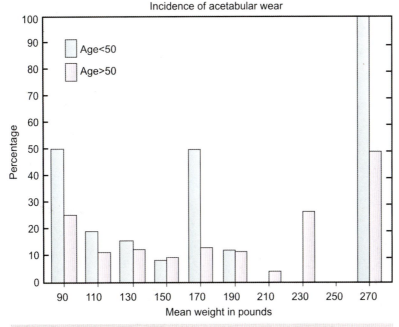

FIG. 55.6

Barograph documenting the degree of wear of polyethylene according to age

have indicated a very low incidence of lysis and wear. It is possible that technical improvement in the manufacturing of the implants has brought about the improved results.

The elimination of motion of the prosthetic components in relation to the underlying bone, brought about by bone ingrowth into the porous surfaces, must be partially responsible for the beneficial effects. Also better locking mechanisms between the modular components have been beneficial. The tendency to eliminate modularity as much as possible has been a healthy development (Fig. 55.9).

In the recent past major efforts have been made by a number of investigators regarding the development of improved polyethylene materials. It appears thus far that cross-linked polyethylenes are superior to the traditional one. I am personally familiar with the work done by Harry McKellop, PhD, from Los Angeles, who for a number of years has studied the subject and has developed a now widely used material. I suspect not enough time has elapsed to allow the making of a final conclusion regarding their long-term performance. As we learned from other experiences, the behavior of materials under laboratory conditions is not always

Section 2

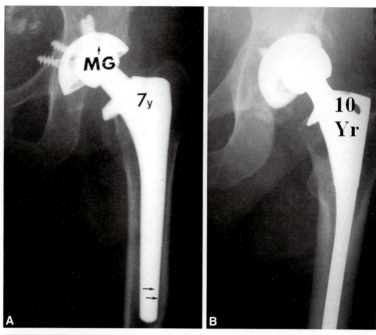

FIGS 55.7A AND B

(A) Noncemented prosthesis showing measurable wear of the polyethylene cup 7 years postoperatively. Notice the accompanying lytic change distally. (B) Non-cemented total hip prosthesis showing significant amount of wear of the polyethylene cup and lysis of the proximal femur

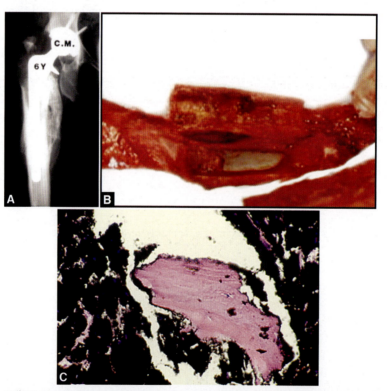

FIGS 55.8A TO C

(A) Radiograph of a noncemented total hip prosthesis in a 34-year-old woman. The procedure was performed as revision surgery for a failed Thompson endoprosthesis performed 5 years earlier. Notice the lysis of the proximal femur. (B) Photograph of the dark-stained tissues surrounding the femoral stem. (C) *Histological slide of the severe metallosis found in the lytic greater trochanter*

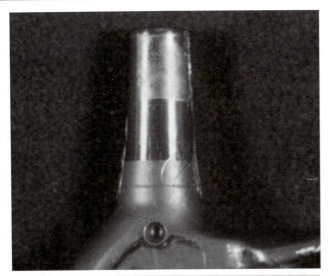

FIG. 55.9

Illustration of corrosion at the junction of the prosthetic head and neck. It is possible that motion between the two components initiated the corrosion process

reproduced *in vivo*. The long-term mechanical properties of cross-linked polyethylenes *in vivo* are not yet known.

The same concerns must be considered regarding other articulating materials currently being used in total hip arthroplasty. *Ceramics seem to offer significant potential benefits due to its excellent wear properties.* However, earlier experiences were associated with occasional breakage of the more brittle material. Improvements have allegedly resulted in an insignificant incidence of breakage. Longer follow-up is necessary before firm conclusions can be drawn.

Recent reports in the literature have indicated that ceramic debris can bring about cytokines responses leading to bone loss, and therefore the loosening of the ceramic implant. Though the clinical experience has not as yet supported the laboratory findings, it would be mistake to ignore the warnings. As I indicated earlier, the same applies to the metal-on-metal prostheses, regarding the presence of chromosomal abnormality in soft tissues affected with metallosis.

Since ceramics are expensive, cost-benefit considerations must be carefully evaluated. Solid and objective data must be analyzed before concluding that its use is justified. If cheaper cross-linked polyethylenes work very well over a long period of time, *it will be difficult to justify the use of more expensive materials, particularly in light of the fact that the vast majority of total hip arthroplasties are and will be performed in older people whose remaining life span is limited to a few years.*

In an effort to improve the wear properties of the articulating surfaces of total hip arthroplasties the concept of using implants where metal-on-metal

surfaces are used has been resurrected. *This system was widely used between 40 and 50 years ago.* The McKee-Farrar arthroplasty gained a great deal of popularity but was eventually eliminated from the armamentarium of the orthopedic surgeon because of the complication rate was higher than those being obtained with the cemented Charnley arthroplasty. The Ring prosthesis, also used in the United Kingdom suffered the same fate (See *64- Metal-on-metal Total Hip Prostheses and 65- Ring Prostheses*).

Metal-on-metal joints have the theoretical advantage of a very low friction between the articulating surfaces, and the argument has been given that the less than satisfactory results with the McKee-Farrar prosthesis was due to manufacturing imperfections that modern technology have overcome. It is possible that the technical and metallurgical improvement justify further experimentation. *However, the fact remains that there is a more important issue to be considered, the long-term effects of metal debris.* Highly sophisticated work conducted by Patrick Case, a distinguished pathologist from Bristol University in England, has demonstrated chromosomal abnormalities in tissues showing metallosis (See *Metal-on-Metal Total Hip Prostheses*).

I am aware of the fact that very good results have been reported with the use of metal-on-metal hip arthroplasty by people of proven honesty and integrity, such as the late Hans Weber, from Switzerland. At this time I perceive pressure on the orthopedic community to embark on the use of metal-on-metal implants from the manufacturing industry and from individuals with major vested commercial interests.

It is most unfortunate that at this time it is extremely difficult to appropriately assess the value, or lack of value, of many "innovations" due to the fact that the whole issue of arthroplasty has become a business matter. *The competition between the many manufacturing companies and the rather superficial nature of many of their investigations preclude the reaching conclusions based on high caliber research.*

Efforts to improve the wear properties of the polyethylene socked were undertaken by many and it appears at this time that progress is being made. However, the various products developed thus far have not been sufficiently tested clinically.

My own experiences with polyethylene sockets in the early 1970's were probably the most rewarding. In my own practice I have been able to confirm that the cemented arthroplasties I performed in those days were the best. I have 109 patients with 15 to 33 years follow-up whose hips look very good and without evidence of wear or with minimal one (See *Long-term Follow-up of Chanrnley Arthroplasties*). The same is not true for subsequent surgeries. *It is possible that the manufacturing and sterilization methods or the intrinsic composition of more recently manufactured cups adversely altered the mechanical and wear properties of the material.* It is puzzling to see active patients who after a period of time show significant wear but no evidence of lysis. Contrari-wise other patients demonstrate no measurable wear but show significant amount of lysis. This phenomenon supports arguments that suggest a chemical/cellular reaction (Figs 55.10 and 55.11).

We had an opportunity to study the behavior of monoblock titanium alloy hip arthroplasties where only the acetabular components had failed and was therefore revised. New acetabula were used and followed for a maximum of 15 years. *At the time of surgery we had noticed the typical "dulling" of cemented titanium prosthetic heads. Surprisingly the speed of wear of the new sockets was slower than that observed following the "virgin" surgery.* Intrigued by this phenomenon, Harry McKellop, PhD, director of our research program, placed old, clinically failed titanium femoral components against new polyethylene cups and

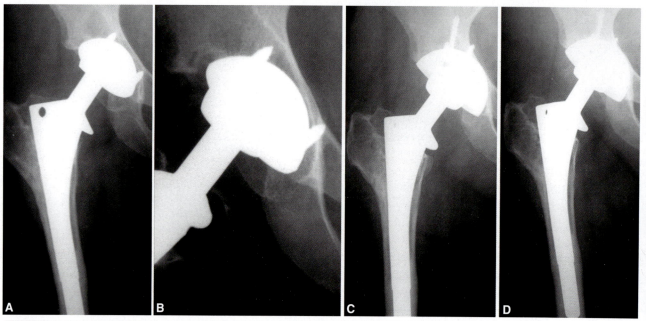

FIGS 55.10A TO D

(A and B) Radiograph of noncemented total hip allegedly performed for the treatment of residuals following slipped capital epiphysis suffered at the age of 13. The arthroplasty was 5 years old when these films were taken. Notice the wear of the polyethylene but no evidence of femoral or acetabular lysis. (C and D) Radiographs taken postrevision and 7 years later

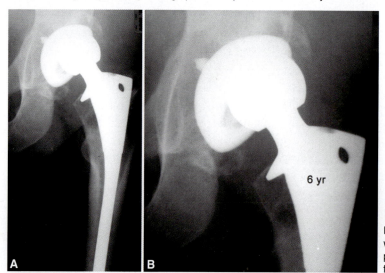

FIGS 55.11A AND B

Radiographs of noncemented total hip in a 67-year-old woman taken ten years after surgery. Notice the significant polyethylene wear, and the lysis in the acetabulum and femoral shaft

subjected them to a wear-testing environment. The wear that the study identified was virtually equal to that seeing with "virgin" prostheses and plastic acetabula. Food for thought (Fig. 55.12) (See *Titanium Implants*).

Charnley described quite clearly the manner in which wear of polyethylene takes place and emphasized the "boring" of the head into the plastic material. The relationship between wear and lysis is not as yet clear. No one questions the fact that debris is found in areas of lysis, but significant wear is not always associated with lysis. Attempts have been made to explain this phenomenon on chemical basis with convincing evidence. I suspect the final verdict has not as yet been rendered. Quite often we see patients with bilateral replacements demonstrating similar degrees of polyethylene wear but marked difference in the degree of lysis (Figs 55.13A and B).

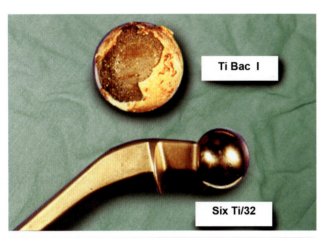

FIG. 55.12

Photograph of an acetabular and femoral component demonstrating the fragmentation of the acrylic cement and its separation from the metallic acetabular surface. It is very likely that particles of cement and metal attached to it are a source of wear when those particles traveled into the joint generating a third-body wear process

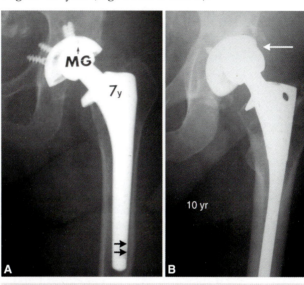

FIGS 55.13A AND B

(A) Noncemented prosthesis showing measurable wear of the polyethylene cup seven years postoperatively. Notice the accompanying lytic change distally. (B) Noncemented total hip prosthesis showing significant amount of wear of the polyethylene cup and lysis of the proximal femur ten years after surgery

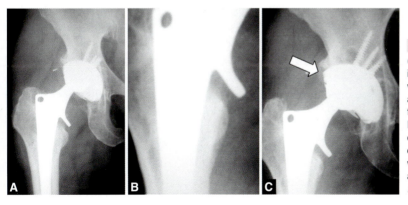

FIGS 55.14A TO C

(A) Radiograph of cemented arthroplasty performed in a woman with osteoarthritis 15 years earlier. She was 36-year-old at the time of surgery. Notice the acetabular wear. (B) Closer view of the resorption of the calcar, probably due to polyethylene lysis. (C) Following an episode of sudden pain the diagnosis of a fractured acetabular component was made. The component was found to be fractured and was revised with a new one. The surgery was performed by another surgeon in another city. *Notice the free metal fragment coming from a stabilizing acetabular prong*

*References**

21, 30, 36, 39, 44, 56, 58, 72, 91, 104

_____

* References provided at the end of the book after annexures.

56

Special and/or Difficult Replacements

I have chosen to write a separate chapter dealing with a group of situations I have designated as *Special and/or Difficult Replacements* simply because, to some extent, they fall within a unique category. These are the instances when standard, well defined criteria do not fit and improvization becomes necessary. These situations range from revision of failed acetabula, failed femoral components or both, as well as massive bone lysis, nonunion of the acetabulum or femur, pre-existing deformity, and others.

The clinical outcomes for these special cases were not always satisfactory. Quite the contrary the failures were many. This experience has helped me to further recognize that good results from total hip replacement cannot be guaranteed; and that its best results are found when it is performed in "virgin" joints where the anatomy of the region is relatively well preserved. *The fact that short-term follow-ups are usually encouraging even in extremely complicated conditions, the fact remains that in situations where that normal anatomy has been lost long-term success is very often elusive.* The revision rate of revised total hip arthroplasties remains very high.

Some 25 years ago, I heard Maurice Muller say that there are situations where it is not possible to find a good solution. He was referring to some major complications from total hip surgery. At the time I questioned his judgment, as I believed that every complication could be overcome. *That's what the arrogance of youth does for us.* It was not until several years later that I realized that attempts to solve every

problem through more and more surgery can be, not only and exercise in futility, but a way to make matters worse. *Too many times I have witnessed surgeons perform all kind of heroic procedures that do nothing but complicate matters even further.*

Other times we operate to treat situations we call problems, when in reality they are not problems. I previously have made reference to a 90-year-old lady I was asked to see in consultation. She was a very elderly person who had several surgical procedures for the care of complications from total hip surgery. She was scheduled for surgery the following week consisting of bone grafting of a nonunion of a femoral fracture. The disturbing feature is that the nonunion was painless and she was, for all practical purposes, a nonambulatory person. The "problem" was an inconsequential radiological finding. The family had been told that "it was good" for the old grandmother if she was 'stood-up every day for a few minutes'. *I never understood how standing up for a few minutes every day, with the help of others, can do any good to anybody. Good for what?*

I concluded that the best thing for the lady was to leave her alone; to accept the "radiological problem" and to allow her to spend undisturbed whatever time she had left in this world. I wrote a pithy note to the surgeon who was about to perform surgery within the next few days that read, "No mas". I was quoting the Panamanian boxer, who in the middle of a fight that he was losing against Leonard suddenly left the ring. "No mas", No more.

The Greek tragedians of antiquity had superb examples of virtually every human condition. They are a pleasure to read and to get an education. While discussing man's ambitions and hubris in his classic tragedy Baccha, written by Euripides, who said, "Far in the air of heaven, the sons of heaven live but they watch the lives of man and what passes for wisdom is not; unwise are those who aspire to outrange the limits of man". Herodotus, the father of history put it in even simpler words, *"God loves to cut short everything that overtops its kind"*.

The first patient I include in this group is not one where I was successful in providing help, just advice, which I suspect was never followed. It represents a situation, where the pathology around the total hip implant was so severe that attempts to overcome the failed surgery were more likely to make matters worse rather than better. This patient got into severe trouble because neither he nor his surgeon realized the importance of regular postoperative follow-up visits. Once he had the surgery he never went back to see his surgeon again. I have long insisted to all my patients to obtain a new X-ray of the operated hip either once a year or every other year regardless of the absence of symptoms, simply, *because very often symptoms around a failed total hip implant do not appear until significant damage to the surrounding bone and soft tissues has occurred.*

The following X-rays belong to a surgeon from Latin America who early in life sustained a fracture of the distal femur that became infected. He suffered from chronic osteomyelitis that required multiple surgical procedures over his entire adolescence. Apparently, drainage finally stopped but by that time his leg was significantly shorter. Later, in his mid-fifties he had the hip replaced in his native country. According to him he did very well and was able to continue the practice of his profession without pain. He never returned to his surgeon who according to the patient, never tried to contact him either. Then pain ensued and the extremity because slightly shorter. By the time he came to see me, was not only the hip dislocated but purulent drainage had developed over the posterolateral aspect of the hip. His knee was particularly painful. He had been using two crutches and had been unable to bear weight on his now severely shortened leg. From looking at the X-ray one can readily surmised that the knee was painful and unstable. Neurologically he was intact (Figs 56.1A to C).

He was most anxious have surgery not only to get rid of the incapacitating pain, but also the gain length and stability. I pondered abut what to do for some time. I first considered a debridement of the entire leg, removal of the implant and excision of the entire femur, and if at all possible lose closure of the skin over large drains, plus massive intravenous antibiotics.

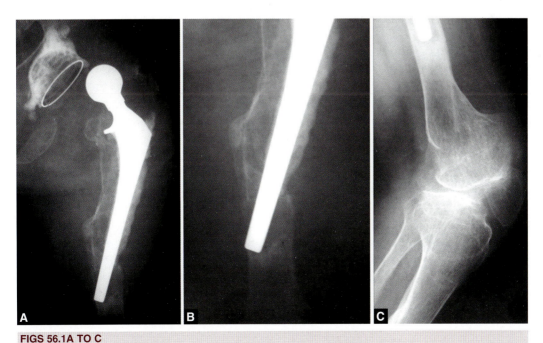

FIGS 56.1A TO C

(A) Massive demineralization and lysis of the femur, along with a dislocated prosthesis, probably secondary to the deep infection. (B) Notice the severe lytic destruction of the femur and the loose implant. (C) The short distal femoral bone shows the postinfectious deformity and the arthritic changes in the knee joint

Section 2

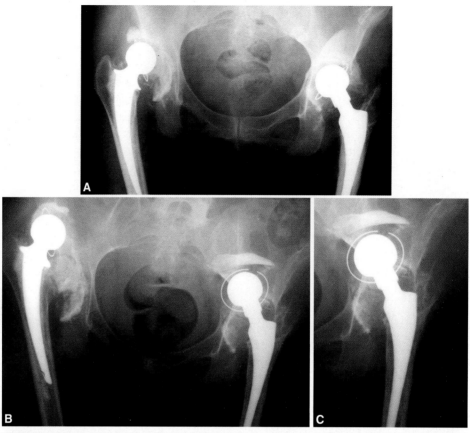

FIGS 56.2A TO C

(A) Earliest radiograph showing the dislocated right acetabular component, and a very shallow acetabulum. (B) Radiograph obtained a few months later demonstrates bilateral superior collapse of the acetabular roof and superior dislocation of the femoral components. (C) A closer view of the left hip demonstrates the dislocated acetabular component and the absence of adequate bony structures. The patient was elderly, obese and diabetic. I advised the patient to accept the current situation; advice she accepted

I had no great illusions about surgery being successful and began to reconsider my tentative plans. If successful, I anticipated the success to be short lived because the condition of the acetabulum, the absence of femur, and the eventual need for replacement of the femur, hip and knee. Gaining length to a significant degree was out of the question.

I came to the conclusion that a disarticulation was the most logical and perhaps the best solution. Readily the patient refused my suggestion. Still sympathetic with the patient's unrealistic hopes and aware of the enormous cost of carrying out the entire surgical management of his problem in the United States, I suggested he should have the debridement in his home country. He agreed to that and had the entire femur removed. The drainage allegedly stopped and he returned to ambulation without pain and without drainage. He still wanted his femur, acetabulum and knee joint reconstructed and his leg made longer.

I refused to be the surgeon. Deep in my heart I knew that anything I did for this 79-year-old man would not give him any help. Quite the contrary, all I could do was to make matters worse.

When I last heard from the patient/doctor, he was still looking for someone to operate on his leg. I once again tried to convince him to accept the disarticulation. I don't think he paid attention to my advice.

The following example (Figs 56.2A to C) of a difficult hip problem is depicted by the X-rays of a 67-year-old obese woman, also a citizen and resident of a rather poor Latin American country. She had been diagnosed as having diabetes and her economic situation was rather precarious. She lives at home and is attended by a young relative of hers. She had bilateral total hip replacement six years earlier, apparently for the treatment of osteoarthritis, secondary to congenital hip disease. Allegedly the surgery never eliminated the pain, though her

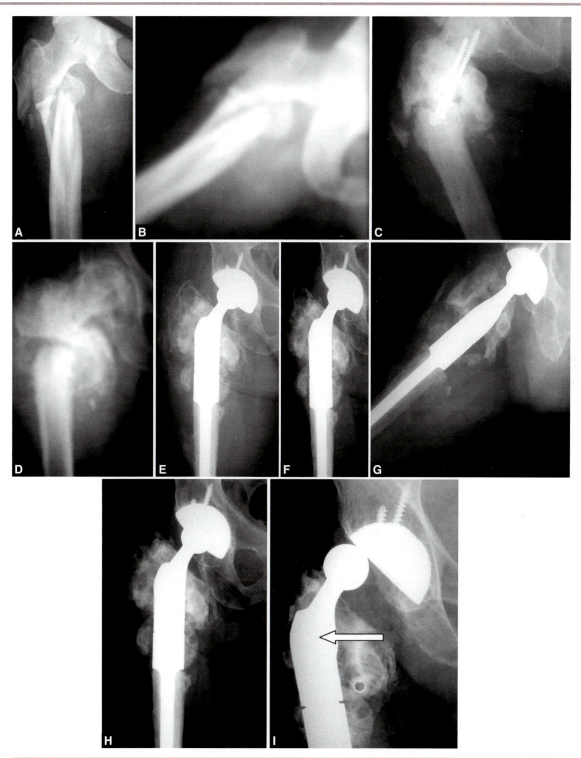

FIGS 56.3A TO J

(A and B) Original radiographs of comminuted intertrochanteric fracture allegedly treated with a nail/plate combination. The fracture failed to unite and a bone grafting procedure was performed, but also eventually failed. (C and D) The internal device was removed and the patient was left with a painful nonunion. (E to G) I removed the femoral head and carried out a total hip replacement arthroplasty. The femoral head was used as a spacer, hoping that union between the proximal femur and distal femur would occur. (H) The femoral head never incorporated into the two fragments, but the patient remains functional and without pain. He walks with an almost unnoticeable limp and minimal shortening of the extremity. (I) Four years after surgery, and while still asymptomatic the hip dislocated. Notice the severe sinking of the prosthesis in the medullary canal. Surgery in the form of an oncology prosthesis is being planned. Revision surgery consisting of reattachment was carried out by Sean Scully, MD in 2007

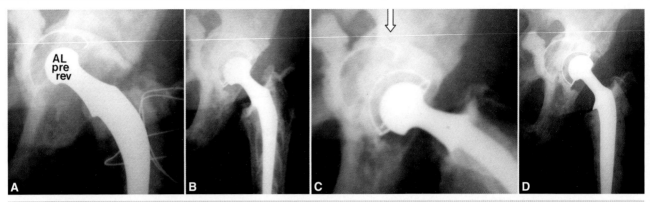

FIGS 56.4A TO D

Radiograph of hip joint of an elderly man who had suffered from Paget's disease for a number of years. He had a hip replacement allegedly a few years before these films were taken. (A) The femoral component failed but the acetabular cup was rigidly fixed against the pelvic bone, despite its migration into the pelvis. (B) *I replaced the femoral component but left the plastic cup in place.* I drilled several holes into the polyethylene over which I pressed acrylic cement. Then I place a polyethylene liner. The length of the leg was restored and the stability of the new hip was satisfactory. (C) Closer view of the hip. (D) Six years later the hip was still painless and functional. The patient expired shortly afterward. *Had I chosen to replace the acetabular component, it is likely that a very large bone graft would have been necessary; a procedure with poor prognosis in light of the nature of the underlying bone*

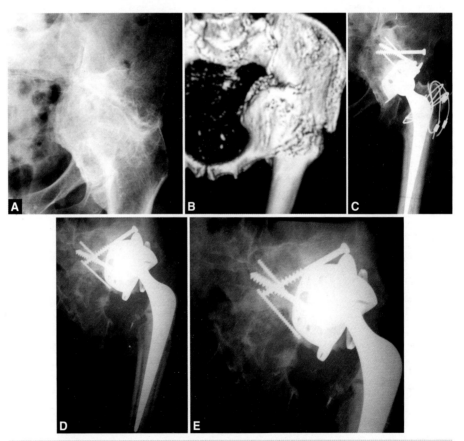

FIGS 56.5A TO E

(A) 35-year-old central dislocation of the hip incurred in an airplane accident. (B) The CT scan shows the relationship of the femoral head in reference to the inner pelvis. (C) *The femoral head was not removed, simply use as a graft to make possible its lateralization. Six years later the hip was functional. And it appears that incorporated with the surrounding bone.* (D and E) Following a dislocation and an episode of septicemia resulting from a gastrointestinal problem a self-constrained acetabulum was performed. Three years later the radiographs began to show loosening of the acetabular component. Then she fell and sustained a fracture of the pubic ramous. The femoral head/graft came completely loose. She is now under the care of another orthopedist

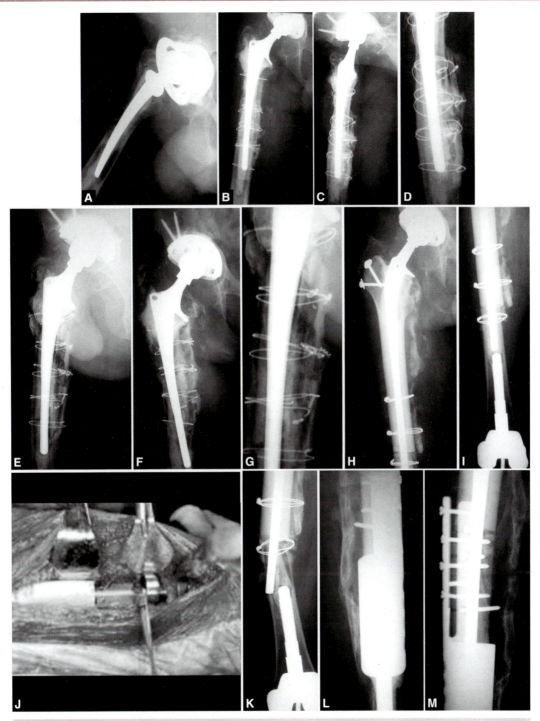

FIGS 56.6A TO M

(A) Radiograph of cemented prosthesis allegedly performed five years earlier in a 33-year-old *rheumatoid man*. The film shows severe femoral lysis. Apparently a metal backed acetabular shell was used. (B and C) I removed the implants and grafted the lytic femoral cortex. (D) The graft appeared to be incorporating. (E) Radiograph showing resorption of the graft three years postoperatively. (F and G) The resorption continued. (H and I) *A large allograph was then used to replace the proximal femur, which was reinforced with a slab of bone graft.* (J and K) Union between the main allograph and the distal femur did not take place and a varus deformity developed. (L) Since the patient already had a total knee implant, a specially made implant was used to connect the distal femoral stem to the knee prosthesis. (M) Radiological appearance of the femur illustrating what appeared to be a stable relationship between the various components. The latest available radiograph.

Note: The last two procedures were performed by my associates James V. Luck, MD and Adolfo Llinas, MD in Los Angeles, CA. I do not have further follow-up beyond the last films shown above)

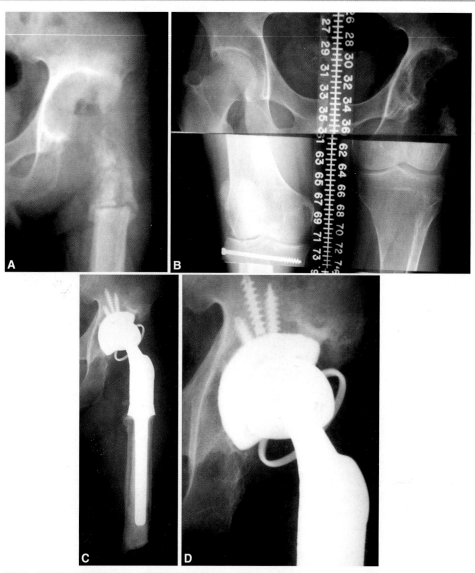

FIGS 56.7A TO D

(A) Radiograph of a 33-year-old man whose total hip replacement allegedly became infected and was treated with removal of the components. (B) Scan studies demonstrate the significant shortening of the leg. (C) With the infection, apparently eliminated, according to sedimentation rate and C-reactive Proteins studies, a cemented, specially designed implant was inserted in the femur. A self-constrained acetabulum was used. Considerable length was gained without producing nerve injury. (D) Radiograph obtained 16 months after surgery. No evidence of complications

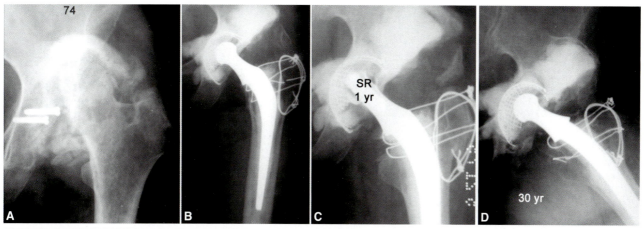

FIGS 56.8A TO D

(A) 10-year-old fracture-dislocation of the hip associated with arthritic changes. (B) Immediate postoperative radiograph showing the large defect on the roof of the acetabulum filled with acrylic cement. (C) Radiograph taken one year after surgery. (D) Radiograph obtained 12 years later, and (E and F) *Radiographs taken 30 years postoperatively*

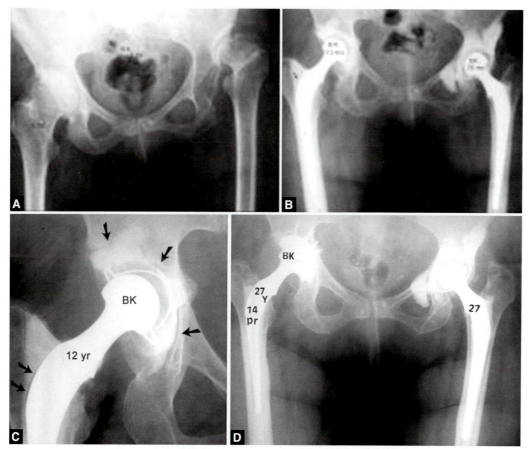

FIGS 56.9A TO D

(A) Radiograph of arthritic hips secondary to hip dysplasia. The right hip is not dislocated, the left hip is. (B) Radiograph taken after bilateral cemented arthroplasties. (C) Radiograph showing early signs of loosening of the right acetabular component. (D) *Radiograph obtained 27 years after the initial surgery and 14 years after revision of the right acetabulum. Radiograph taken 1 year later. Notice the absence of gross wear of the polyethylene acetabula or lysis*

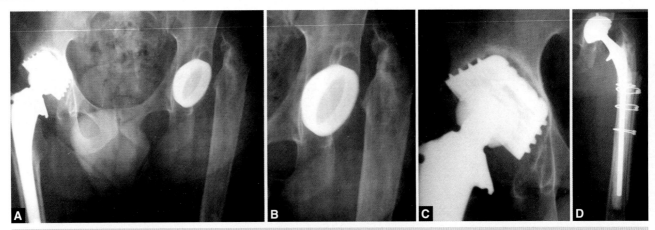

FIGS 56.10A TO D

(A and B) Bilateral total hip arthroplasties in a 50-year-old man. The femoral components had been allegedly removed because of pain and infection three years earlier. (C) After confirming absence of infection in the left hip, a hybrid total hip arthroplasty was performed. The weakened femoral cortex was reinforced with a long bone graft. Long-term follow-up was not available. (D) The right arthroplasty demonstrate loosening of the acetabular component in the typical manner threaded components frequently fail

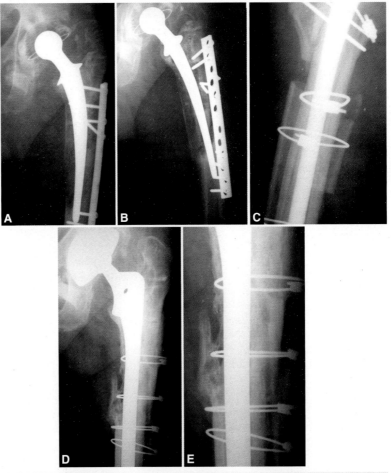

FIGS 56.11A TO E

(A and B) Radiographs of failed cemented total hip arthroplasty demonstrating severe lysis and an insufficiently stabilized femoral fracture. The plate has pulled away from the lytic femur. (C to E) Radiographs obtained after revision arthroplasty. In addition a long and strong bone allograph that was held in place with circular wires. The graft incorporated into the body of the femur in a gradual manner. The last radiograph was obtained two years after surgery

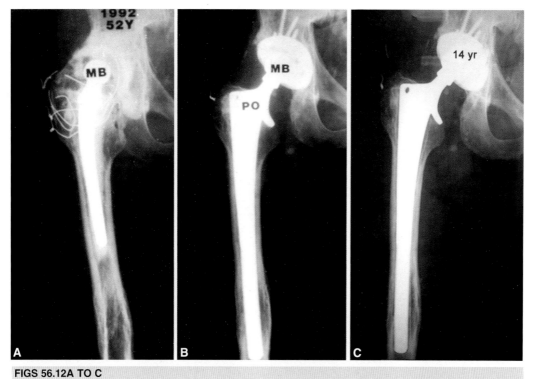

FIGS 56.12A TO C

(A) Failed cemented total hip arthroplasty demonstrating a severe rotational deformity. (B) The failed total hip was revised using a long noncemented stem and acetabulum. (C) Radiograph obtained 14 years later

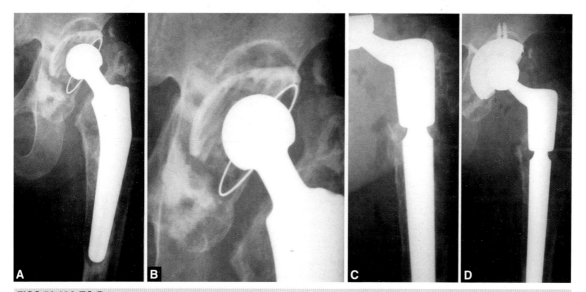

FIGS 56.13A TO D

(A) Radiograph of a hybrid total hip of a 59-year-old man, performed 10 years earlier. The acetabulum had been cemented, while the femur was not. (B) The acetabulum had become loose. (C and D) The revision consisted of insertion of noncemented components: The acetabulum with a conventional porous cup, and the femur with a modular "oncology" implant. No long-term follow-up was available

Section 2

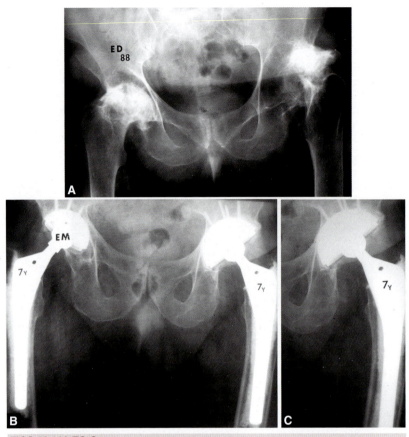

FIGS 56.14A TO C

(A) Radiograph of bilateral hip arthritis in a 62-year-old man suffering from *hypogona-dism secondary to pituitary gland deficiency.* The degree of osteomalacia was severe. (B and C) Radiographs obtained seven years postoperatively showing no evidence of failure. *The hip joints were asymptomatic at the time of his death 9 years after surgery*

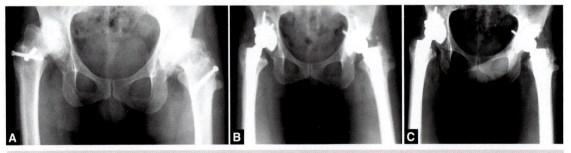

FIGS 56.15A TO C

(A) Radiograph of 30-year-old man with familiar osteochondral dystrophy that affected his hips and shoulders. Patient had poor motion of his hips and shoulder and a fixed flexion contracture of his hips of 35 degrees bilaterally. (B and C) Radiographs obtained immediately postoperatively and four years later. The flexion contracture was reduced to approximately 15 degrees which he compensated well with spine motion

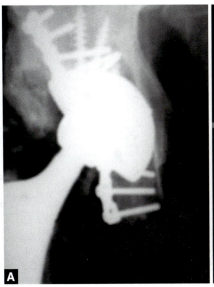

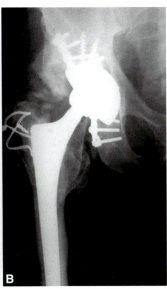

FIGS 56.16A AND B

Prosthetic replacement following internal fixation of an acetabular fracture can be a difficult undertaking when the screws and/or plate preclude reaming of the acetabulum. *In this instance removal of the metallic components was not necessary*

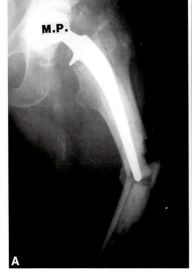

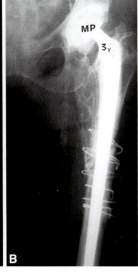

FIGS 56.17A AND B

(A) Transverse fractures at the distal end of the prosthesis are usually the most difficult periprosthetic fractures to treat since stabilization with plates, cables and/or screws is often precarious. *Circumferential wires alone fail to provide rotary stability.* (B) In this instance the femoral component was replaced with a longer one; the fracture site was bridged with long struts of bone

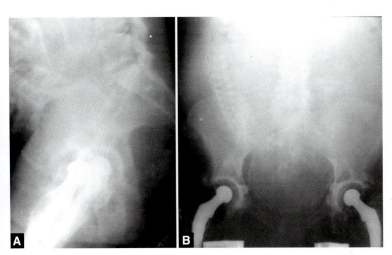

FIGS 56.18A AND B

This particular case does not represent a "difficult" replacement. I have placed it here as an interesting situation. *Notice that the patient is soon to deliver a baby.* Natural delivery took place

Section 2

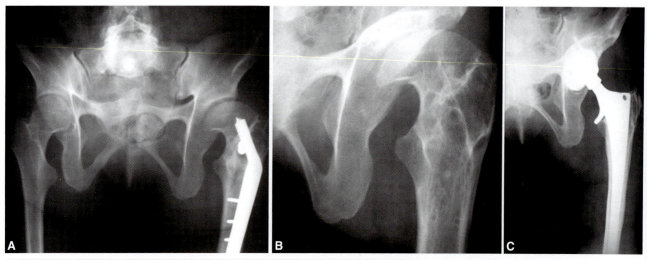

FIGS 56.19A TO C

(A) Severe anteversion of the entire pelvis. Osteotomy of the proximal femur had been performed at the age of 25 years. (B) Closer view of the hip following removal of the nail. (C) Total hip arthroplasty was performed at the age of 38 years. *Orientation of the components was difficult on account of the pelvic deformity*

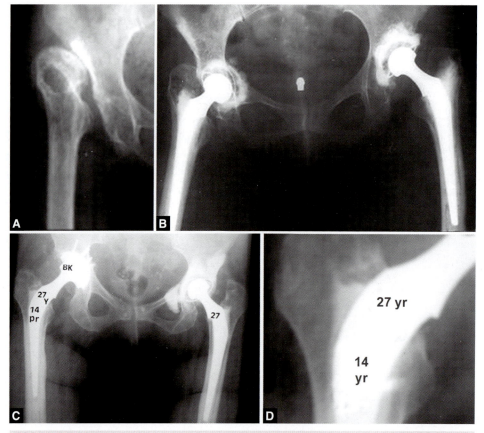

FIGS 56.20A TO C

(A) Congenital dislocation of right hip and secondary osteoarthritis of the left hip. (B) Early postoperative radiograph. (C) Radiograph obtained 27 years later. (D) *The right acetabulum needed replacement 14 years after surgery*

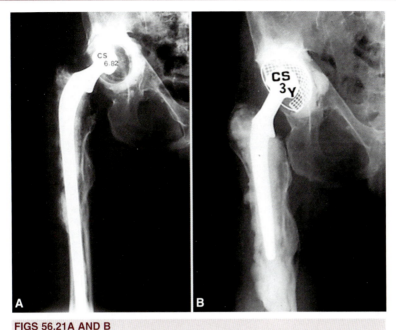

FIGS 56.21A AND B

(A) Failed cemented arthroplasty. (B) The failed revision consisted in the performance of a shorter cemented stem and a cemented acetabulum. Patient was lost to further follow-up

ambulatory abilities were improved. Eventually, the pain recurred and found herself spending virtually all the time sitting in a wheelchair. With difficulty she was able to transfer from bed to chair. She wanted a better lifestyle.

When I was first consulted, the X-rays given to me showed bilateral complications, the right acetabulum being dislodged, but the left one still in place, though associated with signs of loosening. A few months later, when I finally got to examine her I confronted a woman much older than her stated age, relatively comfortable in the chair. It did not take me much time to realize that if surgery was to be performed, it had to be done bilaterally, and not simultaneously. By this time the left acetabular component was also dislocated and the condition of the bony socket was extremely precarious. Obviously the implants had been attached to very shallow bony structures that had further experienced damage over the past years. Surgery would require bone grafts to build deep sockets (Figs 56.1 and 56.2).

I realized the technical aspect of the problems was difficult but not impossible. I had confronted situations by far more difficult than hers. But, what were the changes of success form such surgeries in this obese, diabetic elderly woman? Very slim, I said to myself. I elected then to recommend to her to accept a wheel chair existence as a small price for being alive, being mentally competent and moderately functional. She accepted my advice and returned home. I hope she has adjusted to the limited life style (Fig. 56.21).

Section 2

57

Vascular Injury

During the performance of a total hip arthroplasty I had the terrible experience of piercing one of the obturator vessels with a sharp drill bit. I had anticipated surgery would be uneventful since the patient was a slim, 55-year-old woman who had osteoarthritis with good skeletal structures. I was performing a hybrid replacement and was finishing the acetabular side. Two screws were already in place. As I drilled the last hole a strong stream of blood exploded and hit me in the face. At first, I thought I was dealing with an arterial injury but in retrospect it was a vein. Not knowing what to do under the circumstances, I put my index finger over the screw hole to stop the bleeding. I knew I would be encouraging intrapelvic bleeding, but hoped that tamponade would stop it (Figs 57.1 and 57.2).

We summoned a vascular surgery which the hospital in Los Angeles did not have on-board. The one they eventually found could not be on the scene until 45 minutes later. There was nothing I could do but continue

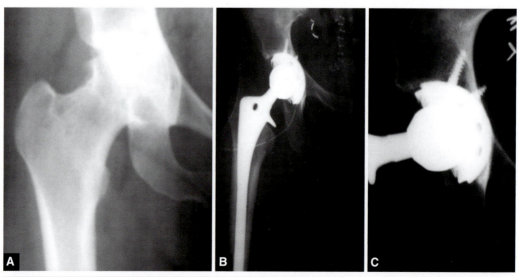

FIGS 57.1A TO C

(A) Radiograph of osteoarthritic hip in a 49-year-old woman with previous history of pelvic inflammatory disease. (B and C) During surgery massive bleeding was encountered when the second hole in the pelvis was made for the insertion of a screw. A laparotomy was performed and a major vein was ligated. Spontaneous homeostasis had already taken place

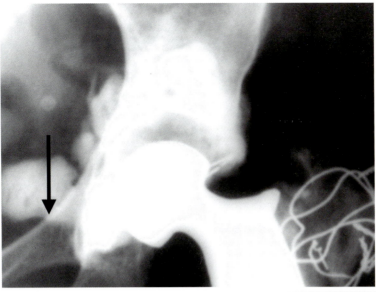

FIG. 57.2

Radiograph of the cemented total hip showing the mass of cement protruding into the pelvis. The removal of this mass at the time of surgery ruptured a small intra-pelvic artery necessitating a laparotomy and ligature of the vessel

to hold my "finger on the dike" and wait, observe the abdomen getting distended and give blood transfusions.

When the vascular surgeon arrived I removed my finger from the screw hole and found that the bleeding had stopped. He opened the abdomen and identified the injured vessel that I had torn by the rotating drill bit. The bleeding had stopped, not from tamponade but from spontaneous homeostasis. *The enlarging abdomen was a product of my imagination: a phantom pregnancy of a sort.*

Trying to determine how the accident occurred we went to the morgue and reproduced the surgical intervention by filling every hole in the acetabular cup but allowing the drill bit and the corresponding screw to penetrate three quarters of an inch beyond the inner wall of the pelvis. The findings were most revealing: protruding drill bits or screws penetrating too deeply can damage important structures such as the sciatic or femoral nerves and major vessels. I suspect that a mild, or not so mild, whipping of the flexible drill might do similar damage.

I also learned from the vascular surgeon that female patients with a history of pelvic inflammatory disease experience scaring and loss of elasticity of tissues on the floor of the pelvis that makes impossible their retraction from an advancing drill or screw.

*Reference**

64

58

Peripheral Nerve Injury

Injury of peripheral nerves during total hip surgery is neither common nor unheard of. I had my share of such complication and have seen it in patients treated by other surgeons. *Its etiology is usually easy to identify since in most instances it is due to direct trauma to the sciatic nerve either from retractors pressing on the nerve or excessive traction applied on its fiber during attempts to gain length to the operated extremity.* In any event it is a very serious complication for the patient but one that tests the character of surgeon to a high degree.

When the sciatic palsy follows a procedure where regaining length was not a serious concern, usually involves both branches of the nerve, and its prognosis is frequently satisfactory. In those instances the etiology is probably compression of the nerve with retractors. *When the surgery required efforts to gain length the palsy is frequently limited to the peroneal branch of the nerve, while the posterior tibial branch remains intact.*

This is the frequent pattern one sees after traumatic dislocation of the hip and can be explained by the fact that the sudden traction on the nerve, not direct compression of the nerve against the pelvis, is tolerated by the posterior tibial nerve because it runs in an uninterrupted distal direction. The peroneal branch, on the other hand, because of its relative fixation at the level of the fibular head experiences traction of a much higher degree. In this instance the sensation over the plantar surface of the foot and the motor function of the planar flexors of the ankle and toes are normal.

If one examines carefully these patients with palsy limited to the peroneal nerve, quite often pain can be elicited from pressure over the peroneal nerve as it crosses the fibular head.

Early in my total hip practice I had a patient who developed bilateral peroneal palsy following an uncomplicated unilateral Charnley arthroplasty. It was created, and promptly recognized, by the straps of the Charnley pillow-splint having been applied too tightly by an aggressive, but not too experienced first year resident, when he was asked to intervene in controlling a very agitated patient complaining of pain in both knees. When I saw the patient the following morning I immediately recognized the problem and identified the marks left by the straps that had unduly compressed the peroneal nerves. We applied bilateral ankle orthosis and recovery of nerve function took place over a three month period.

This patient was the brother of the secretary to the professor of anesthesia at the medical school in Miami. One year later after receiving letters from the "most grateful" patient, he expired from a sudden myocardial infarct. The notification of his death was followed by a letter from his attorney accusing me of malpractice. Nothing came out of it other than my concern about how poorly I would perform before a jury when asked questions regarding heart disease.

Not frequently mentioned in the orthopedic literature is femoral nerve palsy following total hip arthroplasty. However, it does occur. I have three patients on whom I had performed arthroplasties, two through an anterior approach and the third through a posterior approach. The procedures had been uneventful, but paralysis of the quadriceps was recognized when the patients began to ambulate. It took at least seven months before they regained enough control of knee extension to make possible their ambulation without external support. In the two Charnley arthroplasties I identified the etiology of the palsy as thermal injury produced by anterior leaking of the soft polymerizing cement that eventually came in contact with contact with the nerve. I have no idea as to how I injured the femoral nerve when the posterior approach was used.

Waiting for recovery of nerve function is a worrisome time. I usually recommend obtaining a base-line EMG early and having it repeated three months later. Thus far I never experienced the need to re-explore the nerve. While waiting one must avoid the commonly made mistake of not looking for recovery of the first muscles that receive innervation below the level of the injury. This mistake is frequently made in assessing the recovery from a radial nerve palsy. Mistakenly some surgeons first examine the function of the extensors of the fingers, without realizing that those muscles are the last ones to recover.

If the injury to the nerve occurs at mid-arm, long after the elbow extensors are innervated, the first muscle to experience improvement is the brachioradialis, then the extensor of the wrist, and finally the extensors of the fingers and thumb. Likewise when dealing with sciatic or femoral nerve palsy, the first muscles to return are the ones that receive nerve supply just below the lesion.

I am not sure that electrical stimulation helps to expedite recovery of palsies that follow hip surgery, or even surgery of any kind. I suspect that encouraging ambulation and efforts to use recovering muscles is the most effective way to assist "Mother Nature", which in the final analysis will determine whether or not improvement is to be gained spontaneously.

59

Periprosthetic Fractures

Periprosthetic femoral shaft fractures are not uncommon, and it is likely we will see them with greater frequency as we extend the indications for total hip arthroplasty in the younger as well as in the older population. Younger people, engaging in more physically demanding sports following their replacement procedures, might subject their femurs to bending and torsional forces that the bone is not capable of withstanding.

In the case of the elderly the etiology of the periprosthetic fractures is more likely to be the associated pathology that frequently exists in the knee joint. *An arthritic knee, particularly with limited motion, is incapable of responding well to a sudden flexion of this joint. When the forced motion reaches the maximum flexion present in the joint, the stresses are transferred to the proximal femoral shaft to a degree severe enough to fracture the bone.*

The frequency of femoral periprosthetic fractures in patients with an implanted total knee on the ipsilateral side is well-known in orthopedic circles. The reason for its frequency is the same as the one given for the arthritic joint.

Overcoming a femoral periprosthetic fracture may be difficult at times. Whether the fracture is transverse, oblique or spiral in nature, stabilization of the fragments may be problematic. The plate, which is usually the appliance used to hold the fragments together, does not permit in most instances the insertion of screws in the proximal fragment, since the canal is filled with either a cement/prosthetic composite, or with the stem of a noncemented prosthesis.

The preferred treatment today consists of stabilization of the fracture with a plate that is fixed to the distal fragment with screws, but with circular wires to the proximal fragment (Figs 59.1 to 59.8). Such fixation is not mechanically ideal. *Circular wires may provide sufficient bending support, but stabilization against rotary forces is rather poor.* This is why the use of the circular wires around the proximal plate is often reinforced with a long bone graft located over a different surface of the femur and equally held in place with circular wires.

The transverse fracture that occurs just below the tip end of the prosthesis is the most difficult one to manage since rotary forces at the level of the fracture are not lessened in the way oblique and spiral fracture do through friction between the two major fragments.

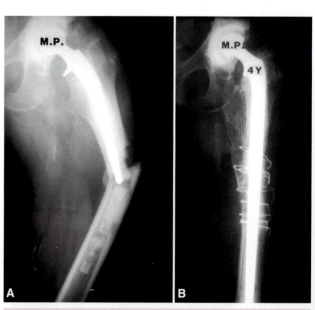

FIGS 59.1A AND B

(A) Transverse fracture at the level of the end of a cemented prosthesis. (B) The facture was stabilized with circular wires and a strut of cortical bone

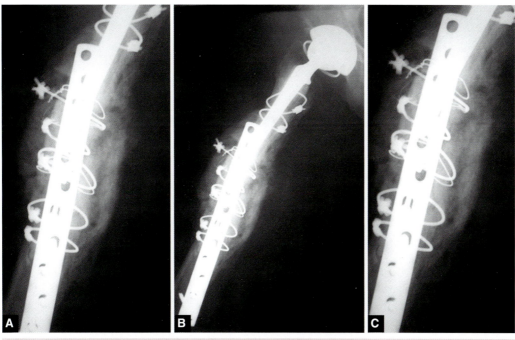

FIGS 59.2A TO C

(A) Allegedly, this patient suffered a fracture of the femoral shaft either intraoperatively or shortly after surgery. The hip also dislocated. The fracture was stabilized with a plate and circular wires. It appears that when the fixation failed a new plate and bone graft were used. A self-constrained acetabulum was inserted. The fractured healed with severe varus. (B and C) The plate was removed and the patient has not as yet decided whether to accept the deformity and associated limp or to undergo further surgery

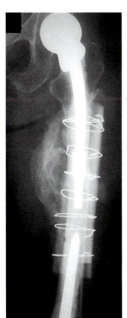

FIG. 59.3

Example of a periprosthetic fracture in a paraplegic patient, treated with two cortical bone struts and circular wires

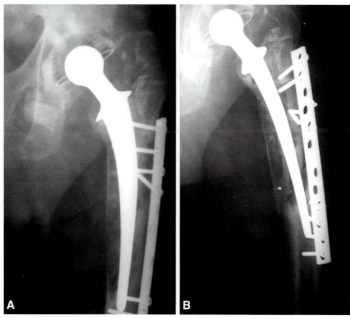

FIGS 59.4A AND B

(A) Periprosthetic fracture treated with a plate, (B) It promptly failed to maintain the reduction

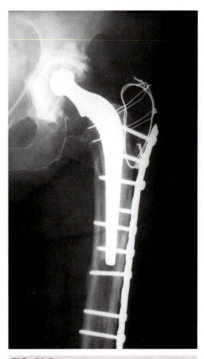

FIG. 59.5

Radiograph of a high oblique periprosthetic
fracture stabilize successfully with a plate
and circular wires

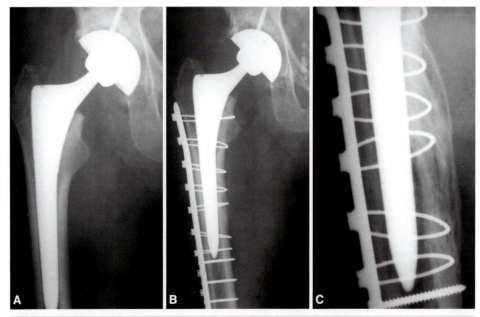

FIGS 59.6A TO C

(A) Radiograph taken shortly after surgery. (B) Shortly afterward he sustained an oblique fracture of the
femoral shaft that was treated with a plate and circular wires. (C) The fracture healed. Peripheral callus
is seen at the end of the fracture suggesting some micromotion at the fracture site at that level. Radiograph
taken 4 years postoperatively shows the large amount of callus

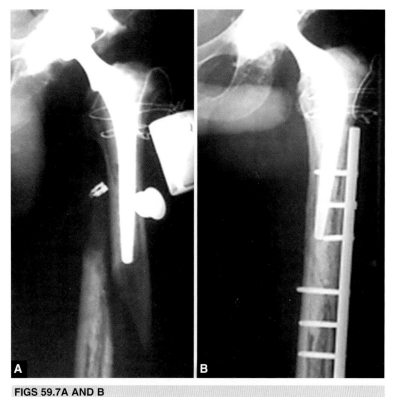

FIGS 59.7A AND B

(A) Long spiral femoral fracture just below the tip end of the prosthesis. (B) This was successfully treated with a plate and circular wires

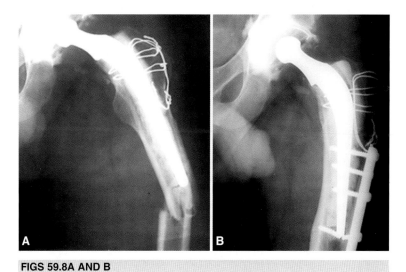

FIGS 59.8A AND B

(A) Transverse fracture at the level of the distal end of the prosthesis. (B) The fracture was treated with a plate. It united, but not before the plate pulled away from the shaft and the prosthesis migrated distally, resulting in a fracture of a screw

When wires are used is best not to utilize filliform ones because they very frequently fragment into smaller pieces, which if close to the joint may travel into the metal/ polyethylene articulation, initiating a dangerous third-body wear process (See *Broken Wires*).

Despite the fact that I have illustrated several instances of successful use of plates and circular wires in a variety of fractures, I still believe that this technique is beset with possible problems due to the poor rotary stability that wires provide. I think that the fixation provided by the plate and wires should be reinforced with an additional cortical bone graft.

There is no doubt that the surgical treatment of periprosthetic fractures is the preferred method till

Section 2

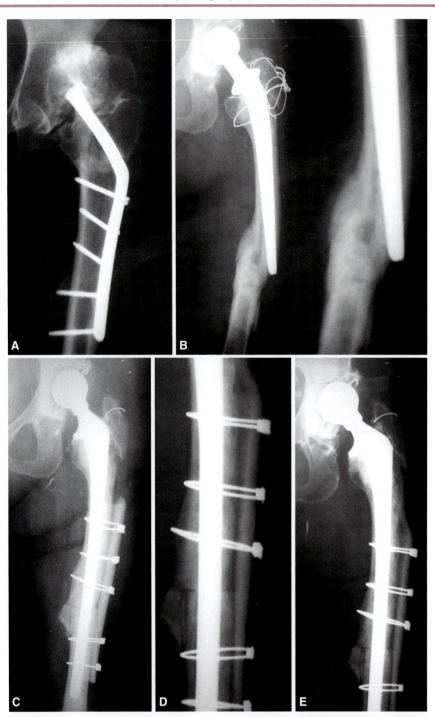

FIGS 59.9A TO E

(A) Radiograph of osteoarthritis that was probably attempted to improve with a subtrochanteric osteotomy. (B) Radiograph obtained allegedly a few days after a prosthetic replacement was performed. From the history I received, it appears that the femur may have broken at the time of surgery. The fracture was treated in traction resulting in a severe varus deformity. (C) The deformity was corrected by osteotomizing the femur. Once the femur was realigned a cemented long-stem prosthesis was inserted. A cortical bone graft was attached to the femur with circular wires. (D) The graft began to incorporate. Notice that the osteotomy is not yet healed. (E) Radiograph showing the complete incorporation of the graft and healing of the osteotomy today. I have treated three (Figs 59.9 and 69.10) periprosthetic fractures by nonsurgical means but for different reasons. Once because I judged that the trauma of surgery would not be tolerated by the elderly and feeble patient suffering from serious heart disease. The fracture healed with an angular deformity that shortened the extremity. This was compensated with a lift in the shoe that she wore until her death a year later. The other two patients refused surgery and healed their fractures uneventfully. Since the fractures had occurred distally in the femur, a brace was applied after three weeks in traction. The resulting deformities were considered inconsequential by me and by the patients.

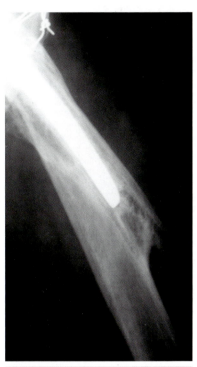

FIG. 59.10

Periprosthetic fracture of the femur treated with traction, resulting in uneventful healing and a mild deformity

*Reference**

115

* Reference provided at the end of the book after annexures.

60

The Broken Stem

Fracture of prosthetic stems rarely occurs at this time. Prostheses are now made of stronger materials therefore reducing the incidence of this complication. The reported frequency of stem fractures (Figs 60.1 and 60.2) in the early 1970s fueled our interest in finding a material capable of better withstanding the enormous stresses to which the implant is subjected during strenuous activities. We, as well as others, had also identified the frequent presence of resorption of the calcar. Both phenomena suggested to me that a stronger metal, but with a lower modulus of elasticity, could effectively address the bony resorption and eliminate the possibility of stem fracture.

These concerns resulted in the eventual use of a Titanium alloy, which was determined to be stronger than stainless steel but with a much lower modulus of elasticity. We inserted the first Titanium prosthesis in the late spring of 1975. The initial experiences were very satisfactory, as we noticed the virtual absence of femoral resorption and fractures. However, after seven years of usage of the Titanium implant we began to notice an increased incidence of femoral lysis. It appears that the alloy was too "soft" and therefore more likely to undergo "scratching" of its surface when exposed to a foreign body that initiates a third body wear process. I eventually discontinued the use of

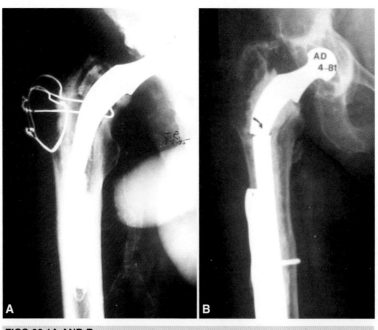

FIGS 60.1A AND B
Radiographs of broken stems

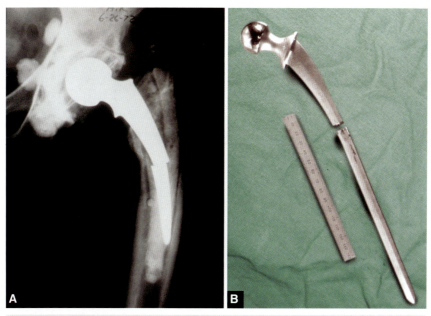

FIGS 60.2A AND B
Representative examples of broken stems

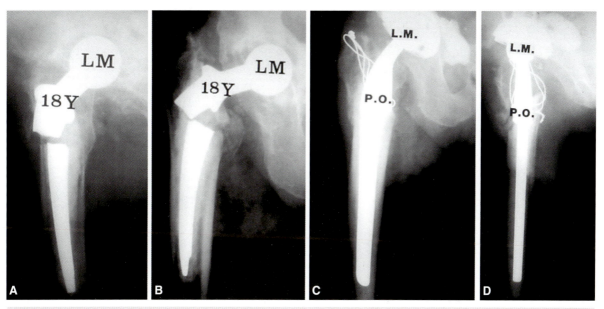

FIGS 60.3A TO D
(A) Broken stem showing only minimal displacement between the two fragments. (B) A few days later the displacement is greater. (C and D) The new implant extended far below the level of the original implant. The greater trochanter had apparently fractured at the time of the breakage of the stem, requiring its reattachment

Titanium alloy implants in hip surgery (See *Titanium Prostheses*).

Solving the problems created by a broken stem may be difficult. If the fracture occurs very proximally, the removal of the proximal fragment is usually uncomplicated, however, even in this instance removal of the distal fragment may be very difficult to accomplish. If the implant was a cemented one it is likely that the distal fragment may be removed by drilling into the surface of the distal fragment, fastening a "screw-like" instrument into it and then driving the component out of the shaft. This is easier said than done. Engaging the screw into the metal may not be possible as the drill slides over a slanted surface. In this instance a window located at the end of the distal stem allows the exposure of the metallic component. With an instrument and heavy blows of the hammer the stem can be removed (Figs 60.3A to D).

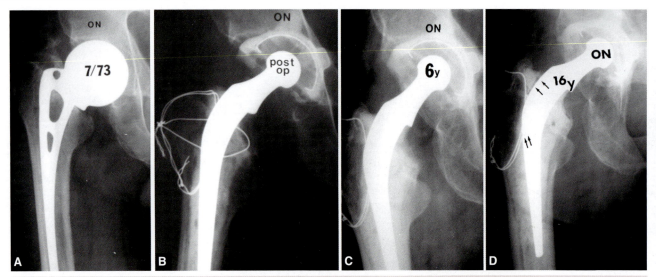

FIGS 60.4A TO D

(A) Radiograph of failed endoprosthesis that had been in place for 5 years. The patient was a muscular man, measuring 6 feet 2 inches in height and weighed 270 lbs. (B) The failed endoprosthesis was revised into a Charnley arthroplasty. (C) Radiograph obtained 6 years postoperatively. (D) Radiograph taken 16 years after surgery shows a fracture of the stem. There was minimal separation between the fragments but the fracture was readily identified in surgery. It is possible that the wire used initially to stabilize the greater trochanter might have scratched the stem, setting the stage for its eventual fracture

If the stem has a porous surface and it is noncemented, the problems multiply manifold. The bone ingrowth into the porous surface prevents it removal. In this instance it is almost always necessary to expose the entire length of the femur to the level of the distal end of the prosthesis through an osteotomy that includes the greater trochanter and the lateral cortex of the femur. The window is put back in its original place and secured with circular wires (Figs 60.4A to D). Wagner, from Germany, described the procedure and I have had the opportunity to use it a few times. The use of a longer stem is usually necessary in order to reduce the stresses at the distal end of the osteotomy.

Section 2

61
Heterotopic Bone

It is well known that heterotopic bone may form in a variety of clinical conditions. Its etiology is not clear. It is seen following burns and often at a distance from the site of the burn. It is not uncommon to see people with burns in the hand developing heterotopic bone about the elbow that may even fuse the joint completely. Its presence is even more common following head injuries. The possibility of some type of metabolic or chemical abnormality triggering the phenomenon has been widely discussed.

I personally believe that the clinical consequences of such a development in the case of total hip surgery have been greatly exaggerated, and that in most instances the presence of some new bone in the area is inconsequential. The degree of limitation of motion of the hip is often minimal. However, it can be severe enough to create serious problems and also predispose to dislocation. I find the frequent use of radiation difficult to justify unless there is a history of previous heterotopic bone formation. *Indocin, taken as a prophylactic measure, seems to be as effective as more radical measures.*

I suspect that in the case of the total hip, a possible cause for the heterotopic bone is the degree of trauma inflicted to the soft tissues during the surgical procedure. Surgery that is performed through a small incision and requires forceful retraction cannot be performed without traumatizing tissues and creating the physiological environment that leads to the formation of new bone. The traumatized tissues are temporarily rendered partially avascular. This brings about changes in the pH of the local medium and therefore the deposition of calcium. A phenomenon probably similar to the one observed around torn conoid and trapezoid ligaments of the shoulder following acromioclavicular

dislocations. This explanation may not suffice since the "bone" seen there is calcification, not ossification.

We should not panic prematurely when we see heterotopic bone form around a total hip replacement. Often the initial limitation of motion improves spontaneously. An illustrated clinical case proves the point. If the limitation of motion is major, it is also a good idea to wait until the active process has been completed. Early attempts to remove the new bone are followed by early recurrence of the pathological process. A cold bone scan is a reliable method to determine when to intervene surgically. *Douglas Garland, from California, who has seriously studied the problems associated with heterotopic bone over the years, has said to me that in the case of the head injured patient, the bone scan activity is not as important as the degree of spasticity at the time of surgery. The spastic patient is more likely to develop new bone following its resection.*

It has been my experience that the presence of bony spurs on the ischial tuberosity prior to surgery is not a reliable predictor of postoperative heterotopic bone. Nor is the disease for which the operation is performed. *I have not found, for example, that patients suffering from ankylosing spondylitis are more prone to develop the complication.*

What I have noticed is that *many of the patients who developed massive amounts of new bone experienced a disproportional degree of pain in the immediate postoperative period.* It is likely that the spasticity provoked by the pain might play a role in the formation of new bone.

In the case of open reduction of fractures of the pelvis it is interesting to note that the heterotopic bone almost always forms over the outer surface of the pelvic bone, even though the soft tissues are stripped from bone on both tables. I suspect that the reason for this phenomenon is that intestinal peristalsis and its resulting pulsatile nature prevents the new bone formation; in the same manner that the intermittent pulsation of an aortic aneurysm pressing against bone dissolves adjacent vertebral bodies.

I have never seen or heard of an artery being occluded by heterotopic bone. This is probably due to the fact that the pulsatile nature of the vessel precludes the occlusion. A similar situation exists in the case of bone placed over the dura during the performance of spine fusion. It is likely that the pulsatile nature of the spinal fluid prevents the growth of bone into the spinal canal. Figures 61.1 to 61.5 are the example of the early appearance of the heterotopic bone.

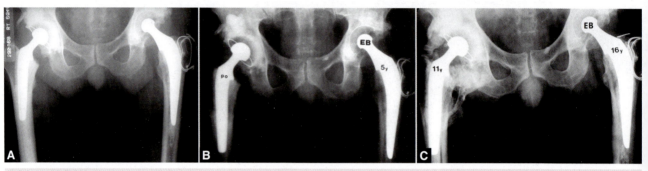

FIGS 61.1A TO C

(A) Radiographs obtained immediately after replacement of the right hip. The left hip had been replaced five years earlier. (B) Radiographs taken 5 and 11 years after arthroplasties of the right and left hips respectively. (C) Radiographs taken 11 and 16 years postoperatively. Despite the massive amount of new bone the range of motion of the hips was almost identical in both hips

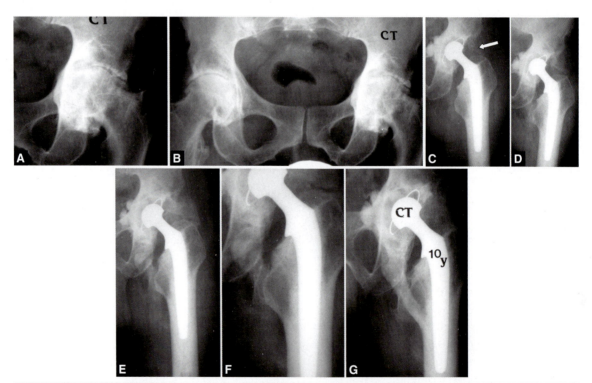

FIGS 61.2A TO G

(A and B) Preoperative radiographs of osteoarthritis of the left hip in a 55-year-old man. (C) Radiograph of total hip that was performed uneventfully and with minimal blood loss. The patient developed considerable amount of pain that lasted one week for which I did not find an explanation. Notice the early appearance of heterotopic bone radiograph obtained two weeks after surgery. (D) Radiograph taken one week later. (E) Radiograph obtained three months later. (F) Radiograph taken two months later. (G) Notice the increased density of the heterotopic bone. Radiograph showing solid fusion of the hip

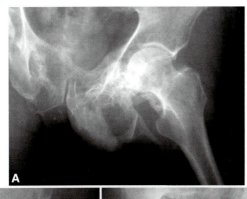

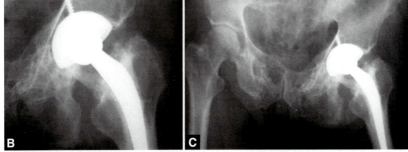

FIGS 61.3A TO C

(A) Radiograph of the pelvis of a patient following a head injury showing the heterotopic bone that formed over his left hip and the severe pelvic obliquity. (B) Radiograph following total hip arthroplasty shortly after surgery. (C) Radiograph obtained two years after surgery. The patient gained addition motion to the point he could sit up straight and walk with a slightly abducted gait. There was no rotation and pain was absent

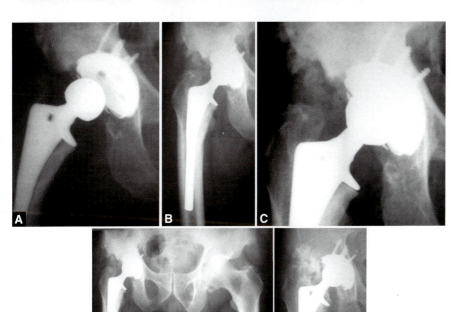

FIGS 61.4A TO E

(A) Radiograph of a dislocated prosthesis performed three days earlier. The patient was a heavy 56-year-old man who experienced significant amount of pain after surgery. Ambulation was initiated 24 hours after surgery. He dislocated his hip as he tried to get out of bed by himself. (B) Radiograph taken three weeks after surgery showing the early formation of heterotopic bone. (C) Radiograph demonstrating the early bone formation. (D) Radiograph showing both hips and the evidence of heterotopic bone formation 3 weeks after surgery. (E) Radiograph showing the large amount of new bone 3 months after surgery. At this time there was significant amount of limitation of motion. However, over the course of the next 12 months the range of motion increased leaving the patient with a hip that flexed to 80 degrees, which he compensated with back flexion. He never regained more than 25 degrees of abduction and probably no more than a few degrees of external rotation

Section 2

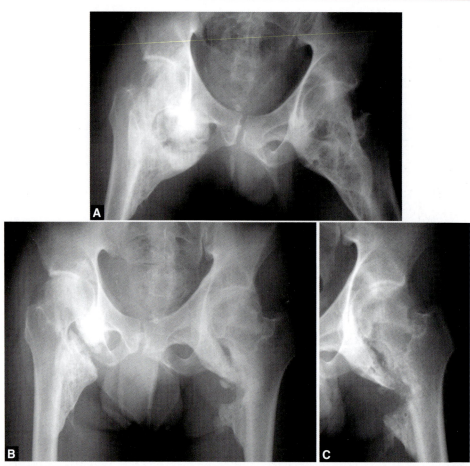

FIGS 61.5A TO C

(A) Radiograph of heterotopic bone in the pelvis of a 19-year-old boy, following a motorcycle accident. An associated head injury left him with severe spasticity, which improved over the next three years. Both hips were solidly fused. (B) Radiograph obtained two years following surgical excision of bilateral heterotopic bone. The clinical improvement was remarkable to the point that the patient was able to sit straight and to ambulate with the aid of one cane and drive an automobile. (C) Close view of left hip. Despite the appearance of fusion the hip can be passively flexed to 80 degrees and abducted approximately 15 degrees. Rotation was never regained

62

Rehabilitation

Among the most interesting changes in the attitude of patients with musculoskeletal conditions toward their postsurgical care in recent years has been their desire to receive supervised rehabilitation for long periods of time. This new attitude has become so pervasive that failure to prescribe such measures places the surgeon under a shadow of suspicion. He or she, is said, is not practicing the best modern medicine. Several times patients cancelled the total hip replacement we had agreed to perform when they were told that I "did not believe in rehabilitation". Obviously, this misinformation was spread around by someone with self-interest motives in the matter, or perhaps some one infected with jealousy, one of the cardinal human flaws. .

When total-hip patients ask me about "how much rehabilitation will be prescribed after being discharged home", I reply that it is very likely that supervised post-discharge rehabilitation will not be necessary, since at that time of discharge he or she will be independent in most activities, and able to carry out the necessary exercises and precautions; furthermore without the pain that produced the incapacitation present before surgery.

To some people this answer is not acceptable. Her friends, who had surgery performed elsewhere, received therapy from a "specialized" physical therapist at home for several weeks. Others traveled to the therapist office where they received therapy also for several weeks. The Health Insurance policy and Medicare pay for that "important" practice. .

The origin of this expensive and unnecessary trend had its beginning at a time when many surgeons had their own physical therapy facilities in their offices or nearby. When this practice was forbidden by the powers-that-be some of them continue to do it through subterfuge and other dubious means.

It is obvious that there are patients who need rehabilitation care following surgery. They should receive it. Those who do not need should not. The post-discharge therapy that is usually given to total hip patients consist in the performance of the same exercises they learned to do in the hospital and can do at home by themselves. A great deal of emphasis is placed on activities aimed at building up "weak muscles". Where did we get the idea that muscles slightly weakened by the preoperative pain need supervised therapy? What is wrong with returning to normal activities and practicing some abduction exercises without someone standing by, while still "supervising" a few other patients doing likewise?

While in the hospital, the physical rehabilitation program begins as soon as possible. Patients being prepared for surgery should learn of the importance of activity throughout the entire recovery period. I place strong emphasis on carrying out isometric exercises of the gluteus maximus and quadriceps as well as isotonic exercises of the ankle and toes. I remind them that failure to do so might result in a pulmonary embolus with possibly catastrophic complications. A number of times I see patients, barely awaken from anesthesia, moving their legs.

The use of the trapeze and the performance of deep-breathing exercises are very useful. However, *perhaps equally as important is the beginning of joint motion while the surgical procedure is being performed.* I expect the assistant in surgery to once in a while move passively the ankle and knee and to avoid, as much as possible, extreme position of flexion and rotation of the hip as well as forced flexion of the knee, since such positions are likely to damage vessels and set the stage for the formation of clots that can become embolus. This possible etiology has been well documented by others (See *Thromboembolic Disease*).

Much importance is frequently given to getting the patient out of bed as soon as possible. I agree with the measure, providing that the sitting position is not prolonged and that during the period of sitting the ankles and knees are exercised. Otherwise, distal-extremity swelling rapidly ensues, leading to possible thromboembolic disease.

Administering routine antithrombotic prophylaxis in all patients following total hip replacement has become an unquestionable ritual heavily promoted by the pharmaceutical industry, which derives enormous profit from such practice. *As far as I am concerned, routine prophylaxis with powerful drugs does more harm than good. The administration of Lovenox, the most common agent, is very expensive and it is associated with complications that can be easily avoided by using inexpensive and more effective drugs, such as aspirin* (See *Thromboembolic Disease*).

Walking instructions should, if at all possible, begin the day after surgery. To do it at the day of surgery is, what I call, "cowboy medicine". Patients need some rest after surgery and a period of recovery from the effects of anesthesia. *It is possible in most instances of primary surgery, and in many instances of revision surgery, for patients to bear weight on the operated extremity.* There is no compelling reason to withhold weight bearing following a properly performed replacement, since the stability of the implant is at its best. A few days later, the stability of the noncemented prosthetic components is less due to cold flow and resorption of devascularized bone. Furthermore, complete curtailment of weight bearing is virtually impossible in elderly patients. The

only way they can walk is if they bear significant weight on the operated leg. *One must remember that the forces sustained by the prosthetic head during partial weight bearing are equal to the ones it experiences in the process of actively elevating the leg while transferring from bed to chair. So, who are we fooling by insisting that prevention of weight bearing is possible?*

With current methods of prosthetic replacement the ambulation protocol for revision surgery is, in many instances, the same used following primary replacement. Therefore the rehabilitation of both patients is usually the same. Special circumstances might require additional precautions for various periods of time. *During the early days following surgery I insist on preceding the onset of ambulation by performing tip-toe exercises for a few seconds.* Walking is first initiated with the aid of a walker and gradually progressed to 2 crutches. *Most younger patients can progress to one cane assistance by the third or 4th day.* Older ones rarely reach this degree of independency that quickly and should be protected with addition support for whatever time seems appropriate.

A large percentage of total-hip patients find it possible to be discharged home around the 4th post-surgery day. Fewer can do it in a shorter period of time. To insist that discharge from the hospital within very short time after surgery is not a sound approach.

Most patients become independent in the basic activities of daily living in the first few postsurgical days. Their routine discharge to a rehabilitation center, I find it unnecessary. Only those people who need that intermediate stage should have it. The ones who have help at home, usually go home directly from the hospital. The help they usually need is minimal, since they are able to get in and out of bed without assistance, dress and walk around the house using a walker, cane or crutches. They conduct the abduction exercises and take the necessary precautions against dislocation on their own.

There is usually no need to establish a precise date for the discontinuance of external support. Like the animal in the wild, humans also sense when they are ready to walk on 3 and then on four legs.

63

Why So Many Total Hips...

Despite the fact that total hip replacement is recognized as one of the major development in the care of the impaired arthritic hip, the success of the operation has not taken place uniformly. Even in those situations where success was attained, in many instances the benefits are short-lived, requiring a "revision" of the failed procedure. The large number of revisions of failed arthroplasties performed world-wide eloquently testifies to that effect. The revisions are being performed not only in implants that had been in place for many years, but also in relatively recently performed surgeries. In other words, not necessarily to replace early cemented prosthetic models, but contemporary noncemented implants as well. I think it is irresponsible for surgeons and/or manufactures to state (as it is being done today) that current implants makes possible for patients to safely indulge in all kind of sport since they will last the rest of their lives. There is no data whatsoever at this time to support such a prediction. Quite the contrary, marketing of such an idea is inappropriate and misleading.

It might be argued with some logic that the success rate with new implants will increase, and the failure rate will decrease as technological improvements are made. No doubt, technological advances will contribute to greater success. However, such a well deserved optimism must be tempered with a strong dose of caution. Recent reports have indicated that the curves illustrating the number of primary hip arthroplasties and the number of revisions are getting closer. In addition, over 50% of revised arthroplasties require additional revisions.

One might suggest that catastrophes such as the one experienced by Charnley with the use of Teflon cannot happen today. This is said with the same confidence that it is expressed when discussing the impossibility of another Depression similar to the Great Depression of the 1930's occurring in an economically advanced country. No one knows with certainty that this confidence can be absolutely guaranteed.

Total hip surgery has witnessed a number of periods of great enthusiasm with new techniques and implants, only to find out after a relatively short period of time that the results expected from the "new and improved" products did not meet the expectations. Legions of patients have found themselves temporarily or permanently damaged, and a large percentage of them had to undergo revision surgeries.

Total joint replacement in its present form is an unphysiological procedure for it simply replaces a biological structure with nonbiological materials, to which the human body sooner or later responds to them in either a salutary or negative way.

The real challenge confronting us is the finding the means to prevent or reduce the incidence of medical conditions for which artificial joint replacement is the answer today. Gene manipulation, which has the entire scientific community energized, might one day reach rheumatoid and osteoarthritis. I doubt very much such a breakthrough will take place in the near future particularly with osteoarthritis, but the effort must continue. Cartilage replacement by biological means is today a major source of investigation and enthusiasm. I remain very skeptical about major breakthroughs in this area as well as in other areas dealing with the musculoskeletal system. *Making acute fractures heal faster is an interesting dream, which may remain a dream never to be realized. The world will not be any worse if the dream remains a dream.*

The noncemented modular acetabulum has been found to be responsible for the production of lysis in a number of instances: from the stabilizing screws rubbing against the convexity of the polyethylene liner, the corrosion of metal from the scratching of the screws against the holes in the metallic cup, the loosening of the anchoring of the liner for the cup, and the ubiquitous wear of current articulating materials. *These features will continue to be important in the production of complications leading to revision surgery.*

From the femoral side we have the problems that may arise from the modular components, the lysis provoked by plastic, ceramics, or metal debris coming from the acetabular side, or the loosening of the implant. *Of the greatest importance is the likely probability that the already recognized chromosomal abnormalities seeing from metallosis may become a clinical reality.*

There is another major factor that has, and probably will continue to have major importance in the incidence of revision surgeries. *It is our innate obsession with the idea that surgical prosthetic implants need to be made stronger and stronger.* One only need to look at the current implants, be it in regards to total joint prostheses, spinal metallic plates or screws, and nails and plates for the treatment of fractures. Every new generation of implants is "stronger" than the previous one.

Such an obsession has led the surgical manufacturing companies, who are in virtual control of research and the design of new implants, to think exclusively on mechanical terms, while disregarding the fundamental biological considerations needed to understand the manner in which the body responds to the presence of foreign materials.

For example, the design of bigger and stronger implants makes them "stiffer". We respond intuitively at the sight of a broken nail, plate or screw by reasoning that if a stronger implant had been used the fracture would have never taken place. What is usually ignored is the fact it was the already "too stiff" nature of the failed implant that brought about the problem. In the case of a fracture of a plate or nail used to stabilize a fracture of a long bone, the failure of the metallic implant simply tells us that the race between healing and metal fatigue was won by the ununited bone. The same applies to plates and screws used in the fusion of vertebral bodies. *In most instances it is not the failure of the implants but the failure of the bone that creates the mechanical failure. Making implants bigger and stiffer simply aggravates the problems we are trying to solve.* We should keep in mind the old aphorism, "The bigger they are the harder they fall". Since the modulus of elasticity of all currently used metals is much higher than that of bone, loosening of the implants is more likely to occur.

In the case of hip implants, the stiffer the material of the prosthesis the greater the degree of stress shielding experienced by the surrounding bone; a phenomenon identical to the atrophy of the cortex observed under plates, particularly with "stiffer" ones.

It is well-known that at this time the Justice Department of the United States is investigating serious allegations of unethical conduct in the relationship between orthopedic surgeons and the implant manufacturing industry. The transgressions consist in most instances on Industry "donating" money to orthopedists in figures amounting to hundreds of thousand or millions of dollars for their "cooperating" with Industry's ventures. This is no longer an occasional happening but a wide-spread one. Needless to say, the surgeons must reciprocate by using implants and marketing them by whatever means become available. Many of them become "peddlers" for industry and travel around the country lecturing on the virtues of the respective products. Successful members of the profession, outside the academic group do likewise. The use of continuing educational courses, as a means to advertise unproven or proven products is part to the scheme. Industry's financial support for residency programs that make possible the recruitment of visiting professors and guest speakers, as well as phony research activities has become a commodity difficult to replace. The resulting "ownership" of large segments of academia and the resulting loss of autonomy is creating major problems. It should go without saying it that among the contributors to the advancement of surgery there are many who are honest, sincere, dedicated individuals. However, the fact remains that the attractiveness of the "deals" extended by industry is enlarging the legion of those with questionable ethical values.

Parallel to the unhappy state of the relationship of orthopedics and industry witnessed at this time is the fact that medicine has began to function as a business and no longer as a profession. This change will probably impede in some degree the future of joint replacement as well as many other areas. The almost pathological obsession with generating an ever increasing amount of money is permeating the medical ranks. The hip "specialists", in particular, have led this new parade. Seeking and getting involvement in the marketing of "new and improved" prostheses seems to be the normal course of events. The more unproven implants reach the market, the greater the number of revisions.

It is not uncommon to see orthopedic surgeons with egomaniac ideas resort to all kind of unprofessional, as well as unethical, practices in order to get public recognition. They advertise their names through every conceivable medium, be it the printed press, the radio, television and throw-away cheap magazines. They ask and get from industry financial support for the development of their own hip or knee implants. It matters not that they have no scientific concepts to identify, what is it that the new implants will do that existing ones do not. The important thing is to have their names on some implant, which if not succeeding in getting acceptance in the orthopedic community, at least they can use in their assembly-line practices. This issue should not be taken lightly since it is highly responsible for the unnecessary plethora of implants and their resulting absurd cost. Obviously, these ventures play a role in the high incidence of revision surgeries.

Two personal anecdotal experience illustrate the boldness the industrial corporate world has found possible to display. During my tenure as Professor and Chairman of Orthopedics at the University of Southern California, I was visited by the vice-president of a major industrial concern, who presented me with a new total hip prosthesis, which according to him was the "Sarmiento Total Hip". The implant, according to him, had been developed by his engineers to represent my "philosophy". After showing me the implant he proceeded to hand me a check in the amount of $250,000. A discussion related to royalties was then to be discussed.

When I informed him that I could not accept having my name attached to an implant I had nothing to do with its design, he apologized. Two months later a picture of the prosthesis appeared in major journals. When I inquired as to the name of the orthopedist "behind" the product I was given the name of a Professor in a major medical school in the North Atlantic, United States. The vendor providing me with the information stated that the prosthesis had been based on the "professor's philosophy".

The second episode took place within the same period of time. I was offered $200 for every total joint replacement performed by the staff of my department. My job was to encourage the surgeons to use their products. Pretending I was mentally trying to figure out how long it would take me to become a millionaire, I asked if the figure of $200 was negotiable. He immediately responded in a positive way. I added, "Instead of $200,can we make it $250?". "That is a deal" he responded. When I refused to "prostitute" myself in that manner, the visiting industrial representative responded, "But we do this all the time."

Remove from the scene the greed and unethical behavior of a few dishonest promoters among our ranks, and the failure rate of total hip implants would precipitously decrease. A tall order, that our discipline, through its organized structures can successfully address. However, their reluctance to forcefully address issues of this nature has contributed to the aggravation of the problem at hand.

I am taking the liberty quoting from an article published recently, which should shed light into the current status of total hip replacements and the cost they represent to the economy of our country.

"A study published in the January issue of the *Journal of Bone and Joint Surgery—American* examines trends in revision total hip arthroplasty (THA). The researchers reviewed data from the Healthcare Cost and Utilization Project Nationwide Inpatient Sample database from 51,345 revision THA procedures performed between October 1, 2005, and December 31, 2006. They found that the most common revision THA procedure was all-component revision (41.1 percent), and the most common causes of revision were instability/dislocation (22.5 percent), mechanical loosening (19.7 percent), and infection (14.8 percent). Revision THA procedures were most commonly performed in large, urban, nonteaching hospitals for Medicare patients aged between 75 to 84-year-old. The average length of hospital stay for all types of revision arthroplasties was 6.2 days, and the average total charges were $54,553, but these varied considerably according to census region, hospital type, and type of revision THA procedure performed."

From an article published in the Journal of Bone and Joint Surgery *The Journal of Bone and Joint Surgery (American)*. 2009;91:128-133, (written by **Kevin J Bozic MD, MBA, Steven M Kurtz PhD, Edmund Lau MS, Kevin Ong PhD, Thomas P Vail MD and Daniel J Berry MD),** I take a few segments which unequivocally demonstrate that statements made by some surgeons and manufacturing companies suggesting that patients with total hip prostheses can safely indulge in all kind of sports since their implants will last the rest of their days, are irresponsible and erroneous. The authors prove that complications from total hip replacement are not infrequent and that abuse of the artificial joint contributes to failure.

References*

84, 87, 88, 103, 108, 110, 119, 120

---

* References provided at the end of the book after annexures.

Section 3

The Fractured Hip

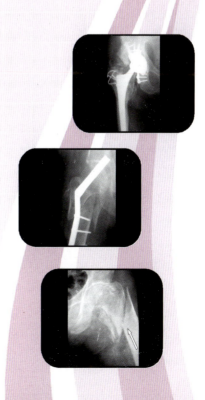

64

Acetabular Fractures

New technology has made possible the surgical treatment of many acetabular fractures in ways not dreamt possible three decades ago. This new opportunity, however, has resulted in an exaggerated emphasis in the technological aspects of treatment, and has given to many orthopedists the impression that all acetabular fractures must be treated by surgical means in order to restore absolute anatomical reduction of the fracture. Any incongruity, is said, is unacceptable, because it inevitably leads to late degenerative changes. To accept the concept that intra-articular fractures with residual incongruity inevitably lead to arthritic changes is wrong. It cannot be true. Thousands, if not millions, of people who sustained acetabular fractures in the past and did not have anatomical repositioning of the fragments, never developed arthritic changes, and among those who developed them, many never became sufficiently symptomatic to require surgery. This statement is made not to suggest that congruity of articular cartilage fractures is not desirable, but to emphasize that other factors must be included in the decision process.

The effect of incongruity in articular cartilage is a subject, which we are just now beginning to understand. Mother Nature spontaneously repairs small step-off defects without leading to arthritic changes. The works of Lansinger, in Sweden, Kristensen, in Denmark and Dietz and Marsh, in Iowa, and our own, are convincing even though they do not deal with the hip but with the knee and ankle joints. Some of these investigators have demonstrated in long-term follow-up studies, that most fractures of the tibial condyles that healed with residual significant incongruity did not develop arthritic changes some 30 years later. Our own laboratory work and clinical experience support their findings. *I have long suspected it is more likely that instability is more important than incongruity as we recently documented in laboratory animals.*

It must be remembered that since many of these fractures are the result of violent impaction of the head of the femur against the acetabulum, the articular cartilage may be irreparably damaged from that moment on. Repositioning the displaced fragments under those circumstances does not change the pathological situation and osteoarthritic changes may ensue. MRI technology will soon be able to share new information, and hopefully will make possible a clear determination of the degree of damage that the various layers of the articular cartilage experience at the time of the initial insult, as well a subsequent pathology not appreciated through simple radiographs.

Senior surgeons have recently reported that long-term follow-up of their patients, indicated that those who had open reduction and internal fixation, developed painful arthritis and required total joint replacement sooner that those whose fractures were treated nonsurgically. One must assess these experiences very carefully. Lumping all acetabular fractures into a single package, may lead to wrong conclusions. There are many fractures that are definitely best managed by surgical means.

Surgical exposure of severely comminuted acetabular fractures requires additional stripping of soft tissue attachment from those fragments, bringing about the associated risk of devascularizing them even further, and setting the stage for the development of heterotopic bone. In addition, even in the best of hands, anatomical reduction is not always attained. Gaps between the many fragments frequently remain.

In the case of the surgically managed patient, the surgeon must worry about infection, sciatic nerve injury, vascular injury and heterotopic bone formation.

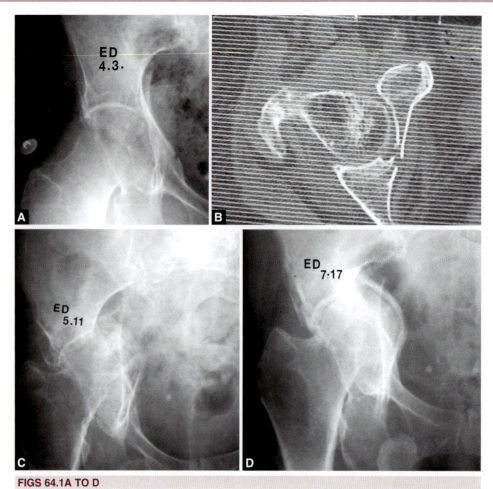

FIGS 64.1A TO D

Unstable acetabular fracture in an 84-year-old woman. The fracture was treated symptomatically. The head migrated into the pelvis within a few days. Three months later patient was minimally symptomatic and ambulatory with the aid of a walker. She died two years later with a hip still asymptomatic

Despite some reports to the contrary, consideration must also be given to the nature of the original injury and the degree of initial displacement of the fragments. I suspect that a fracture produced through a high-energy mechanism behaves differently that one sustained from a fall to the ground after slipping on wet pavement.

I believe that certain acetabular fractures, particularly in the elderly (Figs 64.1A to D), can be treated by non-surgical means in anticipation that if disabling arthritic changes occur, the situation could be remedied with an electively performed total hip replacement. Primary total hip replacement can on occasion be the treatment of choice. I have performed such a procedure a few times. *However, I believe that under this circumstance heterotopic bone is more likely to form.* This also is true for acute fractures of the femoral neck treated primarily with endoprostheses. I have no clear explanation for this phenomenon.

In the case of younger patients, I suspect surgery is not necessary in many instances. Stable fractures that

show minimal incongruity and very mild step-off deformity are likely to lead to good results following nonoperative treatment. Fractures located over the less important weight-bearing area of the dome fall in that category. However, regardless of the type or location, *the presence of floating fragments in the join (easily documented with CT scans) constitutes an ominous sign. If left in place, degenerative changes are almost always inevitable.*

Protection from significant weight bearing for a few weeks (a period probably no longer than the one recommended after surgery) often restores the patient to a very acceptable degree of independence. With surgery or with conservative treatment, patients with these major fractures do not return to normal overnight. Pain lingers for some time (Figs 64.2 and 64.3).

Heterotopic bone develops in the overwhelming majority of instances only on the outer table of the iliac bone, even though stripping of periosteum and muscles is done on both tables. *I have speculated that*

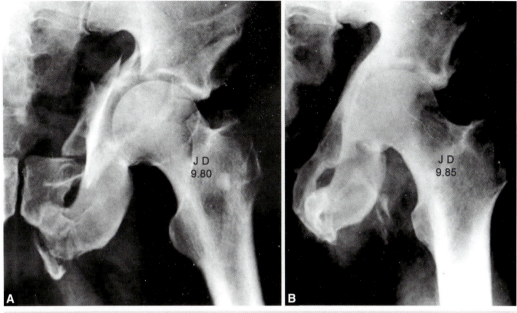

FIGS 64.2A AND B

(A) Comminuted fracture of the acetabulum and pubic and ischial ramous in a 49-year-old man. The fracture was treated with bed rest for a few days followed by protected weight bearing ambulation. (B) Five-year follow-up demonstrates the healed fracture and a fairly well preserved joint space. Though at that time the patient was asymptomatic

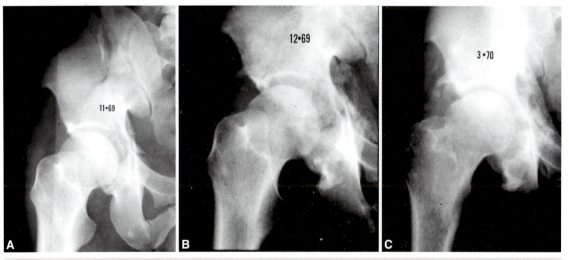

FIGS 64.3A TO C

(A) Pelvic/acetabular fracture treated with bed rest and passive motion of the hip for four weeks. (B) Radiograph obtained at the time of initiation of protected weight-bearing ambulation. (C) Radiograph taken four months later showing the radiologically united fractures and the formation of heterotopic bone. No further follow-up was available. Arthritic changes will probably develop at a later date

the relative absence of heterotopic bone on the inner table is due to the effect of pulsatile peristalsis from the adjacent intestines; a mechanism that resembles the destruction of vertebrae adjacent to an aortic aneurysm. The same reason as to why vessels are rarely obliterated in the callus of the healing fracture (Figs 64.4A to E).

Sciatic nerve injury is commonly associated with fractures of the acetabulum especially if a dislocation occurred at the time of the accident. It should be noted that in many instances the palsy is only of the muscles innervated by the common peroneal nerve. Those, innervated by the posterior tibial branch of the sciatic frequently remain normal. *This suggests that the mechanism of injury that produce the nerve damage is not necessarily a contusion of the sciatic nerve at the level of the pelvis, but a stretching of the nerve at the level of the*

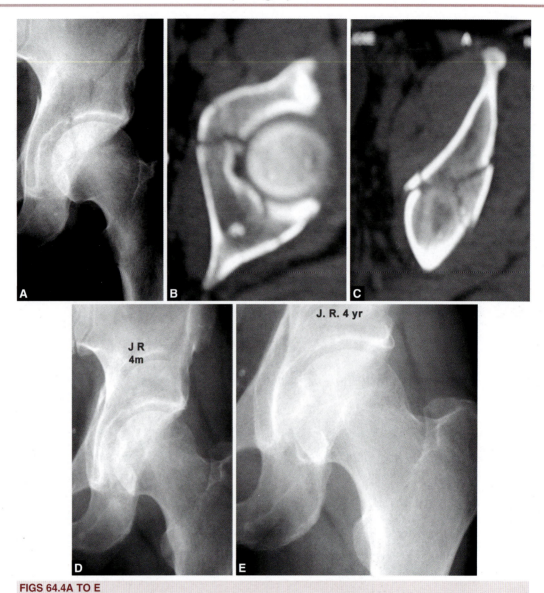

FIGS 64.4A TO E

(A) Minimally displaced, unstable acetabular fracture in a 45-year-old man. (B and C) CT scan illustrating the unstable nature of the fracture. (D) Radiograph taken four months postinjury. (E) Radiograph obtained four years later

knee joint. As the femoral head displaces superiorly in relation to the acetabulum, tension is applied to the sciatic nerve; however, since the common peroneal branch is relatively fixed around the fibular head, it is the tension that produces the paralysis of the peroneal nerves, leaving intact the posterior tibial branch that continues to run into the calf in a unchanged distal direction.

This mechanism is supported by the fact that patients who experience palsy limited to the peroneal nerve, experience pain when the nerve is manually compressed just below the neck of the fibula.

I feel that one of the most difficult total hip replacements is the one that is performed for the treatment of osteoarthritis secondary to a fracture of the acetabulum. The problem is due to the fact that the fracture frequently leaves behind a deformed acetabulum. Trying to create a cavity into which the prosthetic acetabular component can be anchored, is a time-consuming undertaking. The absence of a superior or posterior acetabular wall requires either the fitting of a very large component, a special metallic cage and/or a bone graft. *These are the fractures where initial surgical treatment is often the treatment of choice.*

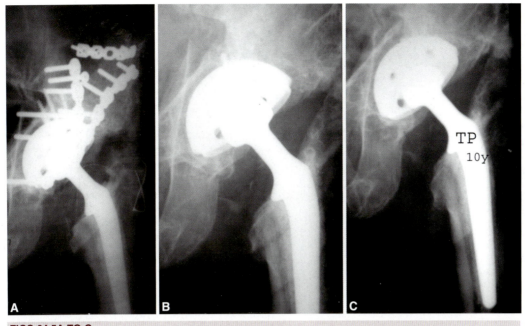

FIGS 64.5A TO C

(A) A severely displaced fracture of the acetabulum treated with multiple plate and screws. (B) The total hip replacement that was successfully performed without removing all the metallic implants. However, heterotopic bone formed, the motion of the joint was very limited and ambulation was painful. (C) The plates and screws were removed and the heterotopic bone was excised. Ten years later the hip was relatively asymptomatic; the good range of motion was maintained; and new bone had not formed

Since a number of acetabular fractures treated by means of internal fixation with either screws and or plates, it is frequently necessary to remove those implants before the acetabular component of a total hip prosthesis can be stabilized in place. When such removal is necessary the surgical incision must be enlarged in a major way. There are times when during the reaming of the acetabulum one encounters screws that preclude the creation of a sufficiently deep cavity (Figs 64.5A to C).

In a few instances (Figs 64.6 to 64.8) I have been able to remove the offending screw or screws without having to remove all the screws and plate.

One of the most unhappy experiences I had in my entire academic career is based on a fracture of the acetabulum (a component of a more serious Malgaine fracture-dislocation of the sacroiliac joint) in a 16-year-old girl who had been hit by an automobile. She was treated initially at another institution and did not come to my attention until several months later. The fracture was allegedly open, but the wound healed spontaneously without complications. In retrospect, I made several errors of judgment that led to grave complications. When I first saw this young woman I recognized a clear evidence of joint damage, with an associated feeble union, or a nonunion at the level of the iliac-ischial level. I sent the films to

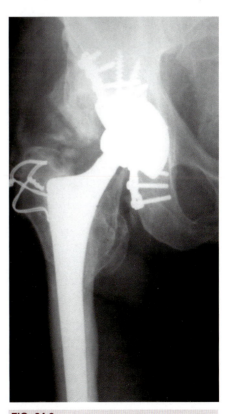

FIG. 64.6

Radiograph showing a noncemented total hip performed without the need to remove the plate and screws

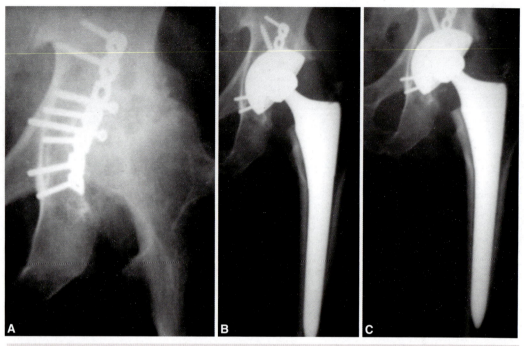

FIGS 64.7A TO C

(A) Osteoarthritic changes following a fracture-dislocation of the hip treated surgically. A partial peroneal palsy never improved. (B) The total hip replacement was performed without removal of the plate. Only 2 screws were removed. (C) Radiograph obtained five years later

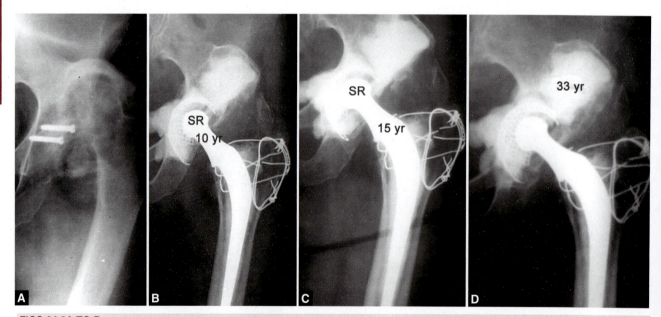

FIGS 64.8A TO D

(A) Radiograph of old untreated fracture dislocation of the hip. (B) The missing bone from the superior and posterior wall of the acetabulum was replaced with acrylic cement, (C) 15 years after surgery the hip was asymptomatic and functional. (D) 34 years after the initial surgery the patients expired. This film was obtained one year earlier

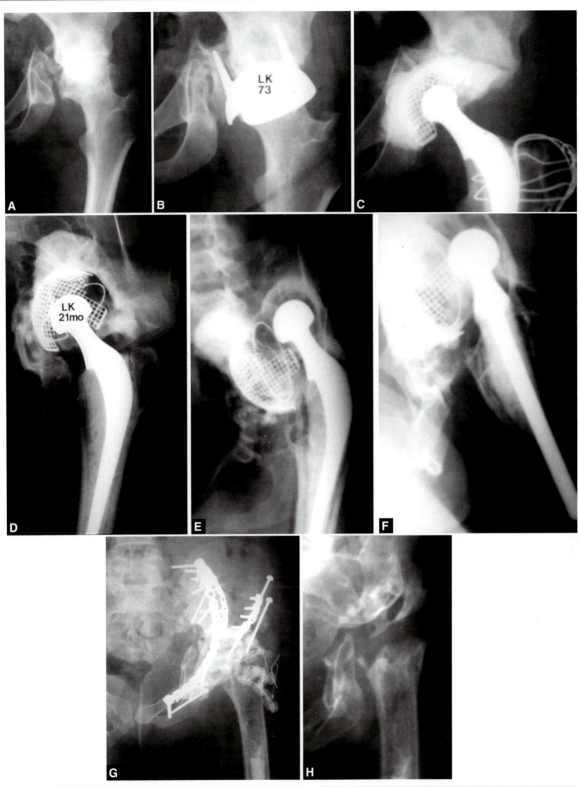

FIGS 64.9A TO H

Surgery was uneventful. No infection was encountered; I could not detect motion between the major fragments at the level of the nonunion, though the bridge between the two major fragments was thin. I grafted the area in order to strengthen what I thought was a weak union. The patient continued to have pain. Accordingly, I talked myself into believing that a total hip arthroplasty was indicated. I performed the surgery uneventfully, and once again I could not identify a nonunion. However, I placed bone graft over the area before pressing the acrylic cement into the two major fragments

Section 3

Sir John Charnley, who said that this problem was the must difficult one he had ever seen. He added that an infection might be present.

I could not understand at the time the uniqueness of the problem. I did not take very long however, to learn that I should have taken Sir John remarks seriously. As I look back at the many years during which time I maintained a close relationship with Sir John, I realize that almost never did he say anything that turned out to be wrong.

Thinking that I could approach the situation through a compromise, I elected to perform a Urist cup arthroplasty (Figs 64.9A to C).

The patient did well. She was by this time 20 years of age. Traveled overseas to finish school; married and had two children. Approximately three years after surgery she informed me that the hip was painless but had noticed that the leg had gotten shorter. The X-ray film showed a complete medial dislocation of the hip along the opening of the nonunion and an exaggeration of the superior displacement of the Malgaine fracture (Fig. 64.9D).

Within a few weeks, the displacement of the fragments got worse (Figs 64.9E and F). By this time the young woman's alcoholism problem had gotten out of hand. The x-ray picture became worse as she took care of pain with the ingestion of alcohol. I proceeded to remove the implants and left her with a Girdlestone hip. I thought that sooner or later I would be able to do something about her worsening problems.

I contemplated the possibility of an open reduction and fusion of the Malgaine dislocation along with massive bone grafting to the nonunited pelvic fracture. However, I was wise enough this time to recognize my limitations and proceeded to contact a prominent hip surgeon from the North Eastern United States. He reviewed the films and made plans to perform surgery on a given date. I was to fly to his city and serve as his assistant. A few days before the planned surgery, the brave surgeon went through the same agony I had just experienced, and cancelled the surgery.

By this time I had already moved to Los Angeles where I became associated with Joel Matta, a member of our faculty at USC. I had seen him in action and observed his extraordinary surgical skills. I presented to him the story of my patient. He felt confident in being able to replace the missing pelvic bone, while stabilizing the sacroiliac joint (Figs 64.9A to H). A massive pelvic allograph was obtained and Matta performed the surgery. I was amazed to see what he had accomplished.

Unfortunately, however, a massive infection developed, requiring removal of the pelvic graft. Nine years later, the infection persisted. She died from cirrhosis of the liver before her fortieth birthday (Figs 64.10A to D).

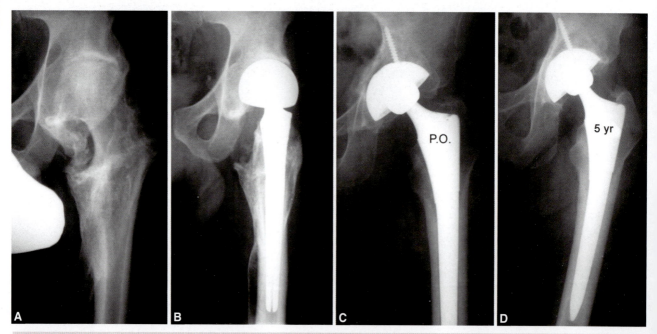

FIGS 64.10A TO D
(A) Radiograph of arthritic hip following a minimally displaced fracture of the acetabulum treated by nonsurgical means. Disabling symptoms were present at 3 years after the initial injury. Notice the associated heterotopic bone. (B) Postoperative films obtained after a bipolar prosthesis was implanted. (C) The hip remained painful, and was then replaced with a noncemented total hip. (D) Five years later the hip was asymptomatic

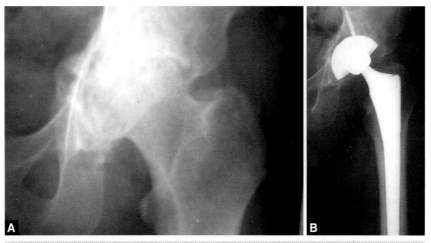

FIGS 64.11A AND B

(A) Acetabular fracture treated nonsurgically. Advanced symptomatic changes were present two years after the initial insult. (B) The hip joint was successfully replaced with a noncemented prosthesis

*References**

18, 27, 41, 52, 63, 97

---

* References provided at the end of the book after annexures.

65

The Intertrochanteric Fracture

The intertrochanteric fracture is a one of the most common fractures in the aged and is associated with high mortality. This latter fact must be kept in mind as treatment is introduced. Heroic procedures, likely to be associated with excessive bleeding are likely to increase mortality and morbidity. In those instances where the changes of short survival are anticipated, i.e. in the debilitated, nonambulatory elderly, the simplest procedure should be chosen. The surgical treatment should be performed simply to provide comfort for whatever remaining lifespan is left.

The relatively recent introduction of closed intramedullary nailing has begun a revolution in the care of these fractures. Though, not a panacea, the new technique has dramatically facilitated the surgical intervention. Whether or not the simpler and less traumatic procedure will prove to have lower mortality and improve the quality of life after surgery has not yet been documented. It is logical to assume that the final verdict will be a positive one.

A number of classifications of intertrochanteric fractures have been described in the literature. However, most of them simply describe the degree of comminution. *I, long ago came to the conclusion that comminution per se is not the determining factor for stability.* The feature that determines most significantly the choice of implant or surgical technique is whether or not the fracture is stable or can be made stable prior to the introduction of the internal fixation device, be a nail-plate or an intramedullary nail (Figs 65.1A to C).

The stability of the intertrochanteric fracture is determined by the degree of contact that can be obtained between the medial cortexes of the two major proximal and distal fragments. It the absence of contact between those fragments, intrinsic stability cannot be obtained; only the stability the internal device can create. Therefore reduction of the two major fractured fragments is essential in obtaining maximum stability. If a stable reduction can not be obtained because comminution of the medial fragments precludes their approximation, or the angle of inclination of the reduced fragments is too high, the only stability the internal fixation accomplishes is the one provided by the implant itself.

In a number of occasions, sliding nails function well, as they permit eventual contact between major fragments, while producing shortening of the extremity. This applies to an almost similar degree to fractures treated with intramedullary nails.

When using fixed nail-plate implants, following adequate re-approximation of the cortices of the two major fragments, the fixation provided by the implant must be sufficient to offset the powerful forces created by weight bearing and muscles contractions. In the absence of sufficient strength of the implant, the nail might bend or break.

The introduction of imaging intensification in the operating room simplified significantly not only the closed intramedullary nailing of trochanteric fractures, but also the performance of open internal fixation. This radiological advance is used worldwide. However,

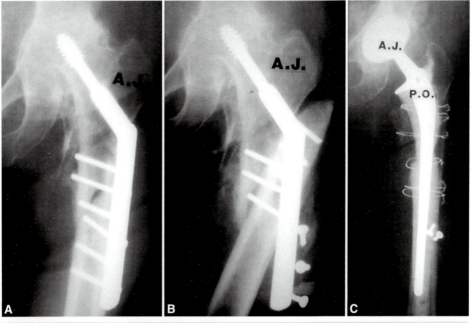

FIGS 65.1A TO C

(A) Intertrochanteric fracture with a subtrochanteric extension that appeared to have been made stable by the adequate reduction and surgical stabilization of the fracture. Such a reduction does not make the fracture stable. (B) Following the introduction of weight bearing, the fracture collapsed as the screws broke and the plate separated from the femoral cortex. (C) Because of the patient's advanced age, I chose to treat the complication with a total hip arthroplasty

there are regions of the world where the expensive method is not yet available. Therefore, the following illustrations (Figs 65.2 to 65.4) are presented in an attempt to prevent pitfalls.

There is controversy concerning the most appropriate angle of a nail-plate. The answer cannot be a simple one, for there are several factors to be considered. One is the prefracture angle between the femoral shaft and the neck of the femur. A proximal femur with a 120 degree of varus angle cannot tolerate a 150 degree nail. Likewise, a fracture with severe comminution, where no contact between the two major fragments can be obtained, and therefore the fracture remains unstable, the nail with a lower angle is better. The sliding of the fragments over the nail is less if the angle is lower, therefore preventing the superior migration of the nail. This consideration applies to rigid, as well as to sliding nails.

We have studied intertrochanteric fractures and have concluded that in the case of stable fractures, which do not have a high degree of verticality, a 150 degree angle nail improves impaction and requires fewer screws to attach the plate against the femoral cortex. We demonstrated that a stable, low-angle fracture allows the nail to withstand forces significantly

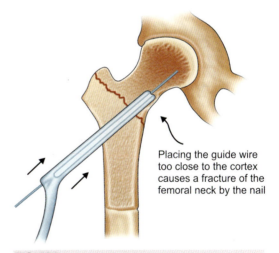

Placing the guide wire too close to the cortex causes a fracture of the femoral neck by the nail

FIG. 65.2

Illustration of inappropriate placement of the nail, capable of producing a fracture of the femoral neck

higher then those required bending or breaking it under laboratory conditions. For example, a 150 degree angle I-beam nail that has a yield point of 250 lbs, can preserve the initially obtained reduction even after 800 lbs of weight had been introduced. This finding was obtained demonstrated with retrieved hip specimens from patients who survived the surgery for only a few days (Figs 65.5 to 65.9).

Section 3

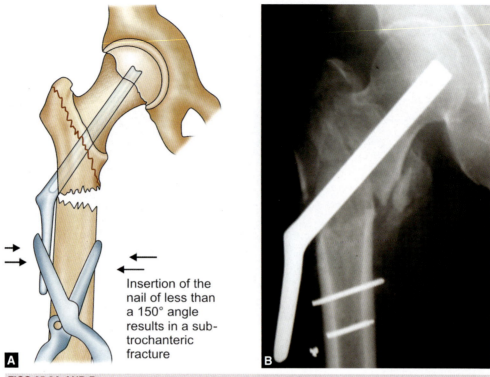

Insertion of the nail of less than a 150° angle results in a subtrochanteric fracture

FIGS 65.3A AND B

If the angle of the nail/plate has not been properly made parallel to the femur, attempts to bring the plate against the femoral shaft may result in the production of a subtrochanteric fracture

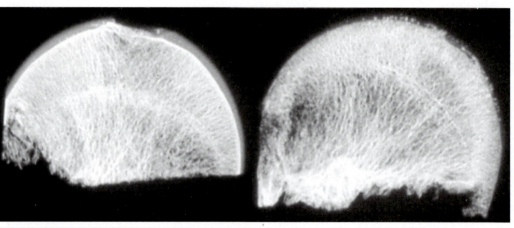

FIG. 65.4

The femoral head is uniformly dense as demonstrated by these femoral heads removed from two patients; one who sustained fracture of the femoral neck; the other suffering from osteoarthritis

There are times when because the severe osteoporosis in very old and feeble patients, is best to reinforce the metallic stabilization with the addition of acrylic cement (Figs 65.10A and B). The routine use of cement in fracture fixation is not recommended. We have conducted laboratory studies that indicated that nonunion is more likely to develop under those circumstances. However, in the nonambulatory, or minimally ambulatory elderly patient, failure to obtain bony union becomes irrelevant. *The importance thing in these instances is to provide relief from pain and to permit mobilization.* Care should be exercised to minimize the contact of the polymerizing cement with the surrounding soft tissue in order to prevent thermic injury to the major nerves.

As indicated early, the angle of inclination of the fracture plays a major role in determining the choice of implant as well as projecting the subsequent course of events. *The vertical intertrochanteric fracture cannot tolerate the weight bearing forces without the fracture collapsing and the nail migrating proximally, even at times when a sliding nail is used (Figs 65.11 to 65.14).*

The recognition of the importance of the angle of inclination of the fracture prompted me a number of years ago to develop a surgical technique that reduces

Yield point of the I-beam is 400 pounds; however, with properly inserted in the bone then bends of approximately 850 pounds

Cross-section

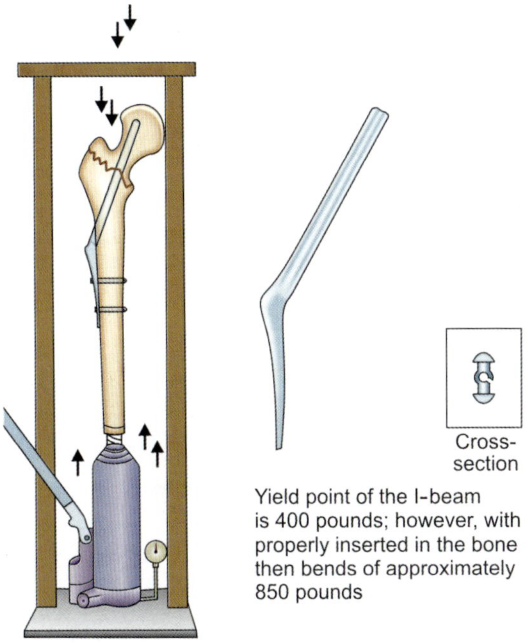

FIG. 65.5

Drawing of the instrument used to test the stability of nailed intertrochanteric fractures

the inclination to an acceptable level, and then brings into contact the two major fragments.

The procedure consists of an osteotomy of the fragment at a 45 degree angle, just below the proximal distal end of the femur, *The surgical cut must begin at approximately one centimeter below the apex of the fracture, in order to shorten the extremity, and in that manner compensate for the additional length gained by the eventual greater valgus of the proximal femur.* The created free fragment is removed exposing the medullary canal of the proximal fragment. A guide wire may be use to ascertain more precisely the appropriate position of the nail (Fig. 65.15).

More vertical fractures, even if anatomically reduced, cannot be subjected to major weight bearing because of the likely possibility that shearing stresses would permit the fragments to displace and the nail to move in an upward direction, eventually cutting through the articular cartilage. This observation prompted me to describe the valgus osteotomy, which for a number of years we used with some success in a large percentage of instances (Figs 65.16 and 65.17).

The following (Figs 65.18 to 65.21) are examples of valgus osteotomies performed in the care of unstable intertrochanteric fractures.

In our series, most of the fractures were stabilized with an I-beam nail in order to enhance fixation. In other instances sliding nails were used. *It should be obvious, that if close approximation of medial/anterior*

Section 3

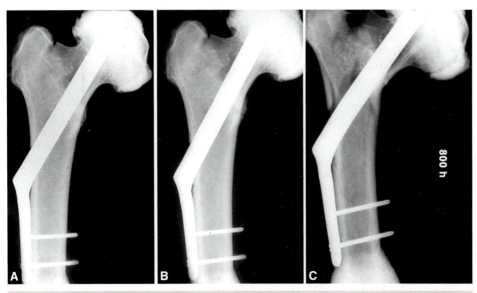

FIGS 65.6A TO C

(A) An anatomically reduced intertrochanteric fracture nailed with a 150 degree angle I-beam nail. The nail itself has a 250 pound yield point. (B) Six-hundred pounds of vertical loading had not produced any changes in the relationship between the fragments. (C) When 800 pounds of pressure were applied the femur broke and the nail cut superiorly

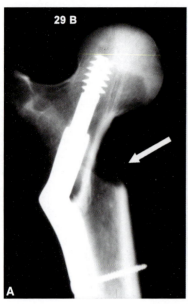

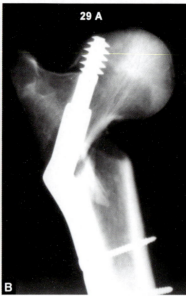

FIGS 65.7A AND B
(A) Illustration of a fracture where contact between the medial cortices of the two major fragments is not present. (B) When subjected to vertical loading a relatively minor vertical loading brought about a collapse of the fracture

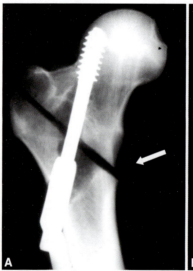

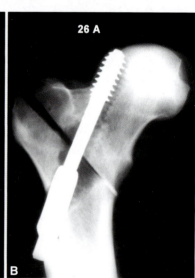

FIGS 65.8A AND B
(A) The imperfect contact between the medial cortices. (B) The gap disappeared under vertical loading but the nail cut out of the head superiorly

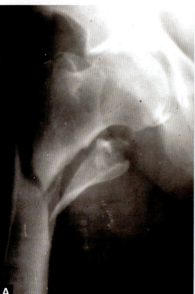

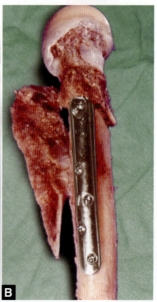

FIGS 65.9A AND B
(A) Radiograph of vertical unstable fracture. (B) The patient expired shortly after surgery. Notice the large size of the fragment that contains the lesser trochanter

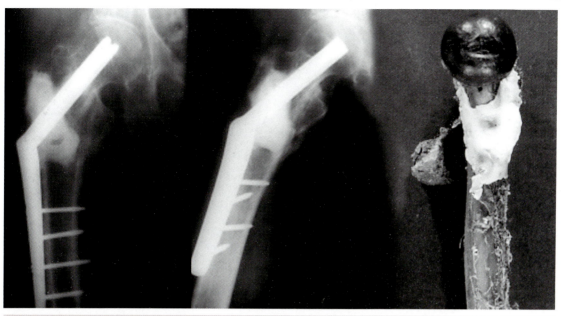

FIG. 65.10

In very elderly and minimally active patients who show severe osteoporosis and anticipated short-term survival, fracture stability may be obtained with acrylic cement. However, such a procedure often prevents fracture healing

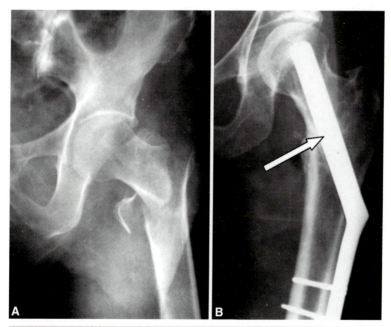

A

B

FIGS 65.11A AND B

(A) Once reduced, the fracture becomes stable, as the cortical wall of the fragments become in contact with each other. Protected weight-bearing ambulation does not result in displacement of the fragments. (B) The fracture healed uneventfully

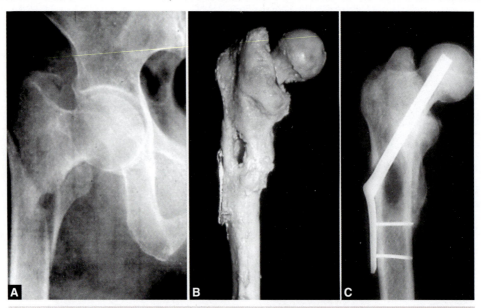

FIGS 65.12A TO C

(A) Radiograph of a comminuted intertrochanteric fracture. (B and C) Photographs of the retrieved femur obtained six months after surgery, and radiograph of the specimen. The patient had expired from heart failure. Notice the adequate medial contact between the two major fragments; the feature that rendered the fracture stable

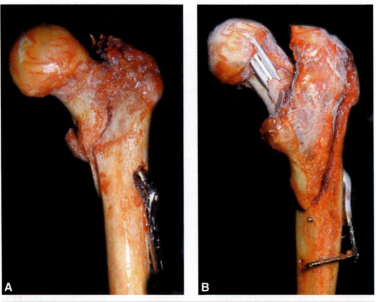

FIGS 65.13A AND B

Specimens of surgically made stable intertrochanteric fracture. The nail, however, cut through the neck of the femur and the most distal screw did not engage the femoral cortex

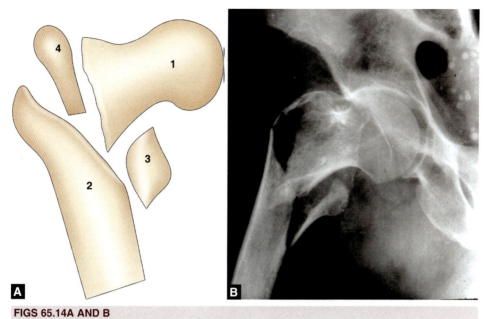

FIGS 65.14A AND B

(A) Schematic drawing of the four-fragment fracture which is frequently an unstable mode due to comminution of the medial cortices. (B) Same as A

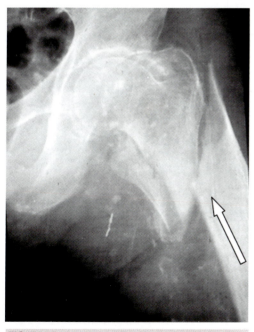

FIG. 65.15

Vertical, slightly comminuted intertrochanteric fracture, which even if reduced anatomically remains unstable because of the high shearing stresses at the fracture site

The I-beam design of a nail guarantees that the nail would not break under weight bearing stresses. *In addition, its configuration provides better rotational stability than the three-flanged nail.* We learned, however, that an I-beam nail does not cut into the hard bone of the femoral head without difficulty, and in the process produce separation between the major fragments. This is why the I-beam nail was modified by retaining the I-beam configuration throughout, minus the most proximal one inch. This one inch of metal was shaped in a T-beam fashion (Figs 65.22A and B). The improvement made surgery easier, the impaction of the major fragments more convenient, while retaining strength and providing additional rotary control

It is usually believed that the proximal end of the nail should be deep into the femoral head and posteriorly. The deep placement engages a greater area of hard bone, above the softer area, called the Ward's triangle. *The concept that posterior placement of the nail in the femoral is desirable lacks documentation. Studies have demonstrated the head is homogeneously dense therefore the stability provided by the tip end of the nail is the same regardless of its location in the head.*

However, the nail should be placed, contrary to popular belief, anteriorly in the neck of the femur, at the level of the fracture. Such a recommendation is based on the fact that during weight bearing, in addition to vertical loading at the fracture site, there are also rotational forces of great magnitude. During the swing phase of

cortical bone is obtained, with or without an osteotomy, a sliding mechanism is not necessary, since cortical bone does provides the necessary stability. The sliding nail is preferable when there is separation between the major fragments is present and some sliding brings about eventual cortical contact without excessive shortening.

Section 3

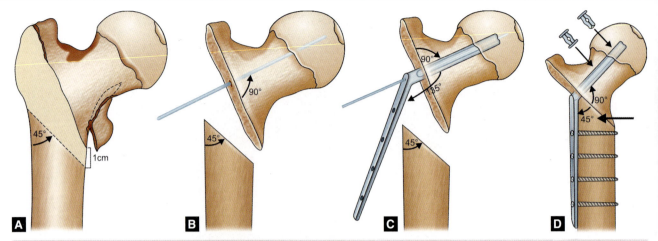

FIGS 65.16A TO D

(A) The femur is osteotomized at a 45 degree angle with its apex terminating one centimeter below the end of the proximal fragment. This one centimeter prevents making the leg too long. (B) The bony segment is excised or displaced and a K wire is driven into the neck and head of the femur entering at a 90 degree angle. (C) Then a 135 degree angle nail is driven over the wire into the neck of the femur. (D) The plate portion of the nail is brought down until contact between the two medial cortexes is obtained

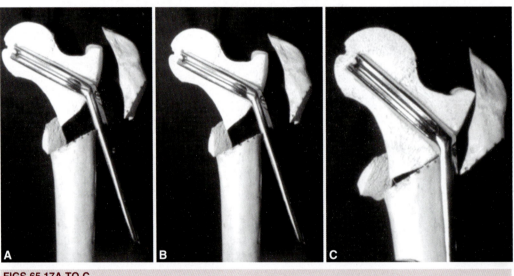

FIGS 65.17A TO C

Same as previous figure

gait the hip rotates internally, however, at heel impact the forces are of an external rotation nature. This means the mail is forced to displace anteriorly. If the nail, at the level of the fracture is already leaning against the anterior cortex of both fragments, displacement of the nail is prevented. If placed away from the anterior wall, it would have to travel a long distance before reaching a stable support from the anterior cortices. It must be kept in mind that, sometimes, by the time the nail has displaced in the femoral neck, the vertical forces would have already produced an axial collapse of the fragments (Figs 65.23A to C).

We never see patients with acute, displaced femoral neck fractures of the femur present to us with X-rays demonstrating a valgus deformity. They all have a varus deformity. Muscular forces working on the fragments must cause the deformity. I had always believed the teaching promulgated in textbooks that were popular in my early career, that is, the varus was produced by the contraction of gluteus medius and minimus. The two muscles, attached to the greater trochanter displace the proximal fragment superiorly without an opposing force.

One day, while observing patients with such fractures, I noticed, as I tried to move the fractured extremity, that the motion least painful was that of additional adduction. The most painful one was abduction. I reasoned that if the two gluteal muscles

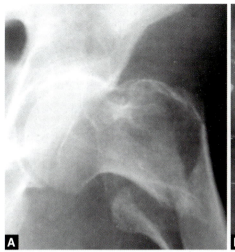
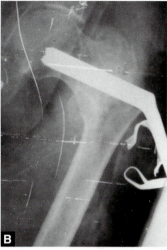
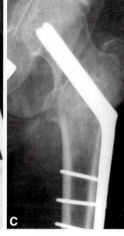

FIGS 65.18A TO C

(A) Intertrochanteric fracture treated with a valgus osteotomy. (B) The position of the nail into the femoral head is confirmed. (C) The completed nailing procedure shows the close contact of the medial cortices of the two main fragments and the less vertical nature of the fracture

FIGS 65.19A TO C

(A) Illustration of an intertrochanteric fracture. (B) The osteotomy was made transverse making the extremity too long. (C) The fracture healed uneventfully

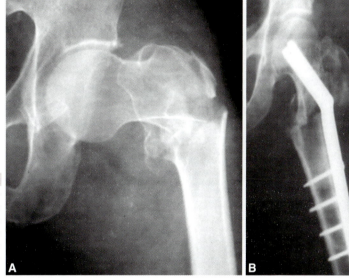
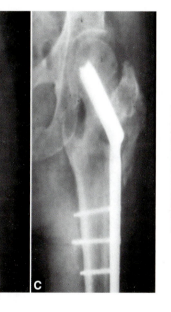

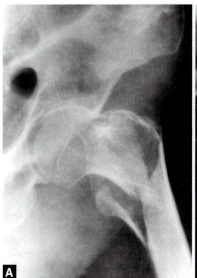
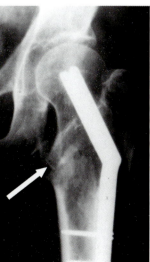
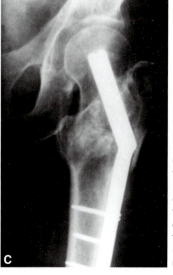

FIGS 65.20A TO C

(A) Vertical, unstable, comminuted intertrochanteric fracture. (B) Appropriately performed valgus osteotomy, that made the fracture less vertical and created contact between the two major fragments. (C) The fracture healed uneventfully

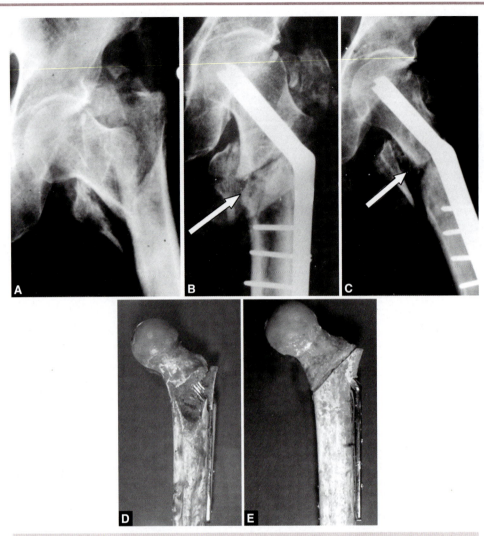

FIGS 65.21A TO E

(A) Unstable, comminuted, vertical intertrochanteric fracture. (B) Anteroposterior radiograph illustrating the conversion of the fracture into a less vertical one. The medial cortices of the two major fragments were brought into contact, making the fracture stable. (C) Lateral radiograph illustrating the contact between the two major fragments. (D) Radiograph showing the relationship between the fragments. (E) The patient expired two weeks after surgery. The posterior view of the proximal femur illustrates the large defect created by the detached lesser trochanter. The front view of the femoral specimen showing the contact between the two major fragments

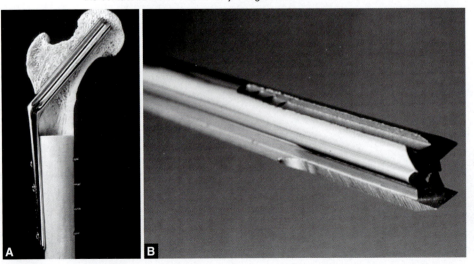

FIGS 65.22A AND B

(A) The I-beam nail. (B) was modified to make its most proximal end shaped as a T beam. This modification results in providing greater rotational stability and an easier introduction of the nail into a dense femoral head

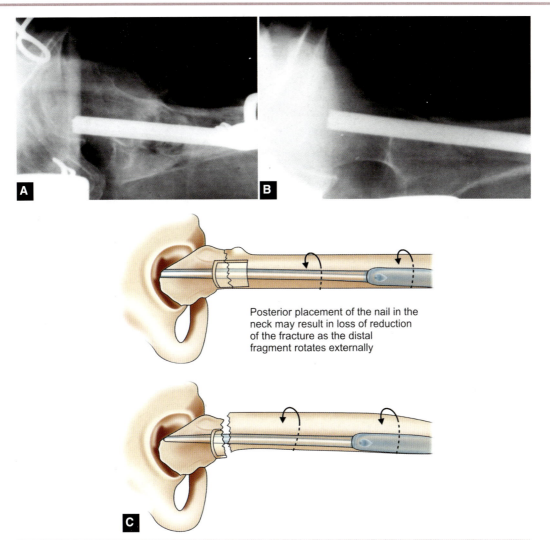

FIGS 65.23A TO C

(A) Illustration of the nail placed posteriorly in the neck and head of the femur. This placement is commonly believed to be the ideal one. However, I suspect it is best if the nail is in contact with the anterior wall at the level of the fracture since the external rotation stresses at the fracture site encourage anterior rather than posterior displacement of the nail. (B) The placement of the nail against the anterior wall of the femur, at the level of the fracture, precludes its anterior displacement from external rotation forces. (C) Illustration depicting the manner in which the posteriorly placed nail permits external rotation forces to displaced the nail anteriorly

were pulling on the greater trochanter additional adduction would be met with resistance and create more pain. The opposite was the case.

I decided then to carryout electromyographic studies. We placed EMG needles into the adductors, abductors, knee extensors and hamstrings. We did not try to study the iliopsoas muscle, first because it would have been difficult to identity with certainty, and secondly, because its possible deforming force was annulled by its frequent separation from the two major fragments of the fracture, in the case of the intertrochanteric fracture.

The EMG studies indicated that contrary to the traditional belief the abductor muscles were silent during the acute stages, but the adductors were in a state of spasticity that lasted until the pain subsided many days later. *In essence, we had mistakenly assumed that the gluteal muscles were responsible for the ubiquitous varus deformity. They are innocent bystanders in the production of the deformity.* The varus deformity seen in femoral neck and intertrochanteric fractures is due to contracture of the adductor musculature rather than from the pull of the "unopposed" abductor mechanism (Fig. 65.24).

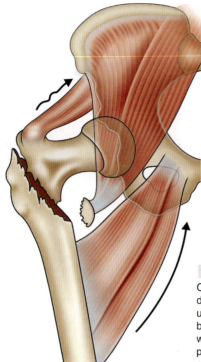

FIG. 65.24

Contrary to popular belief the typical varus deformities that fractures of the proximal femur usually experience, this deformity is created by the strong pull of the adductor muscles which are in a state of spasticity during the painful stages of the condition, rather than that of the abductors, which remain in a state of relaxation for a considerable period of time

References*

2, 5, 6, 7, 9, 13, 14, 16, 18, 26, 29, 38, 41, 49, 53, 79, 110

Section 3

_____

* References provided at the end of the book after annexures.

66

Interlocking Intramedullary Nail

Closed interlocking fixation of femoral shaft and metaphyseal fractures of the femur has proven a most effective method of treatment. Though open intramedullary nailing of the femur has been part of the armamentarium of the orthopedist for more than half a century, the method was limited to diaphyseal fractures. Metaphyseal fractures, because of the sudden enlargement of the medullary canal at this level, precluded its successful use. The use of interlocking nails for the subtrochanteric and intertrochanteric regions, has been also proven to be efficacious.

The same principles I have enunciated in the discussion of nail-plate fixation of intertrochanteric fractures also apply to intramedullary nailing (Figs 66.1A and B). That is, *intrinsic stability of fractures is obtained only if there is contact between the cortices of the two major fragments (Fig. 66.2)*. In the case of the closed intramedullary nailing, however, a stable reduction is less critical in determining the final outcome. However, the introduction of immediate weight bearing ambulation is likely to result in loss of fixation with either breakage of the nail or migration of the nail (Figs 66.3A and B).

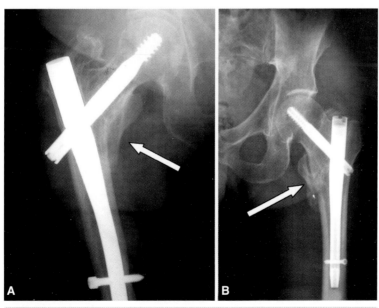

FIGS 66.1A AND B

Appropriate interlocking nailing of intertrochanteric fractures demonstrating approximation of the medial cortices

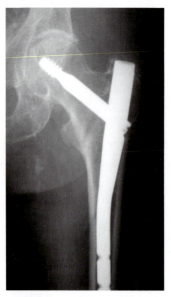

FIG. 66.2

The interlocking nail works very well for most intertrochanteric fractures. However, it requires the reapproximation of the medial cortices of both major fragments. It the absence of bony stability, the stresses are transferred to the nail making possible its proximal migration. Example of intertrochanteric fracture made stable by the reduction of the medial cortices

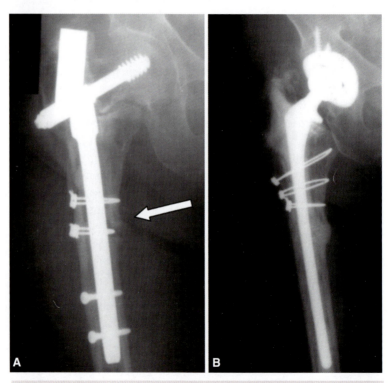

FIGS 66.3A AND B

(A) Failed interlocking fixation of intertrochanteric fracture. The nail broke and the fracture did not unite. Notice the second fracture in the proximal third of the femur. (B) The condition was treated with a cemented total hip arthroplasty

References*

38, 45, 49, 53, 79, 123

* References provided at the end of the book after annexures.

67

Subtrochanteric Fractures

The subtrochanteric fracture of the femur is less frequent than the femoral neck and intertrochanteric fractures. It occurs more frequently in younger people and it is usually the result of injuries of greater magnitude. Prior to the introduction of internal fixation, these fractures were routinely treated in traction. *Attempts to treat this fracture with braces proved unsuccessful because a varus deformity readily developed upon the introduction of weight bearing stresses.*

Experiences with nail-plate appliances in the care of these fractures have been disappointing due to the fact that in a number of instances the nails have either broken, bent or the screws broke, allowing the plate to separate from the femur (Figs 67.1 to 67.3).

Currently the intramedullary nail is the most popular and acceptable method of treatment (Figs 67.4A to C). However, immediate full-weight bearing may lead to complications, such as breakage or bending of the nail

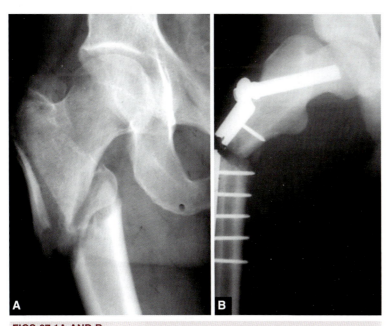

FIGS 67.1A AND B

Subtrochanteric fracture with comminution of the proximal fragment. This feature makes the fracture very unstable. Its fixation with a nail-plate combination often results in loss of fixation or breakage of the nail or plate

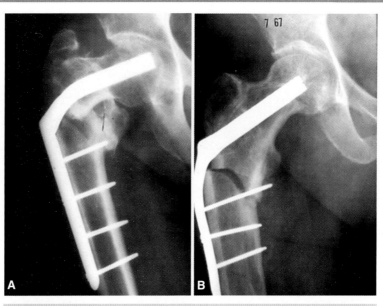

FIGS 67.2A AND B

(A) Illustration of a bent nail produced by the high stresses to which the nail is subjected when bone contact between the major fragments is not obtained prior to the introduction of the nail into the neck and head of the femur. (B) Despite the approximation of the medial cortex of the two major fragments the plate portion of the nail-plate bent upon the initiation of weight-bearing ambulation

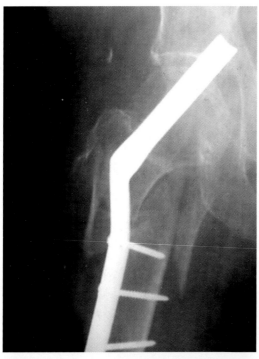

FIG. 67.3

Nail-plate appliances are usually not appropriate in the treatment of subtrochanteric fractures. The stresses on the metallic implant are very significant, leading to breakage or bending of the plate, or to avulsion of the screws

between the two major fragments. The metallic implant alone cannot, under those circumstances, always tolerate the enormous forces at the fracture site that accompany unprotected ambulation.

The subtrochanteric fracture serves as a good example to support my view that the varus deformity that develops in all displaced fractures of the proximal femur is not the result of unopposed muscular forces from the contraction of the abductor musculature, but from the contraction of the powerful adductor muscles. We documented by means of electromyography that during the painful period that follows a fracture, the abductor muscles are silent, while the adductor are in a constant state of spasticity. Obviously, when ambulation is introduced, the greater weight bearing forces become the major deforming forces (see *Intertrochanteric Fractures*).

Complete reliance on the stability provided by the proximal and distal interlocking screws oftentimes proves to be unwise. The screws brake from the enormous weight bearing forces transferred to them.

Though internal fixation is currently the treatment of choice, there are regions of the world where modern technology is not available. Traction remains the only available method of treatment. Many use external fixation, a less expensive method, effectively. A permanent residual varus deformity is often encountered, but it is usually due to insufficient traction or its premature discontinuance (Figs 67.5A and B).

or interlocking screws as well as fractures of the femur below the distal end of the nail when there is comminution that precludes adequate cortical contact

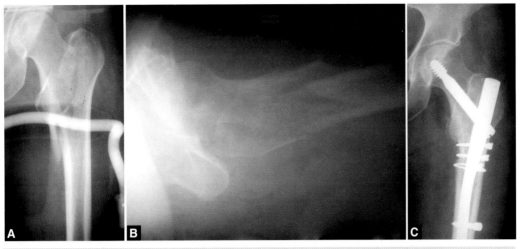

FIGS 67.4A TO C

(A and B) Radiographs of comminuted subtrochanteric fracture of the femur. (C) The fracture was treated with closed intramedullary-interlocking nail. Because of the comminution and the resulting lack of sufficient contact between the two major fragments, circular wires were used to reinforce the fixation. The fracture healed uneventfully. Interlocking nailing has proven to be a most effective method of treatment, providing some degree of initial mechanical stability can be obtained. (*Courtesy:* Jack Cooper, MD)

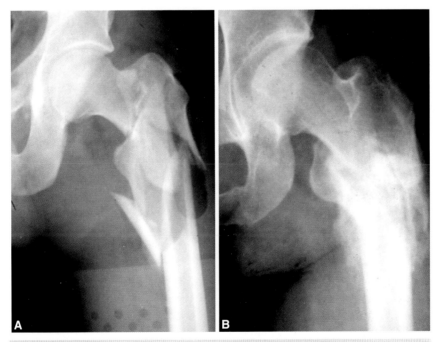

FIGS 67.5A AND B

(A) Comminuted fracture with intertrochanteric and base of the neck components. (B) Due to severe medical complications, surgery was not performed in this instance. The fracture was treated successfully with traction and bedrest

*References**

2, 4, 5, 6, 7, 8, 9, 13, 18, 25, 27, 29, 38, 45, 49, 53, 79, 123

_____

* References provided at the end of the book after annexures.

68

Femoral Head Fractures

Fractures of the femoral head are not very common. A busy trauma center may see no more than a couple every year. Trauma to the hip is more likely to produce a fracture of the neck or metaphysis of the femur, dislocate the joint or fracture the acetabulum or pelvis. When a fracture of the head occurs the prognosis is guarded. The possibility of avascular necrosis becomes very real. With more sophisticated diagnostic imaging tools we will soon be able to determine immediately whether the head is viable or not. At this time we are still obligated to institute for some type of traditional treatment.

Pipkin described the various types of femoral fractures and clearly demonstrated that his Type 4, the one that has the smaller fragments, carries the worst prognosis. Currently, many surgeons consider primary prosthetic replacement the treatment of choice. I agree there are many situations when such an approach is the most rational. However, treating the young in that manner may expose them to the complications that accompany endoprosthetic arthroplasty. The use of a bipolar prosthesis in preference to a traditional prosthesis is not the answer. *As a matter of fact, I think, the bipolar prosthesis is more likely to produce more serious complications. Polyethylene debris from this implant can produce very serious and extensive lysis in the surrounding bony structures* (See *Bi-polar Prostheses*).

Many years ago, I had an opportunity to treat a patient with a Pipkin 4 fracture-dislocation of the femoral head. My attempts to obtain a closed reduction of the dislocated head were unsuccessful. I found it necessary to do an open reduction. Rather than performing a prosthetic replacement I elected to carry out an anatomical reduction of the fragments and to maintain the reduction with metallic screws. I temporarily removed the proximal fragment and created a "trap-door"- like defect on the articular surface of the free articular fragment, as far as I could from the superior dome, into which I partially threaded a screw. I placed another screw at the insertion site of the excised ligamentum teres. This was done under direct vision while the free fragment was on the Mayo table. I then reduced the fracture anatomically and twisted the screws deep into the femoral head (Figs 68.1A to C).

The patient did very well for eight years, when arthritic changes developed necessitating replacement arthroplasty. It is interesting to note that microscopic examination of the removed femoral head specimen did not show evidence of avascular necrosis. The changes observed were those of osteoarthritis. A phenomenon similar to what I observed following synovectomy and partial capsulectomy in osteo-arthritic hips (See *Capsulectomy*).

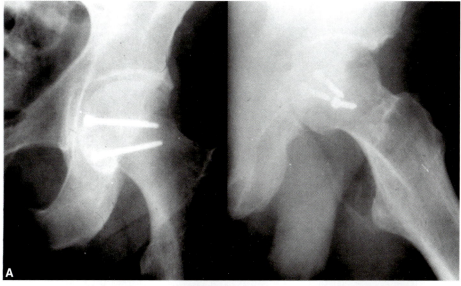

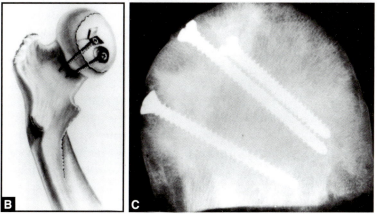

FIGS 68.1A TO C

(A and B) Radiographs of a fracture of the femoral head. The fracture had been openly reduced and stabilized with two screws. (C) Drawing illustrating the placement of the screws. The fracture healed uneventfully and for a period of eight years the patient was relatively asymptomatic. The femoral specimen did not show evidence of avascular necrosis. Notice the virtual disappearance of articular cartilage

References*

12, 105, 123

---

* References provided at the end of the book after annexures.

69

The Femoral Neck Fracture

In 1973, I was invited by Marshal Urist, then editor of Clinical Orthopedics, to serve as editor of a volume devoted of the fractured hip. I recruited some of the best known people to contribute to the issue. Upon reviewing the material I had received, I asked myself how much better off were patients today as a result of advances made in recent years. During my introduction to the edition I remarked, "I cannot help but experience disappointment as I realized that the management and the results obtained from the treatment for these injuries were not significantly better from those of 40 years ago."

Today, 35 years later, I am tempted to say that the same can be said about the lack of progress between that day and today. I fail to see any progress. However, I should limit my criticism to only the femoral neck fracture, because the treatment of the intertrochanteric and subtrochanteric fractures have experienced notable improvements, thanks to the popularization of the closed interlocking intramedullary nail.

It is ironic, however, that had I been better informed in 1973, I would have acknowledged that the closed interlocking operation was already popular in Germany. Kuntscher, from Hamburg, had, during the Second World War, developed a number of different interlocking nails for the treatment of metaphyseal and diaphyseal femoral fractures. My visit to his hospital in 1978 gave me the opportunity to see his museum and to admire his enormous contributions to the field.

Currently, closed interlocking nailing of femoral fractures is a well established method of treatment in virtually all countries of the world, except in those where the financial resources are still very limited.

Progress in the care of femoral neck fractures continues to move at a snail pace. I wonder if there is anyone who seriously believes that today we have a clearer understanding of the factors that may lead to nonunion or avascular necrosis than we did fifty years ago. This in spite of the enormous contribution made in imaging technology and other fields. We still use either Pauwels' or Garner's criteria for their classification, and have accepted the fact that the greater the displacement of the fragments and the more vertical the fracture the worse the prognosis. Then, we debate whether the fracture should be nailed or the head of the femur be replaced with an endoprosthesis, a bipolar prosthesis or a total hip arthroplasty (Figs 69.1 to 69.5).

In the past, some believed that all fractures of the neck of the femur should be nailed. Austin T. Moore, in very persuasive terms stated, "Reduce them well, fix them well and they get well". No one believes that any longer, in spite of the strong evidence presented by the zealous advocates of internal fixation. We have learned that obtaining anatomical reduction of the fracture by closed methods is difficult to achieve and often unsuccessful. That open reduction does not yield better results, and no matter how perfect the reduction is, or what type of internal fixation is used, avascular necrosis frequently takes place, with reports indicating an average of 26%. Reduction in valgus, a technique made popular in the 1960's, eventually lost favor in the orthopedic community. In addition, the need to protect the fracture from full-weight bearing is almost impossible in the older age group. These patients are either incapable of walking without bearing full weight on the extremity, or their memory span is too short to remember the prescribed precautions.

It is commonly believed that avascular necrosis is the result of the sudden severance of the retinacular

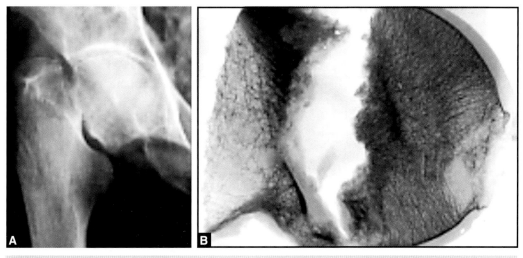

FIGS 69.1A AND B

(A) Radiograph of typical fracture of the femoral neck showing the angle of inclination of the fracture and the varus deformity. The varus deformity, contrary to popular belief, is the result of spastic contracture of the adductor muscles, not the "unopposed abductors". (B) Radiograph of the proximal femur illustrating the irregular nature of the fracture. This is a photograph of the femoral head of the Holy Roman Emperor Charles, given to me by the distinguished Czech surgeon, Ian Bartonicek

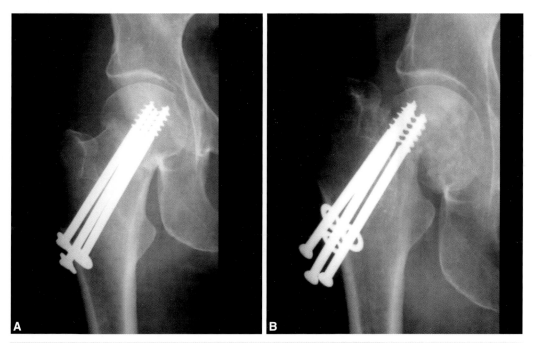

FIGS 69.2A AND B

(A) A radiograph of a well-reduced and appropriately nailed vertical fracture of the femoral neck. (B) Within a few days after the onset of ambulation, the fragments are displaced

vessels at the time of the injury. There is some evidence to suggest that tearing of those important vessels does not always occur. Bach, from Germany, demonstrated in experimental animals, *that the vessels are simply kinked as the femoral shaft displaces superiorly, and in that manner the blood supply of the femoral head fragment is rendered avascular.* If this theory is valid, it should be logical to extrapolate that a displaced fracture of the femoral neck should be reduced as soon as possible to restore circulation through the critical vessels. Others, like Smith, from Oregon, have said that it is the *rotation of the fragments that produces the stoppage of circulation.* Others insist that tamponade, brought about by the intracapsular bleeding, is the culprit.

All these hypotheses indicate that if vascular complications are to be avoided, early reduction of the fracture, aspiration of the joint, and fixation of the fracture are the important steps to be taken. However, there is no data to strongly support them. Perhaps, it is out of frustration that most orthopedists prefer to use endoprosthetic replacement as the initial method of treatment. This treatment, although very effective in many instances, is not a panacea. Many patients never regain the ability to ambulate without pain in spite of satisfactory X-ray pictures. *Loosening of the implant and boring of the femoral prosthesis into the acetabulum are common complications* (See *Endoprostheses*).

In the case of the nondisplaced femoral neck fracture (Figs 69.3A to C), it is also commonly accepted that nailing should be done in order to prevent subsequent displacement. Though there is merit in this argument, I suspect that such a practice is not always necessary. I have seen a number of patients, including my own mother, who recovered well without surgery, after been told to use crutches or a walker for a few weeks. I have come to believe that in the management of nondisplaced, valgus, impacted femoral neck fractures, the severity of pain and its progression can help in determining the need for surgery. If the pain seems to decrease in a few days, chances are that the fragments will not displace. If the amount of pain increases, displacement is likely to occur. In this latter instance, nailing should be done early. However, I would not recommend that approach. Nailing of prosthetic replacement is better.

I am not sure that there are any advantages for the use of the bipolar prosthesis over the traditional monopolar Austin Moore prosthesis. I have no strong feelings whether these implants should be cemented. Relatively very few elderly patients end-up requiring revision to total hip arthroplasty (Figs 69.5A to F); either because they do not live very long after the initial surgery or the symptoms are not severe enough to justify surgery. We must be cognizant of the fact that the one-year mortality following femoral neck fractures is approximately 50%. In the younger patient with displaced femoral neck fractures, I believe, internal fixation is the treatment of choice. I prefer multiple pins to a single screw. The multiple pins must be placed peripherally in order to attain the greatest degree of rotary stability. Some

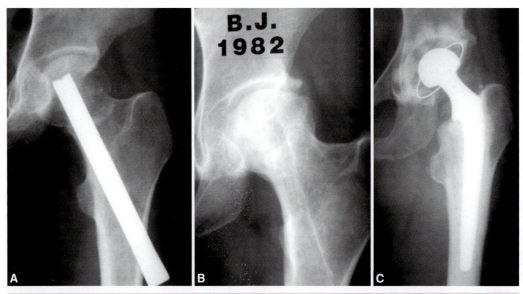

FIGS 69.3A TO C

(A) Radiograph of nailed fracture of the femoral neck in a 34-year-old woman. The fracture was allegedly of the nondisplaced type. (B) Radiographs obtained prior to hip replacement demonstrating avascular necrosis. (C) Radiographs obtained six years postsurgery

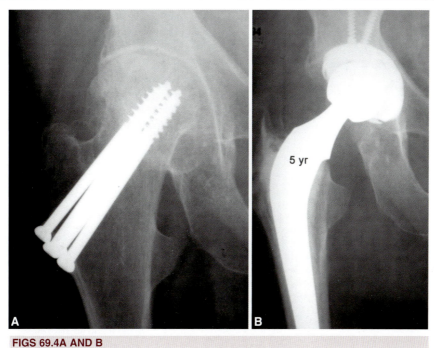

FIGS 69.4A AND B
(A) Radiograph of osteoarthritic hip following a fracture of the femoral neck in a 65-year-old woman. (B) Radiograph obtained 5 years after revision with a total hip titanium prosthesis with a cobalt/chrome prosthetic head

investigators have found no difference in the results according to the type of fixation.

I will now share with the readers an observation perhaps worthy of consideration. In many instances I have noticed that in the process of removing the femoral head in order to insert an endoprosthesis or a total hip implant, difficulties are encountered as a result of a strong ligamentum teres, requiring its section with a sharp instrument. Observation of the severed ligament often shows mild bleeding. This observation runs contrary to the popular belief that after completion of growth the blood supply coming through the ligament ceases to exist. In addition, I have noticed that when the prosthetic replacement is done for the treatment of osteoarthritis, particular if it is advanced, in the overwhelming majority of instances, the ligamentum teres is no longer a barrier to the removal or the femoral head. As a matter of fact, quite often it is no longer present.

These observations beg the question as to whether there is relationship between the underlying arthritic process and the condition of the ligamentum teres. What comes first, the chicken or the egg? Is there a connection between the two entities? Does the damage of the ligament contribute to the arthritic process or the arthritic process brings about damage to the ligament? Although of no practical importance, a scientific answer would be welcome.

In closing the subject of femoral neck fractures, I summarize by saying that a radical and realistic approach to this fracture is necessary in response to the proven high failure of fixation, and more importantly, the fact that the mortality rate is approximately 50% at one year after surgery. That being the case, why don't we approach this fracture in the elderly by performing a primary total hip replacement, using an inexpensive self-constrained prosthesis, preferable of the type that does not require the separate implantation of the acetabulum and femoral components, as in the case of the now defunct Zivash prosthesis. In this manner the need for protection against weight bearing can be eliminated.

Section 3

Section 3

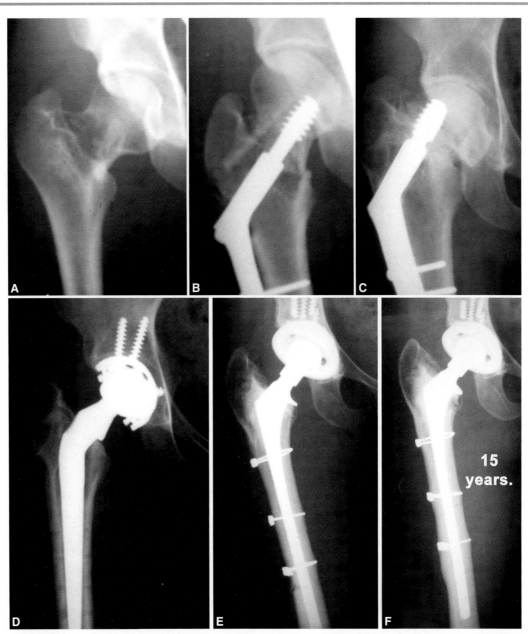

FIGS 69.5A TO F

(A) Radiograph of subcapital fracture of the right femur of in a 25-year-old woman. (B) The fracture was treated with a sliding nail, allegedly after open reduction. (C) The fragments displaced within a few months and a diagnosis of avascular necrosis was made. (D) The condition was apparently treated with a noncemented total hip prosthesis which within two years became painful and loose. The acetabular screws broke. (E and F) A revision arthroplasty consisted of a cemented stem that required the creation of a window to remove the cement, and a noncemented acetabulum. Radiographs obtained eight months and fifteen years postoperatively. The hip has remained asymptomatic

*References**

122, 123

_____

* References provided at the end of the book after annexures.

70

Nonunion of Femoral Neck Fractures

Why is it that avascular necrosis is so common following femoral neck fractures? The usual explanation that I received in my training days has not changed: "The blood supply of the head is permanently damaged at the time of the injury". This gospel-truth has gone relatively unchallenged for generations, apparently without any serious desire to question its scientific validity.

I suspect that in various degrees, various "theories" plays a role in the onset of avascular necrosis. To what extent, if any, still remains unknown to us. It is a sad commentary that despite the sophistication of contemporary techniques such as the MRI, we still remain in the dark, leading to the defeatist mechanical attitude that now governs the care of these fractures.

There are a number of observations that should interest those who wonder why nonunion and avascular necrosis of the femoral head is so common. One is the fact that if one observes the appearance to the femoral head of displaced fracture, which is never reduced and pinned, the fracture obviously never heals. *Even though the head is avascular, it never collapses, and fails to show any of the radiological changes characteristic of avascular necrosis.* If the fracture had been reduced and stabilized, eventually demonstrates the collapse of the head along with the other characteristic features of AVN. *One must conclude that in the absence of compression of the femoral head and without the circulation still present in the distal fragment*

trying to revascularize the head, collapse of the femoral head does not occur (See *Avascular Necrosis*).

There are very few alternatives at this time for the treatment of nonunion of femoral neck fractures. Part of the problem is that in many instance the problems is not limited to lack of union but also to the presence of avascular necrosis. Surgical procedures aimed at obtaining union frequently fail, necessitating at a later date a more definitive procedure, which at this time is a total hip replacement. Nonetheless, efforts should be made to create union through biological means, such as nonvascularized or vascularized bone grafts in the case of the younger individual. I doubt it makes much sense to treat in that manner a nonunited femoral neck fracture in an elderly person. A properly performed total hip arthroplasty is the treatment of choice. Figures 70.1A to E is an example of a vertical, displaced fracture of the femoral neck.

James Urbaniak, from Duke University, has reported most interesting and encouraging observation regarding the use of vascularized fibular grafts in the care of avascular necrosis, whether of a traumatic origin or idiopathic in nature. Despite his reported good results in many instances, the technique has not gained the popularity it deserves. This can probably be partially explained on the technical requirement of the procedure and the general attitude in the orthopedic community regarding procedures that do not provide immediate good results. The grafting

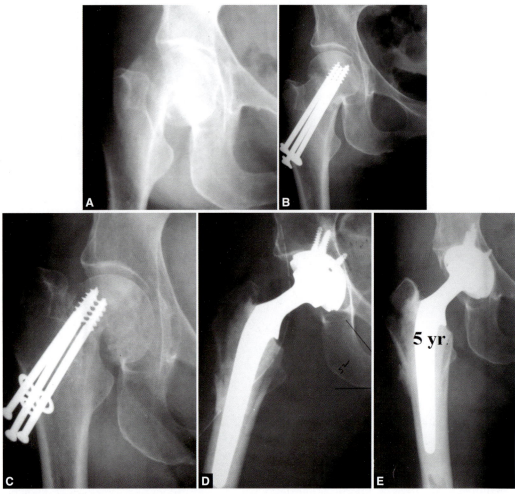

FIGS 70.1A TO E

(A) Vertical, displaced fracture of the femoral neck. (B) Radiograph of the well-reduced and nailed fracture. (C) Within 2 months the fragments displaced. (D and E) Radiographs of hybrid replacement arthroplasty obtained shortly after surgery and five-year later

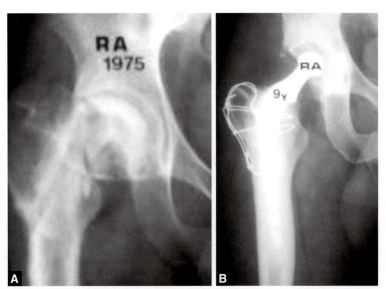

FIGS 70.2A AND B

(A) Ununited fracture of the femoral neck in a 25-year-old man, who had first an unsuccessful pinning of the fracture and secondly a bone grafting procedure. The fracture did not heal. (B) A Charnley prosthesis was used to solve the problem. The procedure was successfull, however, 15 years later the acetabulum had to be revised, and 10 years later the acetabulum and femoral components were subjected to revision

procedure (Figs 70.2A and B) requires a rather long period of observation and a period of protected weight bearing ambulation (See *Avascular Necrosis*).

Osteotomies of various types, designed to modify the impacting forces at the nonunion sites, have not met wide success, despite the logic behind their rationale. They are difficult to perform and not many surgeons possess the skill to carry out the procedure in the desirable way. I had an opportunity to observe Reinhold Ganz in Berne, Switzerland, perform an osteotomy through a nonunited femoral neck fracture in a minimum amount of time and with a precision it would have been impossible for me to display (See *Femoral Osteotomies*).

References*

10, 19, 122

---

* References provided at the end of the book after annexures.

71

Femoral Endoprostheses

Austin Moore's initial experiences with his endoprosthesis were limited to degenerative and neoplastic conditions. As a matter of fact, the first procedure he performed with Harold Bohlman, from Baltimore, was for the management of a malignant giant cell tumor. It was not until later that Moore began to use the prosthesis for the care of unstable femoral neck fractures.

He believed, and rightly so, that the technique for inserting a prosthesis had to be precise and he did not believe in short cuts. The fit of the ball in the acetabulum had to be as perfect as possible. He said, however, that a tight fit was better than a loose one. I wonder how he would feel about that today, when we claim to have so much more knowledge about cartilage's response to friction and pressure. Perhaps his views would have been reinforced. The stem had to fit tightly into the canal, and the collar of the prosthesis rest squarely on the medial cortex of the femur (Figs 71.1A to D).

I was his senior resident when he realized how important was the contact of the prosthesis against the cortical wall of the femur. He, then went to work on the design of his new implant. He determined the various prosthetic sizes by using cadaver specimens in the morgue and filling the femoral medullary canals with "putty". We split the femur and the rubbery "prostheses" were removed, packed and sent to the Austenal Company in New York. Austenal later became Howmedica.

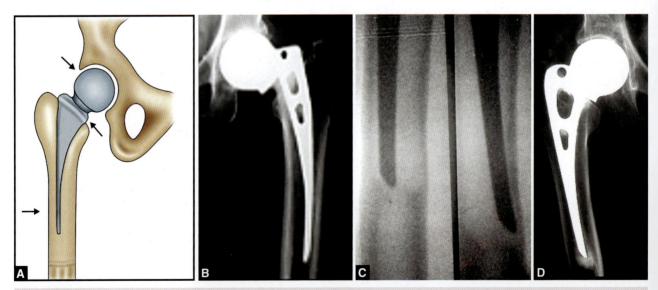

FIGS 71.1A TO D

(A and B) Schematic drawing of an original Austin Moore endoprosthesis suggesting the appropriate fit of the head into the acetabulum; the sitting of the neck of the prosthesis on the femoral neck; and the abutment of the stem against the lateral femoral cortex. These basic concepts have been abandoned in preference for a tight fit of the stem in the canal throughout its entire length. (C) Radiographs of a grossly loose endoprosthesis taken during abduction of the limb and at rest. (D) Characteristic sclerosis and lysis seen in loose endoprosthesis

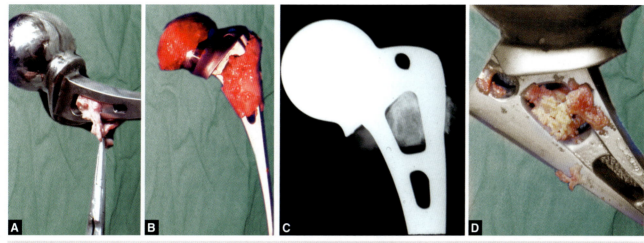

FIGS 71.2A TO D

(A) In grossly loose endoprostheses fibrous connective tissue frequently fill the fenestrations. (B) Thick membrane that formed in the acetabulum and proximal femur in a loose endoprosthesis. (C) New bone that grew into the fenestration on an Austin Moore prosthesis. Rarely is the fenestration completely filled with bone that renders the implant stable. Most often the filling is incomplete allowing "rotation" of the implant. Notice the cortical structure of the bone in its periphery. (D) Bone that grows into the fenestrations of the prosthesis rarely filling the space completely

It has been said that the window in the Austin More prosthesis is there because there was no manufacturing capability to avoid it. This is not true. Austin Moore conceived the idea of the fenestrations as part of his conviction that the new bony bridge, made possible by the window in the metal, would make the implant "part of the living body". *Many years later, I personally studied the quality of the bone that forms in the fenestration and was disappointed to find out that the fenestration, though usually filled with bone, very often has a rather thick membrane separating the bone from the metal.* The thickness of the membrane reached several millimeters in some instances, making the removal of the implant very difficult; often more difficult than removal of an implant where a thick and hard bony bridge has formed. Only on a very few occasions have I seen the fenestration filled completely with bone (Figs 71.2A to D).

I also noticed after examining a large number of post-operative specimens that *motion between the prosthesis and the bone takes place primarily in a rotary plane.* Antero-superior and medial-lateral forces do not always demonstrate motion unless the loosening of the implant is gross. A similar mode of failure has been identified in total hip implants (Fig. 71.3).

Boring of the prosthesis into the acetabulum is commonly seen, and it is claimed to be cause of failure in many instances. It has been assumed that such a phenomenon is due to the difference in the hardness of the acetabulum and that of the prosthesis. This mechanical explanation may be accurate but only to some extent. If the mechanical difference, as currently

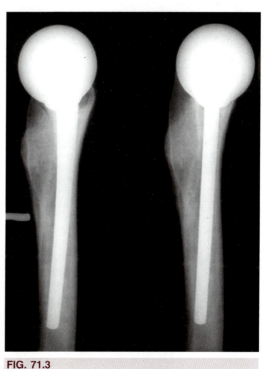

FIG. 71.3

Illustration of the rotational instability that is frequently identified in failed endoprostheses. Inspection during surgery of a loose prosthesis usually shows the bar of bone that has grown into the fenestration of the implant preventing its easy removal. The only motion that seems to be present in all instances is rotational instability. This phenomenon is also the most common mode of failure in total hip arthroplasties

proposed, is the simple and universal explanation for the boring of the implant, then we should see all endoprostheses fail through that mechanism. This is, however, not the case. Many implants have lasted many years without radiological changes on the acetabular side (Fig. 71.4).

I recently reviewed some of my remaining slides of successful endoprostheses and found evidence of large

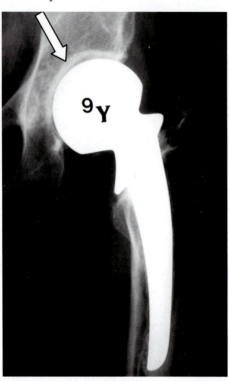

FIG. 71.4

Despite the fact boring of the prosthesis into the acetabulum is a very frequent development, there are instances when the joint space remains intact for many years

amounts of metal on the surface of the acetabulum (Figs 71.5A and B). *I suspect that some of the unusual cases of femoral lysis in the medullary canal are due to metal debris.* Metal debris without secondary polyethylene debris may be a cause of lysis, as we have been able to demonstrate in noncemented total hip arthroplasties. I have come to realize that our explanations for the failure of many endoprostheses was too cavalier; and that we, too quickly, concluded that mechanical conditions would easily explain the failures. Now that we have a much better understanding of the modes of failure of total hip implants, a fresh look at the failure of endoprostheses is desirable. *I suspect that lysis of the articular cartilage, produced by metal debris, is the reason for the boring of the implant into the acetabulum (Figs 71.5A and B). This thesis does not eliminate the role that the difference in the hardness of the two articulating surfaces plays.*

A decrease in the width of the joint space takes place usually in a gradual manner. If the decrease occurs within a short time after the initial implantation and the patient complains of groin pain, the chances are that there is an infection. *If groin pain, rather rapid narrowing of the joint space and heterotopic bone are seen, the diagnosis of a deep infection can be made with almost complete certainty..*

I have reviewed my personal experiences with endoprosthesis in the management of acute fractures as well as in various arthriditis. My reviews were conducted in my younger days without the critical,

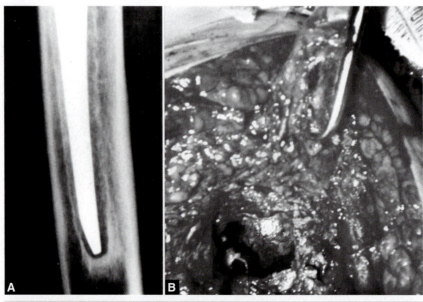

FIGS 71.5A AND B

(A) Lysis around the distal end of the prosthesis associated or created by the metal debris found in the area. (B) Darkened capsular tissues found in a failed endoprosthesis

Section 3

detailed information required in contemporary medical publications. In general, I believe that the procedure is a good one in the treatment of displaced fractures, particularly in the elderly. It is, however, far from being a panacea. Pain does not always disappear and radiological signs of failure are not uncommon. Many "failed" implants are not revised into total hip arthroplasty either because the patients get used to the imperfect joint or we, the surgeons, do not consider them to be suitable candidates for major surgery. Furthermore, the twelve-month mortality following fractures of the femoral neck in the elderly is very high.

Younger patients treated with endoprostheses often require a long period of time before being able to completely eliminate the thigh pain. Some times the pain never disappears and total hip replacement becomes necessary. I have seen, however, a number of patients who after six to nine months of persistent pain spontaneously find themselves free of pain. *Therefore, my practice is not to rush into total hip surgery until the patient has had a relatively long period of observation and protection from full weight bearing with the aid of external support.*

In view of the increasingly good results with noncemented arthroplasty, today I am inclined to perform primary total hip replacement in many patients with displaced, high femoral neck fractures. Further incursion into this area must be done carefully and abuse of the procedure must be prevented if at all possible (See *Femoral Neck Fractures*).

Patients, who receive endoprostheses for the treatment of arthritis or avascular necrosis, an approach common before the advent of total hip arthroplasty, did not do well in many instances. Osteoarthritics did better than rheumatoid arthritics or those suffering from avascular necrosis. A difference that has been identified with total hip treated patients as well (See *Age in Total Hip Surgery*).

The surgical technique used for the implantation of an endoprosthesis requires close attention to details. Good exposure of the head and neck is essential and the severance of the neck should be carried out at the appropriate level in order to avoid making the leg either too short or too long. The collar of the prosthesis must rest firmly on the cortical bone of the femoral neck. The stem should fit tightly against the femoral cortex throughout its entire length (Figs 71.6 to 71.11).

In removal of the membrane that inevitably forms around loose medullary components, it is essential that it be removed in its entirety (Figs 71.12A to C). This is not always easy

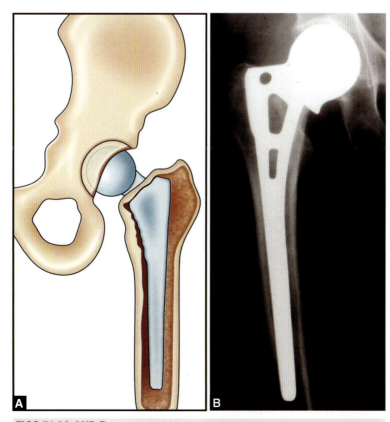

FIGS 71.6A AND B
The endoprosthesis must fit the canal as tightly as possible

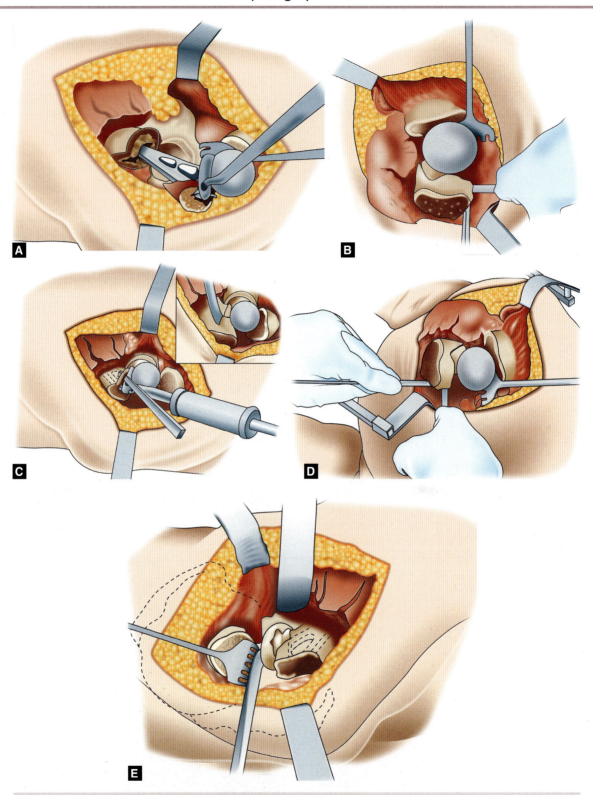

FIGS 71.7A TO E

(A) Since with some frequency the implant subsides into the medullary canal, it is important to ascertain that the greater trochanter is not fractured as the implant exists the canal. (B) Trochanteric osteotomy may be required if the sinking of the prosthesis into the canal is very significant, and attempts to withdraw the implant appear to compromise the integrity of the trochanter. (C) Once the trochanter is moved out of the way the prosthesis is removed. (D and E) Often the bone block that has formed into the fenestration of the prosthesis requires is severance with a thin osteotome introduced close to the metallic implant. Ironically, the difficulties in removing a prosthesis are greater when the fenestration is filled, not with bone, but with a very thick and rather inelastic band of fibrous tissue

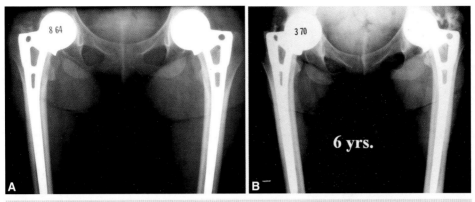

FIGS 71.8A AND B

(A) Bilateral endoprostheses performed for the care of osteoarthritis. (B) Radiograph obtained six years after surgery. The joint space was well preserved

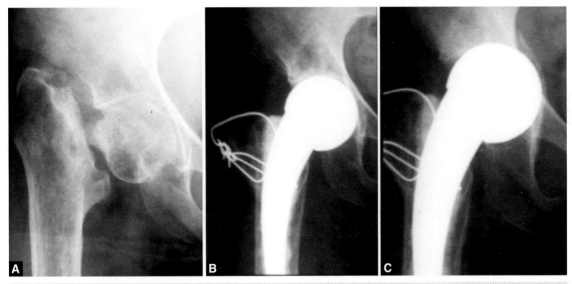

FIGS 71.9A TO C

Typical boring of the prosthetic implant into the acetabulum which is more likely to occur in a rapid fashion when the procedure is performed for a chronic condition

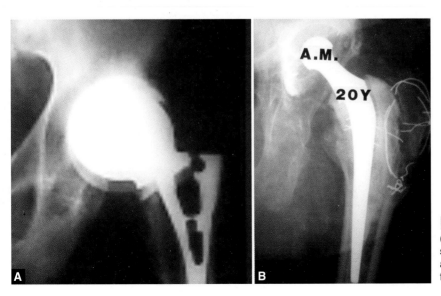

FIGS 71.10A AND B

(A) Superimposed radiographs showing the superior boring of the prosthetic head into the acetabulum. (B) Radiograph obtained 20 years following Charnley arthroplasty

Section 3

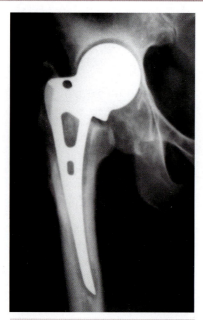

FIG. 71.11

Lytic lesion at the tip end of a prosthesis associated with lysis of the acetabulum characteristic of acute infection

to do. Many times the membrane comes out as a unit when the canal is rasped forcefully. Most of the time, however, it comes in pieces. When I discuss thus issue with residents, I say to them, *"rasp until that you are convinced no more membrane has been left behind; then, start all over again"*.

The membrane left behind will preclude the necessary fixation of the new implant, whether cemented or non-cement. This is probably the reason as to why the results of total hip, when performed for the failure of an arthroplasty, are inferior. One can use the same logic when considering infection following revision into a total hip, thinking that the bacteria form the membrane that contained the bacteria (See *Infection*).

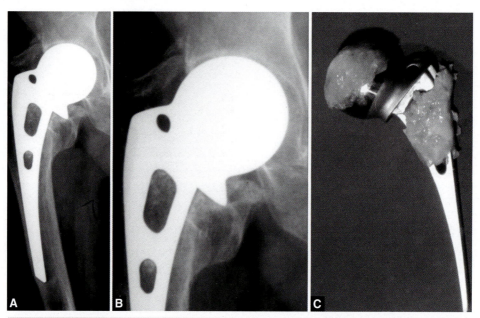

FIGS 71.12A TO C

(A and B) Radiographs of failed painful endoprosthesis demonstrating the narrowing of the joint space; the distal windshield of the prosthesis; and the thinning of the cortex distally. (C) Photo of the thick membrane that had formed around the femoral stem and in the acetabulum. Though gram-stains were negative at the time of surgery, subsequent cultures demonstrated low-grade infection. The patient was kept on intravenous antibiotics for six months. No later infection developed

*References**

1, 3, 10, 19, 26, 32, 34, 43, 60, 61, 66, 90, 103

_____

* References provided at the end of the book after annexures.

72

Bipolar Prostheses

Bipolar prostheses have been popular for at least 30 years and have been used primarily in the treatment of sub-capital fractures of the femoral neck and avascular necrosis in the younger age patient. Some have reported on their successful experiences with the implant in cases of osteoarthritis and for the salvage of failed total hip arthroplasty. My experiences have been mixed. In general, however, I have grown dissatisfied with many of the results. Motion between the articulating surfaces cannot be maintained, suggesting that the advantage of the bipolar concept is rapidly negated. More importantly however, is the fact that I have witnessed a few times very aggressive acetabular osteolysis, particularly in young patients. This is not difficult to understand since the amount of polyethylene debris is higher than from the traditional polyethylene-metal total hip arthroplasty.

Microscopic examination of the debris found in failed bipolar prostheses almost consistently demonstrates polyethylene debris, usually in great amounts (Figs 72.1A to D). The diagnosis of polyethylene debris-induced failure can often be recognized by the development of a large radiolucent space between the metallic cup and the bone rather than the narrowing of the joint space seen in non-bipolar implants. The fact that on occasion metal debris is also found in combination with plastic debris gives credence to my belief that endoprostheses often fail from biological damage to the bony acetabulum and medullary canal created by metal debris (See *Endoprostheses*).

It is likely that my less than enthusiastic interest in bipolar prostheses (Figs 72.2 to 72.4) is due to failure of the femoral component due to its loosening in the medullary canal. However, acetabular changes were also encountered when using noncemented components.

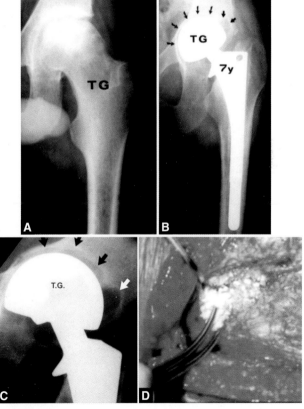

FIGS 72.1A TO D

(A) Radiograph of avascular necrosis of the femoral head. (B and C) Radiographs taken four years later showing medial migration of the cup, and a widened space between the metal cup and the acetabulum. (D) Polyethylene debris filled the space at the bottom of the acetabulum. This is not an infrequent finding in failed bipolar prostheses

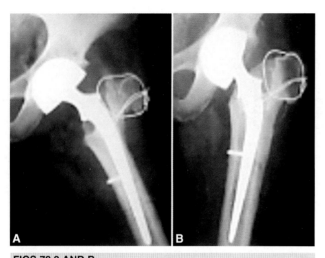

FIGS 72.2 AND B

(A) A Charnley bipolar prosthesis. (B) The cup tilted into valgus and the hip failed

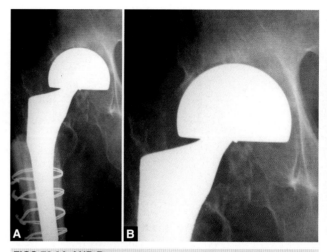

FIGS 72.3A AND B

Radiographs of a bipolar prosthesis that migrated superiorly within a short period of time. An infection was suspected, but ruled out after open inspection of the joint and cultures of the bone and surrounding tissues

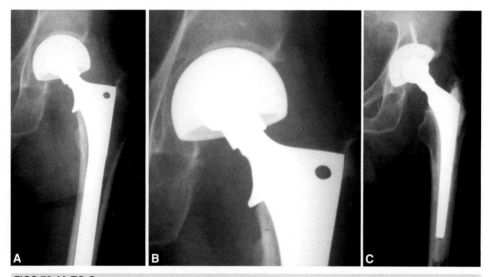

FIGS 72.4A TO C

(A and B) Radiograph of a bipolar prosthesis in a 58-year-old diabetic man. Notice the preservation of the joint space. (C) The hip was revised because of persistence of pain. Radiographs taken three and five years postoperatively

*References**

5, 10, 19, 20, 37, 38, 45, 52, 61, 66, 71, 72

---

* References provided at the end of the book after annexures.

73

Primary Total Hip

Despite the overall progress that has taken place in a multitude of musculoskeletal conditions the fracture of the femoral neck has defied significant healthy change. I suspect the prognosis from the surgical treatment of the displaced varus femoral neck fracture is not a great deal better today than that of fifty years ago. Nonunion and avascular necrosis have remained ubiquitous.

Nailing of these fractures by conventional means or with associated osteotomy or sliding nails of various types have not brought about major improvements. Curtailment of weight bearing after surgery is still required to prevent collapse of the approximated fragments. In addition, such curtailment is often unrealistic, since most elderly patients are not capable of ambulating, bearing no weight on the operated extremity, or if capable of doing so, their shortened memory span precludes the sustaining of such curtailment.

Endoprosthetic replacement appeared a while to be the answer to the problems associated with nailing techniques. However, new problems ensued. Dislocation of the prosthesis due to alleged lack of cooperation from this group of patents was a factor. Loosening of the implant and boring of the metallic head into the bony acetabulum, resulting in pain, were other unhealthy factors.

In-hospital mortality from hip fractures remains high despite the fact that anesthetic and internal medicine advances have reduced it. The death rate during the first postoperative years, though also smaller, is still high. It is likely that further improvement along this line will take place. The patients' age and the natural degenerative diseases that accompany advance age will continue to perpetuate the current problems. While these intractable problems continue to stymie progress in the war against femoral neck fractures, the results from the treatment of arthritic conditions of the hip by means of total hip arthroplasty has been spectacular.

Displaced fractures of the femoral neck in the elderly are, and will continue to be the "unsolved fracture". Further attempts to solve the problem by developing "new and improved" nails will be an exercise in futility. Therefore, a new approach is justifiable. Pretending that perseverance will eventually pay, no longer stands to reason. It is as suggesting that warm compresses can prevent the rupture of an infected appendix.

I suggest that primary total hip arthroplasty should be the treatment of choice for these fractures in the elderly, and perhaps also in the not-so-elderly patient. This approach would virtually eliminate the problems of nonunion and fixation loss, and would permit unprotected weight bearing ambulation immediately after surgery. The dislocation problem could be eliminated by the use of an implant with a constrained acetabulum.

Militating against this approach is the cost of the implant, which at this time is unreasonable high. A commitment made by the manufacturing companies to develop such a prosthesis to be sold at a reasonable price would guarantee wide acceptance of this treatment modality throughout the entire orthopedic profession, as well as among the hospital systems.

*Reference**

---

* Reference provided at the end of the book after annexures.

74

Rehabilitation

Since the vast majority of patients that sustain fractures of the hip are elderly, their rehabilitation may be difficult at times. Fractures of the acetabulum, on the other hand, occur more frequently in the younger age group. A great deal of objectivity is necessary while determining the most appropriate rehabilitation in both groups.

Internal fixation of virtually all hip fractures is the modern standard of care in affluent countries throughout the world. It must be kept in mind that those countries constitute a minority. Nonsurgical methods of treatment still are the only possible option for millions of people. The mortality and complication rates are staggering.

Modern techniques and metallurgical developments have made possible very early and effective rehabilitation of the hip-traumatized patient. It is unfortunate that segments of the orthopedic community have not looked seriously at the issue of rehabilitation of the patient recovering from surgery performed for the care of a hip fracture. The orthopedist performs the surgery most appropriate for a given fracture, and then turns the rehabilitation care of the patient to physical therapist, who in many instances is not aware of the type of procedure performed. At best, the therapist reads a note on the patient's chart recommending that no weight bearing on the operated leg be permitted, or that the amount of weight should be minimal or partial. Furthermore, since the meaningful close academic relationship between orthopedics and physical therapy that existed a couple of decades ago ceased to exist, most physical therapists have minimal or no knowledge of the various fractures and treatments in use. This unawareness precludes a logical individualized approach to rehabilitation.

The idea that a physician specialized in Physical Medicine should be the one to instruct the therapist regarding the modalities used to rehabilitate these patients is not the answer. They are not trained in orthopedics; have never operated on a fracture and are not knowledgeable in the biomechanics of fracture fixation or joint replacement. Therefore, it should be the surgeon who must assume the responsibility for discussing with the therapist the rehabilitation protocol most appropriate for the specific fracture.

Little attention is paid to the fact that the forces transferred to the hip joint from the simple task of lifting the leg in order to get out of bed are identical to the ones experienced during partial weight-bearing ambulation. That being the case, why the attempts to teach a technique that has no practical or physiological value? Add to this the routine practice of patients in rehabilitation units being subjected to muscle strengthening exercises following an internal fixation procedure, an endoprosthetic replacement or a total hip arthroplasty. Why the strengthening exercises? Resumption of ambulation a day or two after surgery will spontaneously restore within a short period of time the strength that may have been lost from the trauma of surgery.

Since at this time, the surgical procedures used in the care of fractures of the femoral neck are limited to either nailing or endoprosthetic replacement, a likely complication following surgery is dislocation when a prosthesis is used. It should be kept in mind that if the surgical approach was an anterior one, the dislocation occurs when the hip joint reaches high degrees of flexion and external rotation. The opposite is true when the posterior approach was use, in which case the dislocation happens when the hip is adducted and internal rotation, particularly if flexion of the hip is introduced.

My awareness of the difficulties encountered in the rehabilitation of the elderly patient with a surgically treated fracture of the femoral neck has led me to conclude that serious consideration should be given to the possibility of making primary total hip replacement the preferred method of treatment. A total hip implant of the self-constrained style would allow patients so treated to bear full weight on the operated leg from the very outset, and transfer from bed to chair without the fear of dislocation.

A limitation to the method is the fact that at this time the cost of a self-constrained prosthesis is ridiculously high, making the procedure very expensive. The likely reduction in the length of hospitalization may not offset the higher cost of the implant. If the implant manufacturing industry were to produce such implants at a reasonable cost, the proposed approach could become a beneficial one. Using bigger head prostheses might help reduce the number of dislocations. However, it would not be the answer. Dislocation following Moore endoprostheses still occurs, even though the prosthetic head are very big.

Another possible complication from hip surgery in the case of the traumatized patient is thromboembolic disease. This topic has been greatly exaggerated to the point that most orthopedists believe that if expensive chemical prophylaxis is not used and thromboembolic disease appears, he or she is subject to malpractice litigation. There is ample evidence in the literature to demonstrate that in the case of total hip arthroplasty, inexpensive prophylactic is more effective and less expensive. My own experience with the use of aspirin and exercises has shown a mortality rate of 0.1% and the incidence of bleeding virtually nonexistent. (See *Thromboembolic Disease*).

References*

3, 5, 6, 10, 82, 92, 99, 102, 106, 109,117

---

* References provided at the end of the book after annexures.

Section 4

Annexures

75

Joint Replacement Registries—The Hurdles Ahead

Fueled by the alleged success of Scandinavian Joint Replacement Registries, interest in the subject in several countries has experienced a crescendo in the recent past. It appears that in the opinion of some, joint replacement registries will settle the many controversies besetting the field by establishing reliable criteria that will chart and guide the future of joint surgery. This radical view might, on the other hand, unintentionally create a system likely to compromise progress.

Despite the attractiveness of joint replacement registries and my sincere desire to see them become a reality, I am of the opinion that there are a number of concerns about their likely success, which, appears to me, have not been addressed as carefully as their need be. Among them are: (1) The credibility of the information submitted to the main repository and, therefore, the subsequent final conclusions; (2) The role the implant manufacturing industry will play in their unfolding.

I will not allow unrewarding personal experiences with orthopedic registries cloud my views, as I realize those experiences took place at a time when the sophistication of computer communications were still in their relative infancy. Nonetheless, I briefly share them with the readers because they might shed some light on the subject at hand.

During my chairmanship of the AAOS Committee on Injuries in 1976 I proposed the establishment of a National Fracture Registry. The Board of Directors approved the project and provided financial support for a pilot study limited to femoral fractures. A handful of major teaching hospitals scattered across the land were to participate in the study. After a very short time it became apparent that the information submitted to the central computer was frequently flawed. I requested the termination of the project.

Shortly afterwards, while serving as president of the Hip Society for two consecutive years, I made the creation of a Hip Registry the centerpiece of my administration. Despite the fact the fellowship at that time was probably no larger than 30 orthopedists I failed to persuade the group of the benefits of a registry. A computer expert met with the Society's fellowship and tried to convince them of the feasibility of the project. He failed in his objective. For a while I felt the reluctance of some members to go along with the idea was the fear they had of losing their already established systems of documentation. This, despite the fact they were assured it was indeed not a possibility. Now I realize that their vision was probably better than mine. They anticipated problems which I had dismissed rather cavalierly.

Just a few years later, Clement Sledge, as newly elected president of the Hip Society, revived the idea and tried to make the registry a reality. He also failed after his efforts to have NIH (National Institutes of Health) fund the project proved futile.

More recently, The AAOS has embarked on a similar endeavor, which has been welcomed with great enthusiasm in some quarters. It is about this venture, and similar ones, that I have reservations, which if not properly addressed at an early state might result in bitter disappointment at the end.

In order to illustrate my concerns, I create several potential scenarios and raise some questions.

1. The Scandinavian joint registries, which have engendered support to the creation of similar registries, have reported data on a relatively small number of implants; definitely smaller than the American registry would require, since the number of different hip joint implants used in the United States is estimated to be over three hundred.

    It has been stated that the Scandinavian Registry has dramatically reduced the number of complications with certain implants, and has cut in half the revision rate of total hip arthroplasties. I doubt the claim that such reduction was solely due to information produced by the registry. It is hard to believe that the literature had failed to report on those complications long before the Registry displayed its findings.

    The Scandinavian countries are smaller and disciplined. Medicine operates under a socialist-like system conducive to the success of registries, since universal or near universal participation is not difficult to achieve. In the United States its more capitalist Laissez-Faire system of healthcare delivery does not permit enforced participation, creating in that manner obstacles the Scandinavians have not experienced. How does the American Registry, and similar registries, propose to overcome this major hurdle? What plans do registries, facing this potential problem, have to obtain broad participation by the thousands of orthopedic surgeons and hospitals throughout the nation? If efforts to gain greater involvement fail, will the project be terminated or be limited to a relatively small number of participants? In this case-scenario, it is likely that a relatively small number of major hospitals and clinics with available funding and already established documentation facilities will constitute the ones feeding data into the registry.

Will this lopsided composition appropriately reflect the status of joint replacement surgery in the general orthopedic community? Since the cost of operating a registry is expensive and time consuming, wide participation is not likely to occur in many nations.

2. The veracity of the data submitted to registries is the seminal and most important issue in the entire subject. To assume every participating surgeon and institution will adhere to high ethical and professional standards is extremely naïve. Will unscrupulous surgeons "and there are some" with their own prostheses generating to them millions of dollars, and others within the same category receiving large kickbacks from industry for using or marketing certain implants, be tempted to provide embellished and false information on successes and failures? How do the registries propose to prevent or deal with this potential scenario? The ongoing investigation of the relationship between orthopedists and industry by the United Sates Justice Department, has already documented the growing degree of wide-spread loss of professionalism in our ranks. Though the number of individuals committing the infractions may be relatively small, many of them are well-known individuals whose influence should not be underestimated.[3,5,6] Greater credibility will be given to pronouncements made by registries, since many readers will assume that these organized institutions are exempt from such flaws. Rather than questioning the accuracy of registries publications, their conclusions will become fiats difficult to challenge once they acquire the odor of sanctity that frequently accompany correct and incorrect dogmas.[2,6]

3. It is reported that the registries provide early warnings regarding trends suggestive of increased risk of failure with various techniques and implants. Will their mechanism of reporting be more effective and expeditious than the existing publications in medical journals, or through presentations at various meetings? Even if it is true "which I doubt" that registries announce complications at an earlier date, I suspect that there will be times when premature disclosure of trends may do more harm than good.

    During the past thirty years, we have witnessed the birth of a number of hip and knee prostheses that because of failures in the hands of some surgeons were soon discredited and many of them removed from the marketplace. That was the fate of unicondylar knee implants, metal-on-metal total hip prostheses, surface replacement arthroplasties, total ankle prostheses and ceramic implants. The orthopedic community learned about the failure rate of those implants through published reports in peer-reviewed journals and from formal presentations at scientific meetings.

Now, many years later, many of these originally discredited concepts are in vogue and some of them quite successfully. What would have happened if registries had been in existence at that time? I assume that if registries had made public the initial alleged bad results, it would have been tantamount to permanent commendation that would have made it very difficult for the original investigators, or their successor, to embark in the development of better implants. In other words, can we extrapolate that registries could unwillingly stymie progress and research?

4. Whether we wish to admit it or not, it is likely that the implant manufacturing industry will do its very best to influence the development and conduct of registries. Because the high cost of running them, financial support from industry will be considered essential by some. If and when industry begins to play a role, how do the registries propose to establish boundaries of involvement to prevent the eventual take-over of the project, in the same manner that industry succeeded in gaining major control of the education of the orthopedist through its almost universal subsidy of continuing education? Some might argue that this scenario can be prevented by marketing surveillance and adherence to Codes of Ethics. However, Codes of Ethics, frequently updated, are ignored by many. The number of ethical violations committed in our profession today is many times greater than three or four decades ago when such codes were documents deeply stapled in the original foundations of the discipline.[1,4,6]

Based on the above concerns and the reality of the current situation, what are the real problems the joint replacement registries attempt to solve? Don't we have enough journals and scientific meetings to make us aware of early failures and successes of implants as it is? Could new methods of publication be established to bring forth on a regular basis summaries of recent data regarding complications and trends of perceived importance?

The leaders of some joint replacement registries are upbeat about the project. However, a precipitous approach to their implementing may not bring about the anticipated results. A sober assessment of a grand narrative would allow them to move forward in a manner more likely to bring success.

I suggest that existing not-for-profit groups, currently studying the results from various documentation centers in a serious and practical manner, be encouraged to continue their work with additional support from the orthopedic community. We should expect them to eventually render a verdict either favorable or unfavorable to formal Joint Replacement Registries.

References

1. Callahan D, Wasumma A. Medicine and the Market. John Hopkins 2006.
2. Carr AJ. Which Research is to be believed? J Bone and Joint Surgery 87B, 2006.
3. Christie C. Five companies in hip and knee replacement industry avoid prosecution by agreeing to compliance rules and monitoring. Public Affairs 2008.
4. Cruess R. Sylvia Cruess. Teaching Medicine as a Profession on the service of Healing. Academic Medicine, 1997;72(11):941-53.
5. Sarmiento A. Medicine and Industry: The Payer, the Piper and the Tune. Royal Canadian Annals of Medicine 2000;33(3):144-9.
6. Sarmiento A. Medicine Challenged. PublishAmerica 2008.

References*

17, 75, 83, 84, 85, 90, 93

Section 4

76

The Hip Society

Having been one of the 20 Founding Members of the Hip Society in 1968 and President of the organization for a two-year period in the 1970s has, hopefully, given me an opportunity to observe its evolution and reach certain conclusions regarding its past, conduct and its possible future. I was further benefited by the fact that for over a six-year period of time I served as the Historian of the Society. My close association with the International Hip Society, where I also was a founding member, has given me additional understanding of the evolution and accomplishments of both organizations.

My loyalty to the organizations has not kept me from being a critic of many of the actions the organization. I have felt that the groups, particularly the American Hip Society, have squandered valuable opportunities and have lacked vision. The Society has failed to be as encompassing in its scope as it should have been. For all practical purposes it addresses only prosthetic replacement of degenerative diseases, while ignoring congenital, developmental and traumatic conditions of the hip. To too great an extent the Society has served simply as a social club where oftentimes a number of self-appointed experts indulge in promoting their new "gadgets" and market their names.

At the annual meeting of the Society in San Francisco in 2004, I gave my report to the assembled group in which I expressed concerns regarding the manner in which the Society had functioned and suggested that changes needed to be made in order to ensure its viability.

A year later my tenure as historian came to an end. I took advantage of the opportunity to summarize my experiences, and once again, warn the fellowship about the growth of unsavory developments that continued to creep into the organization.

These are the written reports I gave at the 2004 and 2005 meetings of the Society in San Francisco and Washington DC respectively.

Report to the Hip Society

(From the Historian: Augusto Sarmiento, MD. San Francisco, CA March, 2004).

Following my election to historian for the Hip Society, I contacted my predecessor requesting any pertinent records. None existed. The role of the historian had been, and has remained for all practical purposes, limited to the reading the names of members of the Society that had expired in the previous six months. The position of "historian" needs to be modified or simply eliminated. I believe it should be preserved. Therefore, as a first step in that direction, I present to the Society an incomplete and brief summary of the development and evolution of the organization over the past 36 years. At a later date, I will submit to the Society a better documented and dated report, provided I am successful in obtaining thus far missing information.

Since the role of a historian should not be limited to the recording of events, but should extent to an interpretation of events, I will present my personal views regarding the Society and will raise a few questions concerning its future viability and the direction it seems to pursue.

The History

Frank E Stinchfield, MD, then professor and chairman of the department of Orthopedics at Columbia University in New York City founded the Hip Society in 1968. The initial group consisted of 21 members. They were: Otto E Aufranc MD, William M Bickle MD, Walter P Blount MD, Mark B Coventry MD, Albert B Ferguson Jr MD, William H Harris, MD, William W Howe MD, Floyd H Jergesen MD, Richard C Johnston MD, Joe W King MD, Carroll B Larson MD, Mark G Lazansky MD, Irvin S Leinbach MD, J Vernon Luck MD, Emmett M Lunceford MD, Augusto Sarmiento MD, Howard B Shorbe MD, Frank E Stinchfield MD, Fred R Thompson MD, Marshall R Urist MD and Philip D Wilson Jr MD.

Only six members survive at this time: Philip D Wilson Jr MD from New York City, Albert B Ferguson Jr MD from Pittsburgh, Pennsylvania, William F Harris MD from Boston Massachusetts, Richard C Johnston MD from Iowa City, Iowa, Mark G Lazansky MD from New York City, and Augusto Sarmiento MD from Miami, Florida (See *list of past-presidents on addendum in the last page of this chapter*).

The Society held its first meeting in Boston in the Fall of 1968. It was a "closed meeting". A good portion of it was devoted to organizational matters; and all scientific presentations were made by local members of the Society. This tradition persisted for several years.

The first "open meeting" was held in conjunction with the AAOS's Annual meeting in Las Vegas in 1973. Sir John Charnley was the guest speaker. After 1973, the Closed Summer and the Open Winter meetings became permanent features; the "closed" one held at the home of the President; and the "open" one in conjunction with the annual meeting of the American Academy of Orthopedic Surgeons.

The closed summer meetings remained informal for several years, but gradually some formality was incorporated. Case presentations, which for sometime were an integral part of the program, were eliminated.

Three awards were established for the best studies dealing with clinical and laboratory investigations. They were identified as the John Charnley Award, the Frank E Stinchfield Award, and the Otto E Aufranc Award.

From 1973 through 1986 the proceeding of the open meetings of the Society were published in hardbound books. Subsequently, the proceeding have been incorporated into the prestigious journal *Clinical Orthopedics and Related Research.*

The initial by-laws of the Society were modified in 1976, and several of the current committees were established. In an attempt to diversify the society's membership a few orthopedists, whose interest included basic sciences and pediatric disabilities, were added to the roster of the society.

During the 1976 and 1977 efforts were made to establish a total hip registry. However, the project failed to generate enthusiasm and support among the then 23 members of the Society.

Initially, the content of the scientific presentations at the two annual meetings consisted primarily of topics dealing with congenital hip problems, developmental disorders, fractures of the hip and pelvis, hematogenous infections, avascular necrosis, mold arthroplasty, endoprosthetic replacement, hip fusion and the then newly introduced total hip replacement arthroplasty. Rapidly, the total hip topic became the main subject for discussion.

The scientific programs of the meetings of the Society during the past 36 years have changed minimally in their format. The presentations made by the Society's members as well as those delivered by the guest speakers have reflected the trends of the times. Ever since total hip replacement established itself as a most revolutionary development, it has dominated the activities of the Society. Initially, the discussions were held around the value of different designs of femoral stems: longer versus shorter stems, round versus square, elliptical, trapezoidal or triangular necks; implants with collars versus those without them; polished versus matted stems. For a short while laminar airflow systems took center stage.

At future meetings the transtrochanteric approach to the hip recommended by Charnley was challenged. The posterior and lateral approaches gained greater acceptance. The issue of dislocation was for a few years a major topic for discussion.

Occasional fractures of stainless-steel stems were reported. Other metals and alloys were then recommended and emphasis was placed in making the stems thicker and stiffer. One such stem was discussed, which was allegedly designed with the aid of the computer. At subsequent meetings it was acknowledge that it was so large that its implantation in human bones was often impossible.

Some recommended ceramics and metal-on-metal components. Others reported initial good results using titanium alloys. Reports submitted a few years later indicated that patients receiving those implants had a higher incidence of complications. Some argued that titanium alloys were contraindicated only with the use of cement while others insisted that it was a potentially harmful material regardless of the type of implant used.

The Charnley arthroplasty continued for several years to be acknowledged as the gold standard. The metal-on-metal designs, represented by the McKee-Farrar and Ring prostheses, retained a few followers.

Within a short time these systems ceased to be popular and were not discussed again for many years.

Similar debates took place over the most appropriate size of the prosthetic head: 22 versus 26, 28, 32, 45 mm. Several investigators presented their results with different diameter heads.

A frequent topic of discussion was thromboembolic disease, a complication frequently encountered following total hip arthroplasties that required prolonged bed rest. It was reported that this complication had been reduced as a result of better prophylaxis, but primarily by the realization that early postoperative mobilization was possible and desirable.

An Italian surgeon described a surface replacement implant that preserved the integrity of the medullary canal. A British surgeon and a few American orthopedists joined the trend and reported some initial encouraging results. However, the enthusiasm with the method decreased when the Europeans and several American surgeons encountered an early high failure rate.

Wear of the polyethylene socket received some attention, and the proposed solution to the problem was addressed primarily by modifications in the size of the prosthetic heads.

The recognition that the acetabular component was more likely to fail prompted the recommendation that the cement column around the plastic component should be reinforced with a metal shell. However, at subsequent meetings the technique was criticized and eventually abandoned.

Emphasis on the importance of proper introduction of cement into the medullary canal led to the description of "second and third generation cementing techniques". Guns of various types were illustrated as well as bone or plastic distal plugs. Pressurization was emphasized. According to some the viscosity of the cement was thought to be important. Low-viscosity cement was introduced. However, it was never discussed at future meetings. Precoated stems were discussed but the innovation ceased to be a topic at subsequent meetings.

The "discovery" of the "cement disease" provoked interesting discussions. The noncemented prosthesis was introduced and heralded as the final solution to all problems surrounding total hip surgery.

At later meetings the enthusiasm created by this novel approach to hip replacement was tempered by reports indicating an increase in the incidence of lysis. It was reported to occur more frequently with non-cemented prostheses.

Isoelastic implants, developed in Europe, were discussed. However, subsequent reports indicated that loosening and lysis were found in a high percentage of patients.

New techniques to ensure permanent fixation of the noncemented acetabular component were discussed, among them the screw-in cup, made of either metal or ceramic. The procedures were not debated at later meetings as alleged evidence showed a high failure rate.

In view of the apparent early failure of the non-cemented prosthesis to prevent bone lysis, the concept of a "hybrid" system was introduced. The non-cemented acetabular component would be preserved but the femoral component would be cemented. Subsequent reports with this approach were mixed. Some surgeons reported an increased incidence of femoral component loosening and increased acetabular wear.

In later years reports indicated significant improvements with noncemented prostheses. The length of the porous surface was thought to be important.

The use of hydroxyapatite to encourage bone ingrowth appeared to provide good mid-term results. Some argued that the initial good results were negated by the discovery of resorption and "fracture" of the coating material.

The genesis of femoral and acetabular lysis was a major topic for discussion for several years. The chemical and histological changes that take place around metal and plastic debris were reported. More recently, attention was also given to chromosomal abnormalities found in areas of metallosis.

As the number of failed arthroplasties increased, primarily as a result of bone lysis, emphasis was placed in developing techniques to salvage failed damaged structures. They were enthusiastically discussed, among them the bone impaction allograph technique. Some reported encouraging reports, while others encountered major difficulties and short-lived good results.

Periprosthetic femoral fractures were frequently discussed. Various techniques to overcome the problem were presented.

Occasional departures from the topic of total hip replacement have consisted primarily of discussions of acetabular osteotomies in the treatment of hip dysplasia and the role the acetabular labrum plays in the genesis of degenerative arthritis. Healthy discussions of this subject have been held in recent years.

At this time the topics occupying significant space in the Society's meetings have dealt with bearing surfaces, such as new polyethylenes, ceramics and metal-on-metal, and the benefits or disadvantages associated with the length of surgical incisions.

During its 36-year history, the Hip Society has not made any contributions that can be traced to its official activities. The progress made in the important arena of hip replacement has been the product of several individuals' independent efforts. Some exceptions must be acknowledged. One is the Society's effort to foster research among young investigators through awards for the best papers dealing with clinical and laboratory investigations. Another exception, though a questionable one, was the Society's failed attempts to develop a Total Hip Registry in the late 1970's and mid-1980's. The ongoing plan to resuscitate the project represents a concerted effort to identify the Society in this regard. Whether or not the proposed Registry proves to be viable and represents a significant contribution is yet to be known. I remain skeptic about its worth.

The Hip Society, by virtue of the popularity and impact of total hip arthroplasty, neglected other very important hip conditions. Neither trauma nor congenital or developmental diseases are discussed in a serious and frequent manner. In very recent years interest in the role of the acetabular labrum in the etiology of osteoarthritis has come forward, as well as the place of acetabular osteotomies in the management of hip dysplasia in the adult. These two items have received the attention of the Society's fellowship.

Society in general and our profession in particular are experiencing profound changes, the outcome of which can only be guessed. What has the Hip Society done, and what is it doing to seek involvement in addressing fundamental issues? None, I believe.

We are witnessing with great discomfort the loss of professionalism within the medical profession. What has the Society done to assist in the correction of the problem? We witness abuses in medicine in general, and know that the same is true in our own sub-discipline. Have we publicly, or even privately, acknowledged the abuse? Not at all. Quite the contrary, with our silence we seem to condone it. We accept, and even encourage, the distasteful practice of advertising private practices through various media, oftentimes in the most egregious and demeaning ways.

It is commonly known that some leading hip surgeons are criticized by the orthopedic community for being "money driven" and for frequently indulging in activities that reflect unprofessional conduct. For example, some hip surgeons advertise through tasteless testimonials from patients. Others make claims of success from techniques and products not yet proven efficacious. What about the obscene number of prosthetic implants that inundate the market (300 different total hip prostheses according to a Harvard report)? Some continuing education courses resemble Persian bazaars. And some surgeons accept "kick-backs" for the use of surgical implants.

The Hip Society impassively observes continuing education of the orthopedist falling under the control of the implant and pharmaceutical industries. Rather than reacting against this domination, the Society implicitly embraces the trend and collaborates with their plans.

We watch some members of our Society functioning as peddlers for pharmaceutical and implant manufacturing industries. Some of them performing as vendors of products in which they have vested commercial interests or simply benefiting financially from the "generosity" of their sponsoring concerns. Is that the response the Society should be giving? If that is case, are we demeaning the dignity of our profession and contributing to its eventual collapse as an ethical and professional entity?

In summary, I suggest that the Society make an effort to address other hip conditions with the same enthusiasm and passion it has displayed regarding total hip arthroplasty. Official cooperation with pediatric orthopedic surgeons, traumatologists and rheumatologists would open new and worthy opportunities.

I suggest the Society establish a mechanism that encourages the maintenance of high professional standards, not only by enforcing admission criteria that look carefully at the character of the individual and his record of professional and ethical conduct in his/her community. As I have observed the evolution of the society over the past 36 years, I sense that, until now, a most important criterion for membership has been the number of total hip replacements the candidate alleges to perform.

In addition, the Society should include in its constitution a mechanism to deal with members whose professional and ethical conduct is found to be inappropriate, allowing for reprimand, temporary suspension or expulsion.

I further suggest that the Hip Society accept the responsibility of including in its agenda discussion of and involvement in social, political and ethical issues

PAST PRESIDENTS OF THE HIP SOCIETY		
1. 1968-1969	William H Harris MD	Boston, MS
2. 1969-1970	Frank E Stinchfield MD	New York, NY
3. 1970-1971	Walter P Blount MD	Milwaukee, WI
4. 1971-1972	Albert B Ferguson MD	Pittsburgh, PA
5. 1972-1973	J Vernon Luck MD	Los Angeles, CA
6. 1973-1974	Mark B Coventry MD	Rochester, MN
7. 1974-1975 1975-1976	Emmett M Lunceford MD None	Columbia, SC
8. 1976-1977	Augusto Sarmiento MD	Miami, FL
9. 1977-1978	Augusto Sarmiento MD	Miami, FL
10. 1978-1979	Marshall R Urist MD	Los Angeles, CA
11. 1979-1980	Harlan C Amstutz MD	Los Angeles, CA
12. 1980-1981	Philip D Wilson Jr MD	New York, NY
13. 1981-1982	Richard C Johnston MD	Iowa City, IA
14. 1982-1983	Clement B Sledge MD	Boston, MA
15. 1983-1984	Floyd H Jergesen MD	San Francisco, CA
16. 1984-1985	C McCollister Evarts MD	Rochester, NY
17. 1985-1986	Jorge O Galante MD	Chicago, IL
18. 1986-1987	Lee H Riley Jr MD	Baltimore, MD
19. 1987-1988	William R Murray MD	San Francisco, CA
20. 1988-1989	Joe Miller MD	Montreal, Canada
21. 1989-1990	Donald McCollum MD	Durham, NC
22. 1990-1991	J Philip Nelson MD	Scottsdale, AZ
23. 1991-1992	Nas Eftekhar MD	New York, NY
24. 1992-1993	William Capello MD	Indianapolis, IN
25. 1993-1994	Robert Fitzgerald Jr MD	Detroit, MI
26. 1994-1995	Mark Lazansky MD	New York, NY
27. 1995-1996	Richard B Welch MD	San Francisco, CA
28. 1996-1997	Dennis K Collis MD	Eugene, OR
29. 1997-1998	Eduardo A Salvati MD	New York, NY
30. 1998-1999	Robert B Bourne MD	London, Ontario
31. 1999-2000	Richard D Coutts MD	San Diego, CA
32. 2000-2001	Leo A Whiteside MD	Saint Louis, MO
33. 2001-2002	Benjamin E Bierbaum MD	Boston, MA
34. 2002-2003	Miguel E Cabanela MD	Rochester, MN
35. 2003-2004	Charles A Engh MD	Alexandria, VA
36. 2004-2005	Richard E White MD	Albuquerque, NM
37. 2005-2006	James D'Antonio MD	Too Township, PA
38. 2006-2007	John Callaghan MD	Iowa City, IA
39. 2007-2008	Larry Dorr	Los Angeles, CA
40. 2008-2009	Wayne Paprosky	Winfield II
41. 2009-2010	William Maloney	Stanford, CA
42. 2010-2011	Chitranjan Ranawat	New York City, NY
43. 2011-2012	Adolph Lombardi	New Albany, OH
44. 2012-2013	David Lewallen	Rochester, MN
45. 2013-2014	Vincent Pellegrini	Baltimore, MD

of importance to the future of our subspecialty and of our profession as a whole.

I suspect that there are some members of the Hip Society who are pleased with the manner in which the Society has functioned, and who would argue that the practices and trends I have questioned are not inappropriate; that "times have changed" and that we must therefore accept the changes. Time might prove them correct, necessitating my retraction from the positions I have taken. However, responding to the responsibilities that my official position as historian for the Society demand, I have attempted, as candidly as possible, to interpret the events I have witnessed, hoping to enhance our pride in the organization.

Upon notification that my long-term tenure as Historian to the Hip Society had expired, I gave my last report to the organization. In it I emphasized the criticism I had voiced in my previous year report and made further recommendations. The following is the entire text of my remarks:

Report to the Hip Society

(From the Historian: Augusto Sarmiento, MD Washington DC February, 2005).

My term in office as Historian for the Hip Society comes to an end after six years of service. It was an honor to hold the position for such a long time and I thank the organization for the support given to me. Last year I summarized for the fellowship the history of the Hip Society and tried to outline the evolution of its educational activities. I ended the report expressing concerns over the direction the Society seemed to be taking and my perception of growing unsavory changes within it. I stated that the Society had, to some extent, squandered some of its potentials and resources while frequently pursuing inconsequential matters. I made some recommendations addressing those concerns. Today, after a year of carefully analyzing the issues I had raised the previous year, I will make additional comments and suggestions. I doubt there are many members of the Hip Society who would not admit that society's moral sphere has broken down; that an exaggerated relativism permeates into the ethos of our culture to the point that a growing number of people feel that everything is OK, therefore implying that there is nothing morally wrong. The obsessive preoccupation with profit, fueled by the expanding globalization of Western culture, is cementing this dangerous pattern.

Medicine, a microcosm of society, has not been immune to the trend, and it is rapidly being stripped of its traditional tenets. To an increasing number of practitioners of the art medicine is "just another business" where profit is the one thing that really matters. As a result of this belief a profound loss of professionalism is eroding our ranks.

Medicine had long claimed to hold- rightly so- the highest professional standards. As an example, physicians' advertising their services was something totally unacceptable and it was considered a demeaning behavior. This no longer seems to be the case. Advertising by physicians is now carried out in the most egregious ways: through every medium available and in manners that even the least sophisticated members of the community find distasteful and even obscene.

Recently, the prestigious *Miami Herald* displayed a half-page whole-body picture of an orthopedist stating that he had the best training in hip and knee replacement in the area; the inventor of unique surgical procedures and instruments; the developer of the minimally invasive total hip replacement technique; his patients become ambulatory four hours after hip replacement; and a host of other falsehoods and exaggerations. I suspect that a third rate used-car salesman would have hesitated to display such a cheap advertisement. Another orthopedist has his own weekly radio-show during which time he is introduced as one of the greatest surgeons in the country; the individual to whom patients and orthopedists from all over the world visit seeking the latest techniques. His telephone number is frequently repeated. The moderator emphasizes that, "If you are being advised by other doctors to have your hip or knee replaced, please pay a visit to the famous doctor, he has the final word". The medical community remains silent before such outrageous displays of unprofessional conduct. It tacitly condones the behavior.

Having been one of the founding members of the Hip Society and having worked and known the other 19 founding members, I am certain that the obscene infractions of professionalism we now observe would not have been tolerated by the likes of Frank Stinchfield, Mark Coventry, Otto Aufranc, Walter Blount, Al Ferguson, Carol Larson, Phil Wilson, Dick Johnston and several others.

I am familiar with the answer frequently given by many in response to the rampant loss of professionalism in medicine and the dangerous surrender of our continuing education and professional autonomy to the manufacturing industry. The ready answer is that "times have changed" and that "new ways" to do business have altered the old system and imprinted a new ethos; that feelings to the contrary are "old fashion" and obsolete. I submit that even if eventually the "old values" prove to be obsolete and disappear into the heap of history, there is not at yet evidence to justify their dismissal at this time, for after all they successfully held together the fabric of society for many a generation.

Despite thoughtless and cavalier responses to the challenges facing medicine, I have concluded that still are many physicians, and lay people as well, who feel the loss of professionalism in medicine is not a healthy development; rather a phenomenon likely to have undesirable unexpected consequences. Ignoring or minimizing the importance of events, some state that nothing that can be done about it because morality cannot be legislated.

Indeed it is true that morals cannot be legislated; however change can take place without specific legislation to effect it. Organizations of various types, possessing no legislative powers, have, over the course of history, brought about changes in behavior and moral conduct to entire societies without coercion or pressure. They did it through example, persuasion and by clearly spelling to their members the principles of conduct expected of them. They emphasized that the maintenance of certain values and behavior were essential for the vitality, growth and dignity that had given birth to their groups.

In suggesting a method to guard against grievous breaches of conduct among the Hip Society fellowship I propose an addendum to our constitution in the form of a document akin to the Bill of Rights that accompanies the American Constitution. A brief addendum that makes clear the expected adherence of its members to a professional behavior that demonstrates honesty and integrity in their professional lives; truth in the reporting of their scientific experiences; and moderation in the manner in which they announce their practices and professional businesses.

I believe such an addendum can be written without causing problems to any one; quite the contrary it would do much good to all parties. If for no other reason, it would serve as a reminder of the need to exercise care during the selection of new members as well as during deliberations regarding the election of officers. The addendum would be interpreted as a subtle threat of exposure of uncalled—for actions before fellow Hip Society members. This in itself is an effective deterrent and a means to encourage compliance.

I conclude saying that if the fellowship of the Hip Society believes that the moral fabric of medicine is unraveling and that a number of disturbing developments are challenging our profession, we should respond through action and begin to address the offending issues in a thoughtful way. Not making a decision to do something about is a decision in itself, which one day might be regretted.

References*

62, 68, 69, 74, 75, 83, 87, 88, 89, 93, 94, 98, 101, 103, 105, 108, 109

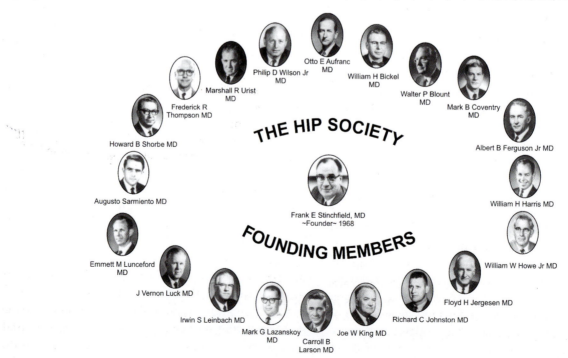

77

The International Hip Society

In the Summer of 1975 a group of members of the Hip Society, attending the meeting of SICOT in Copenhagen, met with several European hip surgeons to discuss the possibility of creating and International Hip Society. We were led by Frank Stinchfield and John Charnley, who had previously agreed that the time was ripe for the establishment of such a group. Among the Americans were Phil Wilson, Mark Coventry, William Harris, Nas Eftekhar, I Leinbach, Harlan Amstutz and I. Representing Europe, in addition to John Charnley, were Maurice Muller, from Switzerland, Michael Freeman and George McKee, form the UK, and Robert Judet and Emile Letournel, from France. A list of other hip surgeons from other countries was tentatively agreed and plans were finalize to hold its first official meeting in Bern, Switzerland, the following year. It was also decided that the Society would hold a meeting during the meetings of SICOT whenever the organization held its meetings.

For several years the meetings of the International Hip Society were held in Bern. Muller had very generously offered to finance the accommodations of its members in his own city, where he had, at the time, the most sophisticated facilities for the live performance of surgery, telecasted into the auditorium. Some 5 years later we began to hold meetings in the country of the president of the Society. We held meetings in London, Paris, Munich, Los Angeles and other cities, whose names I cannot recall at this moment.

The Society has served well as a vehicle for communication between hip surgeons in various parts of the world. The fact that it has held meetings in conjunction with the well attended meetings of SICOT has made possible the reaching of orthopedists from other nations. However, I have questions regarding the overall priorities of the organization over the years, and feel that as in the case of the Hip Society (primarily a North American organization) the International Hip Society has, to some extent, squandered its resources and failed to take advantage of its academic possibilities and moral authority. The meetings it holds, oftentimes, address subjects that do not necessarily concerns the ones the international community needs to learn the most about it. The theme that dominates the open meetings within SICOT is total hip surgery. This is to be anticipated since total hip arthroplasty is the surgical procedure that has replaced many other procedures previously performed for a number of pathological hip conditions. However, other conditions of the hip treated differently, need attention, such as trauma, hematogenous infections, congenital and developmental diseases, adolescent deformities and many others. Little time is devoted their discussion.

I do not know of a simple major development in hip surgery for which either the Hip Society in America or the International Hip Society can claim credit. Any progress that has been made has been the result of individual work carried out independently of the Societies. A partial exception to this perception may be the Scandinavian Hip Registries, though I suspect the birth of these registries took place before the International Hip Society got involved in its their promotion.

In addition, the International Hip Society has not as yet become a truly "international" organization. Its membership is limited to surgeons from the United States and a few European countries. Two or three individuals represent the Far East, but no one is there to contribute to the deliberations of the Society from a number of nations in Europe or Latin America. The traditional "old boys" system that has dominated medical societies for many decades still persists.

I have many good memories of the open and closed meetings of the Society. Vividly stereotyped in my mind is the one held in Bern when 4 of the "great" hip surgeons at the time performed surgery, which the audience was able to observe and discussed, via the radio, with the operating surgeons. They were, Karl Chiari, form Austria, who performed one of his pelvic osteotomies; Maurice Müller, from Switzerland., Robert Judet, from France and John Charnley, from the UK, who demonstrated their skills replacing arthritic joints. It was indeed a memorable occasion!

I have not been able to attend the last two meetings of the organization, but have seen the written programs. The emphasis on hip registries is readily noticed. I have previously raised questions about the problems had beset such projects, despite the fact that in theory they are commendable. I suspect that if hip registries are to become a practical reality in the future, their success will be achieved in small nations, and, hopefully, at a later date in larger ones. Currently, in the United States, efforts to organize and operate a National Total Hip Registry will be, in my opinion, facing difficulties arising from factors, such as the ridiculous number of marketed implants and the frequent release of new ones. Most importantly is the fact that the control that the manufacturing industry has in the education of the orthopedists and the overall practice of medicine has reached the upper echelons of the profession and in that manner is precluding clean and unbiased discussions.

The founding members of the Society were: Frank E Stinchfield, from the United States, John Charnley, from the United Kingdom, Maurice Müller, from Switzerland, Harlan C Amstutz, from the United States, Hans W Buchholz from Germany, Karl Chiari, from Austria, Mark B Coventry, from the United States, Richard L Cruess, from Canada, Nas S, Eftekhar, from the United States, Michael Freeman, from the United Kingdom, William H Harris, from the United States, Floyd H Jergesen, from the United States, Robert Judet, from France, Mark G Lazanski, from the United States, Irwin S Leinbach, from the United States, Emile P Letournel, from France, George K McKee, from the United Kingdom, Soren Pilgaard, from Denmark, Michel Postel, from France, Robert B Salter, from Canada, Augusto Sarmiento, from the United States and Philip D Wilson, from the United States.

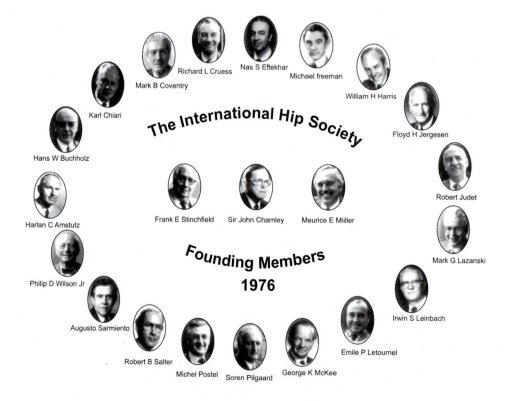

The International Hip Society

Founding Members
1976

Mark B Coventry · Richard L Cruess · Nas S Eftekhar · Michael freeman · William H Harris · Karl Chiari · Floyd H Jergesen · Hans W Buchholz · Robert Judet · Harlan C Amstutz · Frank E Stinchfield · Sir John Charnley · Meurice E Miiller · Mark G Lazanski · Philip D Wilson Jr · Irwin S Leinbach · Augusto Sarmiento · Emile P Letournel · Robert B Salter · Michel Postel · Soren Pilgaard · George K McKee

References

As stated in the introduction, I chose to include only references of publications where I served either as author or as co-author as I realized it would have been impossible for me to include the thousands of references to other people's work. Needless to say, I recognize that with a few exceptions the views I present were vicariously obtained, and even the few ones which I considered original, had most likely been described by others but those contributions were not known to me.

1. Sarmiento A, Grimes HA. The use of the Austin Moore vitallium prosthesis in the treatment of acute fractures and other diseases of the hip. Review of 123 consecutive cases. Clin Orthop & Rel Res 1963;28:120-31.
2. Sarmiento A. Intertrochanteric fractures of the femur. 150 degree angle nail plate fixation and early rehabilitation: a preliminary report of 100 cases. J Bone and Joint Surg 1963;45A:706-22.
3. Sarmiento A, Kalbac JH. Vitallium Austin Moore prosthesis for subcapital fractures of the femur in the aged. Experience with 200 consecutive cases. J Western Pacific Assoc 1964;1:179-88.
4. Mann RJ, Sarmiento A. Two plate fixation of the femoral shaft. Clin Orthop & Rel Res 1965;38:93-9.
5. Sarmiento A, Kalbac JH. The rehabilitation of the fractured hip in the aged. J South Med Assoc 1965;58:428-31.
6. Sarmiento A, McCollough NC. The orthopaedist and rehabilitation. Clin Orthop & Rel Res 1965;41:111-5.
7. Sarmiento A. Avoidance of complications of internal fixation of intertrochanteric fractures: experiences with 250 consecutive cases. Clin Orthop & Rel Res 1967;53.
8. Mariotti JR, Mann RJ, Sarmiento A. Two plate fixation of fractures of the femoral shaft. South Med J 1969;62:11.
9. Sarmiento A, Williams EM. The unstable intertrochanteric fracture: treatment with a valgus osteotomy and I-beam nail plate. J Bone and Joint Surg 1970;52A(7):1309-13.
10. Sarmiento A. Austin Moore prosthesis in the arthritic hip. Clin Orthop & Rel Res 1972;82:14-23.
11. Enis JE, Hall M, Sarmiento A. Methylmethacrylate in neoplastic bone destruction. The hip society. THE HIP, The CV Mosby Company 1973.
12. Sarmiento A, Laird A. Posterior fracture-dislocation of the femoral head. Clin Orthop & Rel Res 1973;92:143-46.
13. Sarmiento A. Unstable intertrochanteric fractures of the femur. Clin Orthop & Rel Res 1973;92:77-85.
14. Sarmiento A. Valgus osteotomy technique for unstable intertrochanteric fractures. Third open scientific meeting of the hip society. THE HIP. The CV Mosby Company 1975;157-69.
15. Jennings JJ, Harris WM H, Sarmiento A. A clinical evaluation of aspirin prophylaxis of thromboembolic disease after total hip arthroplasty. J Bone and Joint Surg 1976;57A(7):926-8.
16. Sarmiento A. Basic problems in hip surgery. Orthop Rev 1977;6(4):43-5.
17. Sarmiento A. Reflections on total hip arthroplasty. Orthop Rev 1977;6(4):83-5.
18. Sarmiento A, Schaeffer JF, Beckerman L, Latta LL, Enis JE. Fracture healing in rat remora as affected by functional weight bearing. J Bone and Joint Surg 1977;59A(3):369-75.
19. Sarmiento A, Gerard FM. Total hip arthroplasty for failed endoprosthesis. Clin Orthop & Rel Res 1978;137.
20. Tarr R, Lewis JL, Jaycox D, Sarmiento A, Schmidt J, Latta LL. The effect of materials, stem geometry, collar-calcar contact on stress distribution on the proximal femur with total hip. Trans Orthop Research Soc 1079;4:24.
21. Sarmiento A, Zych GA, Latta LL, Tarr RR. Clinical experiences with a titanium alloy total hip prosthesis: a posterior approach. Clin Orthop & Rel Res 1979;144.
22. Sarmiento A, Turner TM, Latta LL, Tarr RR. Factors contributing to lysis of the femoral neck in total hip arthroplasty. Clin Orthop & Rel Res 1979;145:208-12.
23. Clarke IC, Gruen TA, Sarmiento A. Finite element analyses studies of total hips versus clinical reality. Proceedings of finite elements in biomechanics. In: Simon BR (Ed). Tucson 1980;2:487-510.
24. Tarr RR, Lewis J, Ghassemi F, Sarmiento A, Clarke IC, Weingarten V. Anatomic three-dimensional finite element model of the proximal femur with total hip prosthesis. Proceedings of finite elements in biomechanics. In: Simon BR (Ed). Tucson 1980;2:511-28.
25. Clarke IC, Gruen TA, Tarr RR, Sarmiento A. Finite element analyses studies of total hips. International conference in finite elements in biomechanics 1980;2:487-511.
26. Tarr RR, Sarmiento A. Anatomic three-dimensional finite element model of the proximal femur with total hip prostheses. International conference in finite elements in biomechanics 1980;146:28-36.
27. Sarmiento A, Mullis DL, Latta LL, Tarr RR, Alvarez R. A quantitative comparative analysis of fracture bracing under the influence of compression plating versus closed weight bearing treatment. Clin Orthop and Related Research 1980;149:232-39.

28. Tarr T, Clarke IE, Gruen T, Sarmiento A. Predictions of cement-bone failure criteria: three-dimensional finite element models versus clinical reality of total hip replacement. In: Gallagher RH (Ed). Finite elements in biomechanics 1980;245-359.

29. Sarmiento A, Latta LL. Periosteal fracture callus mechanics. Moore TM (Ed). In: AAOS symposium on trauma to the leg and its sequelae. The CV Mosby Company 1981;175-86.

30. Clarke I, Gruen T, Gustillo R, Harris LJ, Latta L, Lynch MH, McKellop H, Ranawat C, Rostoker W, Sarmiento A. The use of titanium alloys in orthopaedic medicine. Zimmer 1981;1-40.

31. Clarke I, Espiritu E, Hull D, McKellop H, McGuire P, Okuda R, Sarmiento A. Correction for fluid absorption in sterile polyethylene components. Proceedings 7th annual meeting, society for biomaterials, Troy, New York 1981.

32. Tarr D, Clarke I, Gruen T, Sarmiento A, Espiritu E, Hull D, McGuire P, Sew Hoy A, McKellop H. Total hip femoral component design. Orthopaedic review 1982; 11:23-35.

33. Chandler D, Glousman R, Hall D, McGuire P, Kim I, Clarke I, Sarmiento A. Prosthetic hip range of motion and impingement. The effects of head and neck geometry. Clin Orthop and Related Research 1982; 166:284-91.

34. Tarr RR, Clarke I, Gruen T, Sarmiento A, Espiritu E, Hull D, McGuire P, Sew Hoy A, McKellop H. Total hip femoral component design. Stem characterization, experimental studies, and analytical modeling for orthopaedic surgeons. Orthopaedic Review 1982;11(12).

35. Tarr RR, Clarke IC, Sarmiento A. Analytical model of femoral revision total hip replacement. Trans 28th Annual Orthop Res Soc 1982;7:293.

36. Clarke IC, McKellop HA, McGuire P, Okuda R, Sarmiento A. Wear of Ti-6Al-4V implant alloy and ultrahigh molecular weight polyethylene combinations. Titanium alloys in surgical implants. Luckey/Kubli (Eds), ASTM STP 796 1983;136-47.

37. Tarr RR, Clarke IC, Sarmiento A. Loading behavior of femoral stems of titanium 6Al-4V compared to cobalt-chromium alloys: A 3-D finite element analysis. Titanium alloys in surgical implants. Luckey/Kubli (Eds), ASTM STP 796 1983;88-101.

38. Gruen TA, Sarmiento A. Bone/biomaterial interface in orthopaedic joint implants. Key reference in bio-materials. J Biomed Mat Res 1984;18,577-99.

39. McKellop HA, Hosseinian A, Clarke IC, Sarmiento A. In vitro and in vivo wear of total joint replacements. ACEMB Mtg, Los Angeles, CA 1984.

40. Chandler DR, Tarr RR, Gruen TA, Sarmiento A. Radiographic assessment of acetabular cup orientation: a new design concept. Clin Orthop 1984;186:60-4.

41. Sarmiento A, Latta LL, Tarr RR. The effects of function in fracture healing and stability. AAOS Instructional Course Lectures 1984.

42. Gruen T, Orisek B, Campbell P, Chew S, Bowell W, Hillman D, Sarmiento A. Computerized axial tomography as a new adjunct method for evaluation of postmortem cemented total hip replacement in situ. Trans 2nd World Congress on Biomaterials 1984;7:331.

43. Ebramzadeh W, Clarke IC, Mossessian T, McKellop HA, Gruen TA, Sarmiento A. Cement deformation from cyclic loading of the total hip femoral component. In: Anderson JM (Ed). Trans 2nd World Congress on Biomaterials 1984;7:348.

44. Campbell P, Bloebaum RD, Gruen TA, Sarmiento A. A multifaceted approach to the analysis of the THR implants in a canine model. Trans 2nd World Congress on Biomaterials 1984;7:138.

45. McKellop HA, Glousman R, Clarke IC, Sarmiento A. A plastic bone model for the evaluation of femoral fracture fixation. Trans 2nd World Congress on Biomaterials 1984;7:240.

46. Sarmiento A, Gruen T. Radiographic analysis of a low-modulus titanium-alloy femoral total hip component. Two-to-six year follow-up. J Bone Joint 1985;67(1):48-56.

47. Bloebaum R, Sarmiento A. A study on the effects of cement intrusion in cancellous bone. An USC Internal Publication 1985.

48. Bloebaum RD, McLaren AC, Campbell P, Chew S, Sarmiento A. Comparative thin section histology on composite and titanium THR interfaces. Orthop Trans, J Bone and Joint Surg 1985;9(2):151-2.

49. McKellop H, Ebramzadeh E, Matta J, Wiss D, Sarmiento A. Stability of femoral fractures with interlocking intramedullary rods. Trans Orthop Res Soc 1986;11:319.

50. Valos N, Sarmiento A. A bone/cement/porous metal experimental technique for stabilization of cemented total hip arthroplasty. Internal publication Dept of Orthopaedics University of Southern California 1986.

51. Sarmiento A, Nataranjan V, Gruen TA, McMahon M. Radiographic performance of two different total hip cemented arthroplasties. Orthop Clin 1988;1-11.

52. Shanfield S, Campbell P, Baumgarten M, Bloebaum R, Sarmiento A. Synovial fluid osmolality in osteoarthritis and rheumatoid arthritis. Clin Orthop & Rel Res 1988; 235:289-95.

53. McKellop H, Ebramzadeh E, Fortune J, Sarmiento A. Stability of subtrochanteric femoral fractures fixed with interlocking intramedullary rods. In: JP Harvey, AU Daniels, RF Games (Eds). Femoral intramedullary rods: clinical performance and related laboratory testing. ASTM STP 1008. ASTM, Philadelphia 1988.

54. Ebramzadeh E, McKellop H, Wilson M, Sarmiento A. Design factors affecting micromotion of porous coated and low modulus hip prostheses. Trans Orthop Res 1988;13:351.

55. Sarmiento A, Ebramzadeh E, Gogan W, McKellop H. Effect of stem size and positioning on performance of total hip prostheses. SIROT 1990.

56. McKellop HA, Sarmiento A, Schwinn CP, Ebramzadeh E. In vivo wear of titanium alloy hip prosthesis. J Bone and Joint Surg 1990;72A(4):512-17.

57. Sarmiento A, Ebramzadeh E, Gogan WJ, McKellop HA. Acetabular cup containment and orientation in cemented total hip arthroplasties. J Bone and Joint Surg 1990;72B(6):996-1002.

58. Sarmiento A, Ebramzadeh E, Gogan WJ, McKellop HA. Total hip arthroplasty with cement: A long-term radiographic analysis in patients who are older than fifty years. J Bone and Joint Surg 1990;72A:1470-6.

59. Sarmiento A, Ebramzadeh E, Llinas A, Gogan W, McKellop H. Correlation of patient's sex and weight with the long-term performance of cemented total hip replacements. SICOT 1990.

60. McKellop H, Ebramzadeh E, Neiderer PG, Sarmiento A. Comparison of the stability of press-fit hip prostheses using a synthetic model femur. J Orthop Res 1991;9:297-305.

61. Llinas A, Sarmiento A, Ebramzadeh E, Gogan WJ, McKellop HA. Total hip replacement after failed hemiarthroplasty or mould arthroplasty. J Bone & Joint Surg 1991;73B:912-17.

62. Sarmiento A. Staying the course. AAOS. First vice president's address. J Bone & Joint Surg 1991;73A:479-83.

63. Llinas A, Park SH, McKellop H, Marshall G, Sarmiento A. Evaluation of a polylactic acid biodegradable cortical screw in a rabbit model. Trans Soc Biomaterials 1991; 14:220.

64. Brien W, Sarmiento A. Vascular injury during cementless total hip arthroplasty. Orthopaedics 1992; 15(1):54-6.

65. Sigholm G, Gendler E, McKellop H, Marshall GJ, Sarmiento A. Early healing of four different ethylene oxide processed bone. Preparations in rabbit ulnar segmental defects. Acta Orthop Scand 1992;63(2):177-82.

66. McKellop HA, Sarmiento A, Brien W, Park S. Interface corrosion of a modular head total hip prosthesis. J Arthroplasty 1992;7(3):291-4.

67. Llinas A, McKellop H, Marshall J, Sharpe F, Lu B, Kirchen M, Sarmiento A. Healing and remodeling of articular incongruities in a rabbit fracture model. J Bone & Joint Surg 1993;75A(10):1508-23.

68. Sarmiento A. An agenda for surgeons and industry. Orthopaedic Network News 1993;4(1).

69. Sarmiento A. Editorial orthopaedics at a crossroads. J Bone & Joint Surg 1993;75A(2):159-61.

70. Ebramzadeh E, Sarmiento A, McKellop H, Llinas A, Gogan W. The cement mantle in total hip arthroplasty: Analysis of long-term radiographic results. J Bone & Joint Surg 1994;76A(1):77-87.

71. Ebramzadeh E, McKellop H, Dorey F, Sarmiento A. Challenging the validity of conclusions based on p-values alone: A critique of contemporary clinical research design and methods. American Academy of Orthopedic Surgeons. Instructional Course Lectures 1994.

72. McKellop H, Campbell P, Park S-H, Schmalzried T, Grigoris P, Amstutz H, Sarmiento A. The origin of submicron polyethylene wear debris in total hip arthroplasty. Clin Ortho & Rel Res, 1995;(311).

73. Lu Z, Ebramzadeh E, McKellop H, Sarmiento A. Stable partial debonding of the cement interfaces indicated by a finite element model of a total hip prosthesis. J Orthop Res 1996;14:238-44.

74. Sarmiento A. The role of industry in orthopaedic education. J Orthopaedics 1997;20(2):100-3.

75. Sarmiento A. Orthopaedics and industry. Point counter point. Orthopaedics 1997.

76. Sarmiento A, Ebramzadeh E. The stainless steel and titanium alloy femoral prostheses total hip arthroplasty outcomes. In: Finerman et al (Eds). Churchill Livingston 1997;41-53.

77. Sarmiento A, Ebramzadeh E, Llinas A, Reflections on a 25 year experience with total hip arthroplasty. In: Finerman G, Grigoris P, Dorey F, McKellop H (Eds). Total hip arthroplasty outcomes. Churchill livingston, New York, NY 1997.

78. Sarmiento A. Commentary: Responding to change. Journal of Bone and Joint Surg. JBJS 1998;80A(4):601-3.

79. Park, Sang-Hyun, O'Connor K, McKellop H, Sarmiento A. The influence of active shear or fracture healing. Journal of Bone and Joint Surg 1998;80A(6):868-78.

80. Goswami A, Sarmiento A. A review of infections in total hip arthroplasty. A university of southern california internal publication.

81. Llinas A, Sarmiento A, Ebramzadeh E, Park SH, McKellop H, Campbell P. Mechanism of failure with an uncemented, all polyethylene socket. Clin Orthop Rel Research 1999;#362:145-55.

82. Sarmiento A, Goswami DK. Thromboembolic prophylaxis with use of aspirin, exercise and graded elastic stockings or intermittent compression devices in patients managed with total hip arthroplasty. Journal of bone and joint surgery 1999;81A(3):339.

83. Sarmiento A. Responding to change. Journal of Bone and Joint Surg 1999;81A(9):1346-8.

84. Sarmiento A. Medicine and industry: The payer, the piper and the tune. Royal canadian annals of medicine 2000;33(3):144-9.

85. Sarmiento A. Academic medicine and industry—the ethical dilemma. Iowa Orthop J 2000;20:87-90.

86. Sarmiento A. Don't shun the non-surgical treatment of Fractures. AAOS 113. Bulletin 2000.

87. Sarmiento A. On the future of orthopaedics—I am concerned. Journal of Orthopaedic Science 2000; 5:425-30.

88. Sarmiento A. Thoughts on the impact of technology on orthopaedics. J Bone Joint Surg 2000;82B:942-2.

89. Sarmiento A. The future of our specialty. Acta Orthopedica Scandinavica 2000;71(6):574-9.

90. Sarmiento A. On the education of the orthopaedic resident. Clin Orthopaedics 2002;400:259-63.

91. McKellop H, Rostlund T, Ebramzadeh E, Sarmiento A. Wear of titanium 6-4 alloy in laboratory tests and in retrieved human joint replacements. Titanium n Medicine. In: DM Brunette at al (Eds). Springer 2001;748-70.

92. Sarmiento MD. Antithrombotic therapy. Letter to the editor. Journal American College of Surgeons 2001; 193(4):465-6.

93. Sarmiento A. Thoughts on the role of orthopaedics in basic Research. Jour Bone and Joint Surg (A) 2001;83A: 1002-4.

94. Sarmiento A. Ethical concerns regarding the orthopaedic relationship with industry. British Orthopaedic News. A bridged version of AOA talk, 2001.

95. Sarmiento A. Letter to the editor. Industry and medicine. JAMA 2001;186(3):302.

96. Sarmiento A. Antithrombotic therapy. J AM Col Surg Oct 2001;193(4):465-6.

97. Lovasz G, Prk SH, Ebramzadeh E, Benya PD, Llinas A, Bellyei A, Luck J, Sarmiento A. Characteristic of degeneration in an unstable knee with a coronal surface step-off. J Bone Joint (BR) 2001;83(3):428-36.

98. Sarmiento A. The pharmaceutical industry and continuing education. JAMA July 18; 286(3):302; author reply 2001;303-4.

99. Sarmiento A. Anti-thrombotic therapy. J Am Coll Surg 2001;193:465-6.

100. Sarmiento A. Letter to the editor. Is titanium so bad? JBJS 2002;84B(6):931.

101. Sarmiento A. A joint replacement registry. A letter to the editor of the academy bulletin 2002.

102. Sarmiento A. Letter to the editor JBJS-A. Prophylaxis against venous thromboembolic disease: Cost and controversy. J Bone Joint Surg 2002;84A(12):2305-6.

103. Sarmiento A. Have we lost objectivity? J Bone and Joint Surgery 2002;84A(7):1254-8.

104. Ebrmzadeh E, Norman P, Sangiorgio S, Llinas A, Gruen T, McKellop, H, Sarmiento A. Long-term radiographic changes in cemented total hip arthroplasty with six designs of femoral components. J of Biomaterials 2003; 2:335-6.

105. Sarmiento A. Subspecialization. Has it been all for the better? Journal of Bone and Joint Surg 2003;85A(2):369-73.

106. Sarmiento A. The geriatric patients. Fractures and osteoporosis. Orthopaedic Today International 2004.

107. Sarmiento A. The future of specialization in orthopaedics. Letter to the editor JBJS. Ref. Article by James H. Herndon JBJS 2004;86:2560-6.

108. Sarmiento A. Bare Bones. Prometheus 2004.

109. Sarmiento A, Goswami AK. Thromboembolic disease prophylaxis in total hip arthroplasty. Clinic Orthop 2005;436:138-43.

110. Sarmiento A, Latta LL. A surgical technique to prevent lysis in cemented total hip arthroplasty. Submitted for publication 2006.

111. Martinez A, Sarmiento A, Latta LL. Experiences with a rapid failure rate of a hybrid total hip arthroplasty. Submitted for publication 2006.

112. Goswami A, Sarmiento A. A review of bilateral simultaneous total hip arthroplasties. A university of Southern California Internal Publication 1989.

113. Malagon V, Malagon JM, Sarmiento A. Displasia del desarrollo de la cadera. (Hip Dysplasia. Its Evolution). Celsus 2006.

114. Sarmiento A, Latta LL. The evolution of functional fracture bracing. J Bone and Joint Surg (B) 2006;88-8(2):141-48.

115. Sarmiento A. Ethics in orthopaedics. Letter to the editor, ethics in orthopaedic surgery, and which research is to be believed? JBJS (B) 2006;88B(3):416.

116. Sarmiento A, Latta, LL. A radiographic review of 135 total hip Charnley arthroplasties followed between 15 and 35 years. Acta Chirurgiae Orthopaedicae et Traumatologiae Cechosl 2006;73:145-50.

117. Sarmiento A. Is Socrates dying? J Bone and Joint Surg (A) 2008.

118. Sarmiento A. On exaggerated subspecialization. Orthopaedics Today 2008.

119. Sarmiento A. Medicine challenged. Publish America 2008.

120. Sarmiento A. Our system is broken. Let's fix it. AAOS Now 2008.

121. Sarmiento A. Cemented knee prostheses should have more study. Orthopaedics Today 2009;5.

122. Sarmiento A, Latta LL. The interlocking nail. A perspective. Current Orthopaedic Practice 2010;l(21):1-3.

123. Sarmiento A. The stability of intertrochanteric fractures. Submitted to Current Orthopaedic Practice 2011 (To be published).

Index